WISDOM AND COMPASSION IN PSYCHOTHERAPY

Wisdom and Compassion in Psychotherapy

Deepening Mindfulness in Clinical Practice

Edited by
Christopher K. Germer
Ronald D. Siegel

Foreword by His Holiness the Dalai Lama

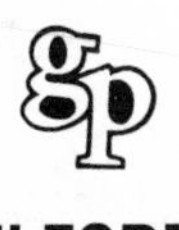

THE GUILFORD PRESS
New York London

by The Guilford Press
n of Guilford Publications, Inc.
g Street, New York, NY 10012
iilford.com

Printed in the United States of America

This book is printed on acid-free paper.

Last digit is print number: 9 8 7 6 5 4 3 2 1

The authors have checked with sources believed to be reliable in their efforts to provide information that is complete and generally in accord with the standards of practice that are accepted at the time of publication. However, in view of the possibility of human error or changes in behavioral, mental health, or medical sciences, neither the authors, nor the editors and publisher, nor any other party who has been involved in the preparation or publication of this work warrants that the information contained herein is in every respect accurate or complete, and they are not responsible for any errors or omissions or the results obtained from the use of such information. Readers are encouraged to confirm the information contained in this book with other sources.

Library of Congress Cataloging-in-Publication Data

Wisdom and compassion in psychotherapy : deepening mindfulness in clinical practice / edited by Christopher K. Germer, Ronald D. Siegel.
p. cm.
Includes bibliographical references and index.
ISBN 978-1-4625-0376-6 (hardcover)
1. Mindfulness-based cognitive therapy. 2. Compassion—Religious aspect—Buddhism. I. Germer, Christopher K. II. Siegel, Ronald D.
RC489.M55W57 2012
616.89′1425—dc23

2011037134

In memory of G. Alan Marlatt

About the Editors

Christopher K. Germer, PhD, is a clinical psychologist in private practice, specializing in mindfulness, acceptance, and compassion-based treatment. He has been integrating the principles and practices of meditation into psychotherapy since 1978. Dr. Germer is Clinical Instructor in Psychology at Harvard Medical School and a founding member of the Institute for Meditation and Psychotherapy. He lectures internationally on mindfulness and self-compassion, is coeditor (with Ronald D. Siegel and Paul R. Fulton) of the professional book *Mindfulness and Psychotherapy*, and is author of *The Mindful Path to Self-Compassion: Freeing Yourself from Destructive Thoughts and Emotions.*

Ronald D. Siegel, PsyD, is Assistant Clinical Professor of Psychology at Harvard Medical School, where he has taught since 1984. He is a long-time student of mindfulness meditation and serves on the board of directors and faculty of the Institute for Meditation and Psychotherapy. Dr. Siegel teaches internationally about mindfulness and psychotherapy and mind–body treatment, while maintaining a private clinical practice in Lincoln, Massachusetts. He is author of *The Mindfulness Solution: Everyday Practices for Everyday Problems* and coeditor of *Mindfulness and Psychotherapy.*

Contributors

Antra K. Borofsky, EdM, is a marriage and family therapist in private practice in Cambridge, Massachusetts. She is a contributing author to *On Intimate Ground: Gestalt Approaches to Working with Couples* and *Joyful Wedding: A Spiritual Path to the Altar.* Along with her husband, Richard, she is codirector of the Center for the Study of Relationship, where they offer workshops and retreats for couples. She is also on the faculty of the Omega Institute, Kripalu, and the Rowe Conference Center. She has been a Zen student since the 1990s.

Richard Borofsky, EdD, is a clinical psychologist in private practice in Cambridge, Massachusetts, specializing in couples therapy. He is a contributing author to *On Intimate Ground: Gestalt Approaches to Working with Couples, Right Here with You: Bringing Mindful Awareness into Our Relationships,* and *Joyful Wedding: A Spiritual Path to the Altar.* Along with his wife, Antra, Dr. Borofsky is codirector of the Center for the Study of Relationship, where they offer workshops and retreats for couples. He is also on the faculty of the Omega Institute, Kripalu, and the Rowe Conference Center. He has been a Zen student since the 1980s.

Sarah Bowen, PhD, is a research scientist at the Addictive Behaviors Research Center at the University of Washington, where she received her doctoral degree under the mentorship of the late G. Alan Marlatt. Her research has focused primarily on mindfulness-based therapies for addictive behaviors, with a specific focus on mechanisms of change. In addition to numerous papers and book chapters in this area, Dr. Bowen is lead author of *Mindfulness-Based Relapse Prevention for Addictive Behaviors: A Clinician's Guide.* She has facilitated mindfulness-based relapse prevention groups in private and government treatment agencies, and has offered training to researchers and clinicians in the United States and internationally. Dr. Bowen has a particular interest in mindfulness-based treatment for dual-diagnosis populations.

Tara Brach, PhD, is a clinical psychologist and a leading Western teacher of Buddhist meditation, emotional healing, and spiritual awakening. She has practiced and taught meditation since the 1970s and is the senior teacher and founder of the Insight Meditation Community of Washington. Dr. Brach is the author of

Radical Acceptance: Embracing Your Life with the Heart of the Buddha and the forthcoming *True Refuge: Three Gateways to a Fearless Heart.*

John Briere, PhD, is Associate Professor of Psychiatry, Keck School of Medicine, University of Southern California; Director, Psychological Trauma Program, Los Angeles County–USC Medical Center; and Past President, International Society for Traumatic Stress Studies. He received the Award for Outstanding Contributions to the Science of Trauma Psychology from the American Psychological Association and was designated as Highly Cited Researcher (Behavioral Sciences) by the Institute for Scientific Information. Dr. Briere's recent books include *Principles of Trauma Therapy: A Guide to Symptoms, Evaluation, and Treatment*; *Therapy for Adults Molested as Children: Beyond Survival*; *Psychological Assessment of Adult Post-traumatic States: Phenomenology, Diagnosis, and Measurement*; and *Treating Complex Trauma in Adolescents and Young Adults.*

B. Rael Cahn, MD, PhD, is Resident Physician and Research Fellow, University of California, Irvine, Department of Psychiatry, and Scientific Co-Director of the Meditation Research Institute, Rishikesh, India. He researches the clinical and neurobiological effects of the spectrum of meditative practices.

Richard J. Davidson, PhD, is the William James and Vilas Research Professor of Psychology and Psychiatry; Founder and Chair, Center for Investigating Healthy Minds at the Waisman Center; and Director, Waisman Laboratory for Brain Imaging and Behavior and the Laboratory for Affective Neuroscience, University of Wisconsin–Madison. Dr. Davidson is the recipient of numerous awards, including the Distinguished Scientific Contribution Award from the American Psychological Association; the National Institute of Mental Health Research Scientist Award; membership, American Academy of Arts and Sciences; one of the 100 most influential people in the world, *Time* magazine; and Person of the Year, *Madison Magazine*. He is the author of over 275 publications, including *Training the Brain*, *Visions of Compassion*, and *Anxiety, Depression, and Emotion*.

Elissa Ely, MD, is a psychiatrist at the Massachusetts Mental Health Center who has written monthly over the past three decades for *The Boston Globe*. She has also written for *The New York Times*, and for many years was a commentator on NPR's *All Things Considered*. Through the Department of Mental Health, Dr. Ely sees patients with major mental illness, including residents of several homeless shelters in the Boston area.

Jack Engler, PhD, is Clinical Instructor in Psychology, Harvard Medical School, and in private practice in Cambridge, Massachusetts. He is coauthor of *The Consumer's Guide to Psychotherapy: Transformations of Consciousness* and *Conventional and Contemplative Perspectives on Development*, and is a contributing author in *Psychoanalysis and Buddhism: An Unfolding Dialogue*. Dr. Engler was a founder, board member, and teacher at the Insight Meditation Society and the Barre Center for Buddhist Studies in Barre, Massachusetts.

Carol Ann Faigin, PhD, is a clinical psychologist in private practice in central Maine, specializing in the treatment of posttraumatic stress disorder and other trauma-related disorders. She has lectured and coauthored book chapters and articles on the topic of spirituality and psychological wellness. Dr. Faigin is an active contributor to the U.S. Army's Comprehensive Soldier Fitness Program: Spiritual Resilience Initiative, which is being administered to U.S. Army soldiers. She plans to continue developing interventions that integrate psychology and spirituality.

Barbara L. Fredrickson, PhD, is a Kenan Distinguished Professor of Psychology and Director of the Positive Emotions and Psychophysiology Laboratory at the University of North Carolina at Chapel Hill. She is a leading scholar within social psychology, affective science, and positive psychology. Dr. Fredrickson's research and teaching have been recognized with numerous honors, including the 2000 Templeton Prize in Positive Psychology from the American Psychological Association and the 2005 Career Trajectory Award from the Society for Experimental Social Psychology. She is the author of *Positivity*, a general-audience book that draws on her own research and that of other social scientists.

Paul R. Fulton, EdD, is former Director of Mental Health, Tufts Health Plan; former president, founding member, and director of the Certificate Program, Institute for Meditation and Psychotherapy; former member of the board of directors, Barre Center for Buddhist Studies; and member of the Advisory Committee, Garrison Institute Trauma Recovery Initiative. He maintains a private clinical practice in Newton, Massachusetts, is coeditor of *Mindfulness and Psychotherapy*, and is a contributor to *Mindfulness and the Therapeutic Relationship* and *Clinical Handbook of Mindfulness.*

Christopher K. Germer (see "About the Editors").

Paul Gilbert, PhD, is Professor of Clinical Psychology at the University of Derby, England, and head of the research unit. He was made a fellow of the British Psychological Society for contributions to psychological knowledge in 1993 and is Past President of the British Association for Cognitive and Behavioral Psychotherapy. Dr. Gilbert has also served on the U.K. NICE guideline committee on depression. He has published and edited 18 books, the most recent being *The Compassionate Mind,* and over 100 academic papers and book chapters. In 2010, Dr. Gilbert was conferred the honor of Order of the British Empire.

Trudy Goodman, PhD, is the executive director and founding teacher of InsightLA, a nonprofit organization for *vipassana* (insight) meditation training and secular mindfulness education. She was a psychotherapist in private practice for 25 years and studied Buddhist meditation for 38 years with Asian and Western teachers. Ms. Goodman was one of the original mindfulness-based stress reduction teachers with Jon Kabat-Zinn, and she cofounded the Institute for Meditation and Psychotherapy in Cambridge, Massachusetts, as well as two family mindfulness programs: Family Path and Growing Spirit (with Susan Kaiser Greenland). She teaches meditation retreats and workshops nationwide, and is a contributing author to the *Clinical Handbook of Mindfulness* and *Mindfulness and Psychotherapy*.

Susan Kaiser Greenland, JD, is author of the Inner Kids mindful awareness program; cofounder and former executive director of the Inner Kids Foundation; founding member of the Leadership Council, Garrison Institute Initiative on Contemplation and Education; and former co-investigator on a multiyear, multisite research study at MARC/UCLA's Semel Institute on the impact of mindfulness in education. She is also author of *The Mindful Child: How to Help Your Kid Manage Stress and Become Happier, Kinder, and More Compassionate* and coauthor of a study on the Inner Kids program conducted by the Mindful Awareness Research Center at UCLA.

Dilip V. Jeste, MD, is Estelle and Edgar Levi Chair in Aging; Distinguished Professor of Psychiatry and Neurosciences; Director, Sam and Rose Stein Institute for Research on Aging; and Chief of the Geriatric Psychiatry Division, University of California, San Diego. He is also President of the American Psychiatric Association.

Judith V. Jordan, PhD, is Founding Scholar and Director of the Jean Baker Miller Training Institute, Wellesley Centers for Women, Wellesley College, and Assistant Professor of Psychology, Department of Psychiatry, Harvard Medical School. Dr. Jordan received the Career Achievement Award for Outstanding Contribution to the Advancement of Psychology from the Massachusetts Psychological Association and the Distinguished Psychologist Award from the American Psychological Association. Her publications include *Women's Growth in Connection; The Complexity of Connection; Women's Growth in Diversity; Relational–Cultural Therapy; The Power of Connection;* and over 40 articles and chapters on relational–cultural practices, mutuality, and empathy. She has presented at over 1,500 conferences nationally and internationally and is a lifelong practitioner of insight meditation.

Marsha M. Linehan, PhD, is Director of the Behavioral Research and Therapy Clinics and Professor of Psychology and of Psychiatry and Behavioral Sciences, University of Washington, Seattle. She is the recipient of numerous awards, including the Louis I. Dublin Award for lifetime achievement in the field of suicide prevention from the American Association of Suicidology, the Distinguished Award for Contributions to the Science and Profession of Clinical Psychology from the American Psychological Association, and the Outstanding Clinician Award from the Association for Behavioral and Cognitive Therapies. Dr. Linehan is Past President of the Society for Clinical Psychology and the Association for Behavioral and Cognitive Therapies, and is author of *Cognitive-Behavioral Treatment for Borderline Personality Disorder*; *Skills Training Manual for Treating Borderline Personality Disorder*; and *Dialectical Behavior Therapy for Suicidal Adolescents.* She is also a Zen teacher in both the Leere Wolke/Empty Cloud lineage and the

Diamond Sangha, and focuses her teaching primarily on Zen and mindfulness practices for psychotherapists.

Anita Lungu, PhD (in computer science), is pursuing doctoral studies in clinical psychology at the University of Washington under Marsha M. Linehan, with a focus on developing and transferring effective treatments to those with severe and life-threatening mental disorders.

M. Kathleen B. Lustyk, PhD, is Professor of Psychology at Seattle Pacific University (SPU) and Affiliate Associate Professor of Psychology and Nursing at the University of Washington (UW). She is the developer and Primary Investigator of the SPU Women's Health Lab and, in collaboration with scholars at the UW Addictive Behaviors Research Center, is investigating brain activation and physiological responses to mindfulness-based relapse prevention therapy. Dr. Lustyk received the Professor of the Year Award in 2009 and 2010 from the SPU School of Psychology. In 2002, she received the Outstanding Research Article Award from the Society of Gastroenterology Nurses and Associates.

John Makransky, PhD, is Associate Professor of Buddhism and Comparative Theology at Boston College, a senior faculty advisor for Chokyi Nyima Rinpoche's Centre for Buddhist Studies in Nepal, cochair of the Buddhist Critical–Constructive Group in the American Academy of Religion, and guiding meditation teacher for the Foundation for Active Compassion. He is the author of *Awakening through Love: Unveiling Your Deepest Goodness* and *Buddhahood Embodied: Sources of Controversy in India and Tibet*, and coeditor of *Buddhist Theology: Critical Reflections by Contemporary Buddhist Scholars*.

G. Alan Marlatt, PhD, until his death in 2011, was Director of the Addictive Behaviors Research Center and Professor of Psychology at the University of Washington. For over 30 years, Dr. Marlatt conducted pioneering work on understanding and preventing relapse in substance abuse treatment and was a leading proponent of the harm reduction approach to treating addictive behaviors. He was a recipient of many honors, including the Jellinek Memorial Award for outstanding contributions to knowledge in the field of alcohol studies, the Robert Wood Johnson Foundation's Innovators Combating Substance Abuse Award, the Research Society on Alcoholism's Distinguished Research Award, and the Career/Lifetime Achievement Award from the Association for Behavioral and Cognitive Therapies.

Thomas W. Meeks, MD, is Assistant Clinical Professor, Division of Geriatric Psychiatry, University of California, San Diego. He has published several articles in the field of geriatric psychiatry, and coauthored the 2009 article "Neurobiology of Wisdom: A Literature Overview" in the *Archives of General Psychiatry*.

Stephanie P. Morgan, MSW, PsyD, is on the faculty of the Institute for Meditation and Psychotherapy. She maintains a private clinical practice in Manchester, Massachusetts, and is a contributing author to *Mindfulness and Psychotherapy*.

Kristin D. Neff, PhD, is Associate Professor in Human Development and Culture at the University of Texas at Austin. She was one of the first scholars to define and measure self-compassion in an academic context, has written numerous research articles on the psychological benefits of self-compassion, and is a codeveloper of an empirically supported, 8-week mindful self-compassion training program. Dr. Neff is the author of *Self-Compassion: Stop Beating Yourself Up and Leave Insecurity Behind*. She is featured in the award-winning book and documentary *The Horse Boy*, which chronicles her family's adventure with autism.

Andrew Olendzki, PhD, is Executive Director and Senior Scholar at the Barre Center for Buddhist Studies. He is the author of *Unlimiting Mind: The Radically Experiential Psychology of Buddhism* and the editor of *Insight Journal*.

Susan M. Orsillo, PhD, is Professor of Psychology, Suffolk University; coauthor of *Mindfulness- and Acceptance-Based Behavioral Therapies in Practice* and *The Mindful Way through Anxiety*; and coeditor of *Acceptance- and Mindfulness-Based Approaches to Anxiety: Conceptualization and Treatment*. She has authored over 70 publications that reflect a program of research, conducted collaboratively with her doctoral students and Drs. Lizabeth Roemer and Sarah Hayes-Skelton, aimed at developing and evaluating the efficacy and underlying mechanisms of acceptance-based behavioral therapies that address problems such as sexual revictimization, relational aggression, and anxiety. Dr. Orsillo regularly conducts workshops and trainings on applying acceptance-based strategies in clinical practice.

Kenneth I. Pargament, PhD, is Visiting Distinguished Scholar at the Institute for Spirituality and Health at the Texas Medical Center and Professor of Clinical Psychology at Bowling Green State University. He has published over 200 articles on religion and mental health and is the author of *The Psychology of Religion and Coping: Theory, Research, Practice* and *Spiritually Integrated Psychotherapy: Understanding and Addressing the Sacred*. Dr. Pargament is editor-in-chief of the forthcoming two-volume *APA Handbook of Psychology, Religion, and Spirituality*. He was awarded the 2009 Oskar Pfitzer Award from the American Psychiatric Association in recognition of his work in the area of religion and mental health.

Lizabeth Roemer, PhD, is Professor of Psychology, University of Massachusetts at Boston. She is coauthor of *The Mindful Way through Anxiety: Break Free from Anxiety and Reclaim Your Life*, *Mindfulness- and Acceptance-Based Behavioral Therapies in Practice*, and *Behavior Therapy;* and coeditor of *Acceptance- and Mindfulness-Based Approaches to Anxiety: Conceptualization and Treatment*. Dr. Roemer's research, in collaboration with her clinical psychology doctoral students and Drs. Susan M. Orsillo and Sarah Hayes-Skelton, uses both experimental and treatment outcome methodology to examine mechanisms, processes, and outcomes of mindfulness- and acceptance-based interventions targeting anxiety, emotion regulation difficulties, and racial stress. She has published over 70 journal articles and regularly teaches workshops in mindfulness- and acceptance-based behavioral therapies.

Daniel J. Siegel, MD, is Clinical Professor of Psychiatry at the UCLA School of Medicine; faculty member of the Center for Culture, Brain, and Development; and codirector of the Mindful Awareness Research Center. He is a Distinguished Fellow of the American Psychiatric Association and recipient of several other honorary fellowships. Dr. Siegel is also Executive Director of the Mindsight Institute, an educational organization that focuses on the interface of human relationships and basic biological processes. He is the coeditor of a handbook on psychiatry, the editor of the Norton Series on Interpersonal Neurobiology, and author of numerous articles, chapters, and books, including *The Mindful Brain, Mindsight, The Mindful Therapist,* and *The Developing Mind.*

Ronald D. Siegel (see "About the Editors").

Robert J. Sternberg, PhD, is Provost and Senior Vice President, Oklahoma State University, and Honorary Professor of Psychology in the Department of Psychology at the University of Heidelberg, Heidelberg, Germany. He is listed in the *APA Monitor on Psychology* as one of the top 100 psychologists of the 20th century and by the Institute for Scientific Information as one of its most highly cited authors in psychology and psychiatry, and is the author of about 1,200 journal articles, book chapters, and books, including *Beyond IQ: A Triarchic Theory of Human Intelligence; Metaphors of Mind: Conceptions of the Nature of Intelligence; Successful Intelligence;* and *Wisdom, Intelligence, and Creativity Synthesized.* He is editor of *Wisdom: Its Nature, Origins, and Development.*

Janet Surrey, PhD, is Founding Scholar of the Jean Baker Miller Training Institute at the Stone Center, Wellesley College, and a faculty member of Andover–Newton Theological School and of the Institute for Meditation and Psychotherapy. She has been consulting and teaching relational–cultural theory nationally and internationally since the 1990s, working to synthesize Buddhist and relational psychology. Dr. Surrey is coauthor or coeditor of *Women's Growth in Connection, Women's Growth in Diversity, Mothering Against the Odds: Diverse Voices of Contemporary Mothers, We Have to Talk: Healing Dialogues between Women and Men,* and *Bill W. and Dr. Bob: The Story of the Founding of Alcoholics Anonymous.*

Foreword

Everyone wishes to be happy. Economic progress and technological development are necessary for human advancement, so it is easy to imagine that lasting happiness can come from material success or physical comfort alone, but this is a mistake. Both the Buddhist mind-training tradition and Western psychotherapeutic tradition teach that our attitude toward our experience is often far more important to our happiness, and the happiness of those around us, than our fleeting good or bad fortune.

In recent years, Western researchers and psychotherapists have discovered that principles and practices drawn from Buddhist psychology can be very helpful in alleviating the stress of modern life. Therapies that include mindfulness and acceptance are being widely and successfully used to treat a broad range of physical and mental ailments. As interest in the Buddhist understanding of the mind grows in the medical and psychological community, many scientists and therapists are studying Buddhist teachings and cultivating the practice of meditation. They are learning that these teachings and practices have the potential to radically alter our understanding of ourselves and of one another, and can help us do our work more effectively.

In the Buddhist tradition, there are two qualities seen as essential both to our own well-being and to being able to be of appropriate help to others. These are compassion and wisdom. They are said to be like the two wings of a bird or the two wheels of a cart, for the bird cannot fly and the cart cannot roll with only one. Compassion involves wishing to free someone else from suffering, recognizing that she or he wishes to be happy and to avoid distress and misery just as we do. Wisdom involves seeing things as they are, with clear, open eyes, appreciating the interdependence and constantly changing nature of people, things, and events.

In May 2009, I took part in a conference at Harvard Medical School that explored the roles of compassion and wisdom in psychotherapy. We discussed how compassion and wisdom might be developed, how they might benefit therapists in their work, and how helping patients to cultivate these qualities themselves might help them overcome their problems. This book came about as a result of that conference and expands on many of the ideas we began exploring there. In addition to the contributions of many of the conference participants, it includes interesting perspectives from other innovative researchers and clinicians.

I am very happy to see that ancient teachings and practices from the Buddhist tradition can be of benefit today when they are employed by Western scientists and therapists. In today's world, many people turn to psychotherapy to understand what is making them unhappy, and to discover how to live a more meaningful life. I believe that as they come to understand compassion and wisdom more deeply, psychotherapists will be better able to help their patients and so contribute to greater peace and happiness in the world.

His Holiness the Dalai Lama

Acknowledgments

Seen through the eyes of wisdom and compassion, this section of the book could easily be the largest. Just as the universe is implicated in a single sheet of paper—the earth and sun that nourished the tree that made the paper, the oil that generated the electricity that propelled the presses, the trucker and the truck that brought this book to you—each contributor to this book had a universe of support for his or her own efforts. We therefore offer thanks to these many helping hands, visible and invisible.

The editors would particularly like to thank His Holiness the Dalai Lama for his unstinting efforts to bring compassion and wisdom to our global community. His presence at the Meditation and Psychotherapy Conference at Harvard Medical School in 2009 was the main catalyst for this book. The Conference also would not have occurred without the remarkable skills of Judy Reiner Platt, our co-organizer of the event, and Lobsang Sangay at the Harvard Law School, who is currently the Prime Minister of the Tibetan Government in Exile.

We live in circles within circles of supporters. Every editor needs an editor, and we are indebted to Jim Nageotte for his vision, deep feeling, and skillful guidance throughout this project, and to his entirely trustworthy collaborators at The Guilford Press. Many of our contributing authors also had some assistance with their chapters. In this regard, we'd like to particularly acknowledge Christa Smith, clinical psychologist, who skillfully transposed Richard Davidson's conference talk into the written word for this book. And then there are our beloved friends and colleagues at the Institute for Meditation and Psychotherapy, some of whom contributed chapters to this book and all of whom supported our efforts. Each of them lives in some corner of our hearts, smiling.

Editing a book is a learning adventure, and we're grateful to our brilliant authors who moved our understanding of compassion and wisdom immeasurably beyond where it began. In particular, we honor

G. Alan Marlatt, who passed away shortly after he and his colleagues completed their chapter. Alan was a pioneer in the integration of Buddhist psychology and empirically supported psychotherapy, and championed meditation retreats and deeper practice for transforming our view of the world. This book is therefore dedicated to his memory.

We also wish to acknowledge our formal teachers—H. H. the Dalai Lama, Thich Nhat Hanh, Sharon Salzberg, Joseph Goldstein, Jack Kornfield, and Jon Kabat-Zinn, among others—embodiments of the wisdom and compassion that permeate this book; as well as our many clinical colleagues, instructors, and supervisors who have helped us to understand the art and science of psychotherapy. However, perhaps our most important teachers are our patients, who trust us with their secret lives every day, hoping to be truly understood and embraced just as they are, and guided through difficult times. They are the reason this book was conceived, and they are the renewable source of energy behind the undertaking. Although our patients deserve the limelight, their identities have been disguised to protect confidentiality.

Finally, we offer warm hugs and kisses to our families that offered so much, and endured so much, so that we could do what it takes to birth a book. We're always looking for ways to repay their innumerable day-to-day kindnesses.

Contents

Introduction

Christopher K. Germer
Ronald D. Siegel

What personal attributes and qualifications do we look for in a psychotherapist? When we're in emotional pain, the answer likely will not depend upon academic knowledge, training in a particular approach, or even life experience. Instead, we probably want someone who's compassionate (able to relate empathically to suffering, with good will) and wise (has a deep understanding of how to live life well). Indeed, it's difficult to imagine benefiting from a therapist who is *un*wise or *un*compassionate. Although mental health professionals don't generally discuss compassion and wisdom, nor do they try to explicitly cultivate these qualities in themselves or their patients, we nonetheless assume that wisdom and compassion are important elements of all good treatment.

But what exactly is compassion? What is wisdom? A groundbreaking conference took place at Harvard Medical School in May 2009—Cultivating Compassion and Wisdom in Psychotherapy—with His Holiness the Dalai Lama and prominent therapists, scientists, and scholars from around the United States. It was a fascinating exchange, punctuated by good-hearted laughter, moments of confusion, and deep insights into how to live with suffering, the sine qua non of psychotherapy. Many more questions were raised than answered at that meeting. For example:

- Are compassion and wisdom indeed valuable attributes of a psychotherapist?
- Can wisdom and compassion actually be cultivated? If so, how?
- Do ancient traditions that purport to develop compassion and wisdom have anything to offer modern clinicians?

- Are compassion and wisdom important to psychological well-being? If so, should they be integrated into treatment planning and goal setting?
- Is it possible for patients to learn wisdom and compassion in the course of psychotherapy?
- What is the state of psychological research on wisdom and compassion, and what can clinicians learn from it?
- Is there a distinctive neurobiology of wisdom or compassion?
- Are there objective ways of measuring compassion and wisdom, or of recognizing these qualities in the consultation room?
- Are compassion and wisdom mediators of therapeutic change? If so, how do they work?
- What gets in the way of clinicians expressing/acting with compassion and wisdom in their work? What gets in the way for patients in cultivating these qualities in their lives?
- How are compassion and wisdom related to particular clinical conditions such as depression, anxiety, trauma, substance abuse, or relationship conflict?

This book addresses these questions. The authors are all leaders in their fields. Each was given the challenge of offering his or her insights on compassion or wisdom in a relatively short chapter. Many struggled to communicate their ideas without portraying themselves as an "expert" on compassion or wisdom—which, in the true spirit of the subject, none felt qualified to be. As editors, we hope you'll agree that the authors achieved their goals admirably.

Wisdom and compassion have been fundamental to Buddhist psychology and other introspective traditions for at least the past 2,500 years, both as core concepts and as practical paths to liberation from suffering. Over the last two decades, Buddhist psychology in particular has converged with modern psychotherapy to a remarkable extent, primarily in the form of empirically supported mindfulness- and acceptance-based treatments. As the personal and professional practice of mindfulness ripens for many therapists, interest in finding new ways to understand and see our way through complex life circumstances (wisdom) and open our hearts to suffering (compassion) is also growing. Indeed, wisdom and compassion may be seen as the fruition of mindfulness practice.

His Holiness the Dalai Lama was the inspiration for the Harvard psychotherapy conference as well as for this book. Not only is he a brilliant teacher of wisdom and compassion, but he also embodies these qualities in his life. As was pointed out at the conference, "His Holiness makes us proud to be human beings." The Dalai Lama also works tirelessly with scientists around the world to explore how wisdom and compassion can help to alleviate individual and collective suffering in modern times. His approach is unconventional for a religious leader, as his comment in a 2005 presentation reveals:

> . . . empirical evidence should triumph over scriptural authority, no matter how deeply venerated a scripture may be. Even in the case of knowledge derived through reason or inference, its validity must derive ultimately from some observed facts of experience.

This book is informed by insights from Buddhist psychology and practice, as well as by Western psychotherapeutic and scientific discoveries. As we experienced at the conference, the exchange between these differing worldviews can be simultaneously exciting, puzzling, and fruitful.

Psychotherapy and Buddhist mind training share a common objective: overcoming emotional suffering. Compassion and wisdom are qualities of mind that allow us to tolerate, accept, and even grow from suffering. For example, when we empathize with our patients' pain but don't simultaneously nourish the positive, altruistic attitude of compassion, or when we exclude ourselves from our circle of compassion, we're likely to develop compassion fatigue. Wisdom also helps. It allows us to view problems from many different angles, realize that circumstances are constantly changing, and understand that how we *relate* to our experience (tenderly–harshly, accepting–resisting, curious–avoidant) affects our sense of well-being even more than the conditions of our lives. With compassion and wisdom, there's always hope.

Wisdom and compassion are also inseparable; one simply cannot exist without the other. Most of us notice that when we have a multilayered understanding of a patient's problem, our hearts open. Conversely, when we feel warmly toward a client, our minds can see many more treatment possibilities. This book explores how wisdom and compassion comingle at both the relative level—in the day-to-day experience of psychotherapy—and at the absolute level—in our fundamental, unconditioned nature. Depending on our perspective, we may say that compassion emerges out of wisdom or that wisdom emerges out of compassion, but either way, these two qualities are indistinguishable at the deepest level of experience and understanding.

The most surprising discovery for many people is that wisdom and compassion are actually *skills* that we can deliberately cultivate. For example, peering quietly into our inner life in mindfulness meditation, we can develop wisdom about how the mind works as well as about our personal idiosyncrasies. We notice how particular thoughts and emotions snag our awareness and drag us into unconscious, often stressful rumination. We can also develop compassion—shifting the conversation from self-criticism to self-encouragement—by practicing specific exercises, many of which are described in this book. Interestingly, in the intimate dance of a therapeutic relationship, wisdom and compassion often arise simultaneously in the minds and hearts of the therapist and client who are empathically attuned. By exploring the nature of these abilities and how they develop, we can learn to further cultivate them in our personal and professional lives.

A unique feature of Buddhist mind training is the *bodhisattva* ideal. A bodhisattva is a person dedicated to the welfare of others. Most psychotherapists fall into this category, at least some of the time. The traditional bodhisattva "vow" is a commitment to seek enlightenment not only for ourselves, but to continue on until all beings are liberated from suffering—for how can we possibly be free from suffering when we encounter someone who is struggling? Therefore, the path of compassion and wisdom is a group effort. It is in this spirit that we offer this book to our dear friends and colleagues around the world.

May we be open to suffering, with wisdom and compassion.
May we accept ourselves and others, just as we are.
May we know our deepest nature.
May we be free.

PART I

What Are Wisdom and Compassion? Why Should We Care?

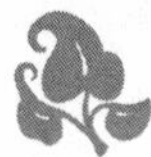

Many clinicians currently have some understanding of mindfulness. Although it is essentially a preconceptual experience, efforts to define and measure mindfulness have contributed to robust research across diagnostic and theoretical boundaries. Over time and with deeper practice, the direct experience of mindfulness yields related experiences such as wisdom and compassion. These concepts are less well understood, even though efforts to describe them have existed as long as recorded history. They, too, can inform clinical research and the practice of psychotherapy.

Chapter 1 begins to explore the meaning of compassion and wisdom, East and West, as well as their intimate relationship to each other and to mindfulness. Chapter 2 provides a model with which therapists can establish mindful presence—a repository of wisdom and compassion—even when their lives become difficult. Then, in Chapter 3, we see how positive emotions such as love and compassion can become a base for opening the mind and expanding awareness, leading to the establishment of wisdom and compassion as personality traits.

We invite you to try practicing the exercises in these chapters and throughout the book, and to evaluate the ideas you encounter on the basis of your own personal experience.

CHAPTER 1

Wisdom and Compassion

Two Wings of a Bird

Ronald D. Siegel
Christopher K. Germer

> Ultimately, the reason why love and compassion bring the greatest happiness is simply that our nature cherishes them above all else. The need for love lies at the very foundation of human existence. It results from the profound interdependence we all share with one another.
>
> —TENZIN GYATSO, the 14th Dalai Lama (2011)

Carmen had suffered from anxiety since she was 9. She panicked in school during a science presentation and soon after felt nauseous at the mere thought of standing up in front of people. When Carmen came to therapy at age 27, she and her well-informed parents (who both also suffered from anxiety) had tried every medication and psychotherapy imaginable. She was virtually housebound due to fear of vomiting, and quite depressed as she watched her friends move forward in their professional and personal lives while she couldn't even go to the hairdresser.

In psychotherapy with a mindfulness-oriented therapist, Carmen discovered that fighting her feelings of nausea simply increased the likelihood that she would vomit in public. In the office, she learned to anchor her attention in the soles of her feet when anticipating a social encounter and to surf the waves of anxiety that coursed through her body. Nothing worked in real-life social situations, however; every sensation of nausea left Carmen overwhelmed and exhausted. Anxious genes and a lifetime of conditioning couldn't be overcome. Carmen and her therapist agreed that her situation was hopeless . . . almost.

Carmen began to speak candidly about her struggle with social phobia and panic disorder: "I'm broken—I'm pathetic!" She and her therapist wondered aloud, might telling someone about her fear of vomiting reverse the shame she felt about her condition? In desperation, Carmen took a chance and told her hairdresser. She was amazed at how quickly her fear melted away. A month later, however, the fear and nausea returned in full force because Carmen was too embarrassed to tell her hairdresser that she *still* suffered from panic. Depressed, Carmen stopped therapy for several months.

When Carmen returned to treatment, she presented a handwritten note describing what she wanted to do in therapy. It contained a three-pronged approach that included: (1) exposure, (2) mindfulness and acceptance, and (3) self-compassion. Taking day trips away from home would decondition her fears; anchoring her attention in present-moment sensory experiences, such as the soles of her feet contacting the ground, would help her tolerate the sensation of nausea, letting it come and go; and telling people about her difficulties would help dissolve her shame. She called the whole plan "internal acceptance"—learning to accept her experience and herself wherever she went. Her therapist felt gratified that some part of Carmen had been listening during the previous year of apparently zero progress.

The following week, Carmen proudly returned to therapy having completed more *in vivo* exposure (shopping, visiting friends, jogging) than ever before. During the next 2 years, she gradually overcame her many fears. It was a rocky road, but when Carmen couldn't accomplish what she planned, she reminded herself that she was "not to blame." When she started feeling nauseous, she pulled out an airline bag and waited for the sensation to pass. Eventually she volunteered at her church's soup kitchen, the first of many steps to building a new life.

What happened here? This case illustrates the power of compassion and wisdom in psychotherapy. Carmen couldn't stop fighting her fear of vomiting, which only made it worse, until she felt the fullness of despair about her situation and responded to her misery with warmth and encouragement rather than with self-criticism, shame, and withdrawal. For Carmen, like many other patients who feel fragile or defective, first she had to begin to accept *herself* in her brokenness before she could face what she feared—in this case, panic and vomiting in social settings. Compassion was the missing link. In the midst of her frustration and despair, Carmen felt the compassionate attitude of her therapist. This gave her courage to tell her hairdresser about her panic, who also responded sympathetically. Finally, Carmen was able to give kindness and understanding to *herself.*

Wisdom also played a key role. Wisdom allowed her therapist to feel Carmen's despair without considering himself a bad therapist, to resonate with Carmen's pain while maintaining perspective and hope, to work neither too much nor too little, and to let Carmen be the expert on her own life. He helped create an atmosphere of curiosity, ease with uncertainty, and mutual regard. Carmen's own wisdom unfolded in multiple ways: She began to look at her problem from a new, broader perspective; recognize the catastrophic, unrealistic meanings that vomiting had acquired; take her frightened, self-critical thoughts less seriously; tolerate discomfort as "not me"; see setbacks and failure as part of life; and commit herself to meaningful activity with others.

But what exactly are *wisdom* and *compassion*? Why are they important in psychotherapy? In this chapter we attempt to define these elusive concepts; to briefly outline the conceptual, scientific, and historical context of the terms in Western and Buddhist traditions; and to discuss how compassion and wisdom are inextricably related to one another. We also begin to examine the relevance of these qualities for clinical work, which is the topic of the rest of the book.

MINDFULNESS: A FOUNDATION FOR WISDOM AND COMPASSION

Interest in incorporating mindfulness into the practice of psychotherapy has grown steadily over the past 25 years. Mindfulness- and acceptance-based treatment is considered the "third wave" of behavior therapy (Baer, 2006; Hayes, Follette, & Linehan, 2004; Hayes, Villatte, Levin, & Hildebrandt, 2011; Hoffman & Asmundson, 2008), following behavioral and cognitive approaches, and mindfulness is influencing a wide range of other treatment models, including psychodynamic (Epstein, 1995; Hick & Bien, 2008; Safran, 2003), humanistic (Johanson, 2009; Khong & Mruk, 2009), and family therapy approaches (Carson, Carson, Gil, & Baucom, 2004; Gambrel & Keeling, 2010; Gehart & McCollum, 2007). In mindfulness-oriented therapy, we're less interested in changing the *content* of our personal experience than in changing our moment-to-moment *relationship* to our sensations, thoughts, emotions, and behavior. This new relationship is characterized by *mindfulness*: "(1) awareness, (2) of the present moment, (3) with acceptance" (Germer, 2005b, p. 7) or "the awareness that emerges through paying attention on purpose, and nonjudgmentally, to the unfolding of experience moment to moment" (Kabat-Zinn, 2003, p. 145). It particularly emphasizes *acceptance*: "active nonjudgmental embracing of experience in the here and now" (Hayes, 2004, p. 21). The opposite of mindfulness and acceptance is resistance or experiential avoidance—warding off unpleasant experience by tensing our bodies, getting stuck in our thoughts, avoiding distressing situations, or blocking out our feelings with psychological defenses. Although such reactions may reduce emotional discomfort in the short run, they tend to amplify distress in the long run (Fledderus, Bohlmeijer, & Pieterse, 2010; Kingston, Clarke, & Remington, 2010).

Research on mindfulness is growing exponentially. As of December 2011, there are over 1,760 peer-reviewed articles in PsycINFO using the word *mindfulness*, whereas in 2005 there were only 364 citations, in 2000 there were 125, and in 1985 there were 24. The most researched mindfulness training program is mindfulness-based stress reduction (MBSR; Kabat-Zinn, 1990; Stahl & Goldstein, 2010). Other empirically supported, widely adopted programs include the MBSR-derived mindfulness-based cognitive therapy (MBCT; Segal, Williams, & Teasdale, 2002; Williams, Teasdale, Segal, & Kabat-Zinn, 2007), dialectical behavior therapy (DBT; Linehan, 1993a, 1993b; see also Chapter 15), and acceptance and commitment therapy (ACT; Harris, 2009; Hayes, Strosahl, & Wilson, 1999). While increasing empirical evidence for the efficacy of mindfulness- and acceptance-based treatments is contributing to their popularity, mindfulness is also now recognized as a transtheoretical and transdiagnostic change process—a mechanism of action underlying diverse forms of treatment for a wide range of conditions (Baer, 2010a; Hölzel, Lazar, et al., 2011). Mindfulness has the potential not only to link different schools of therapy, but also to bridge clinical research and practice and to integrate the personal and professional lives of therapists (Germer, Siegel, & Fulton, 2005).

Cultivating a kinder, more compassionate relationship toward oneself and others is included, explicitly or implicitly, in the mindfulness training programs mentioned above, and research has demonstrated that mindfulness training increases self-compassion (Birnie, Speca, & Carlson, 2010; Krüger, 2010; Shapiro, Astin, Bishop, & Cordova, 2005; Shapiro, Brown, & Biegal, 2007). Although the influence of mindfulness practice on the development of wisdom has not yet been studied experimentally, its primary purpose within the Buddhist tradition has been to develop penetrating insight into the nature of the mind and, by extension, life itself (see Chapter 9). In fact, what Western psychotherapists call "mindfulness meditation" is also known in Buddhist traditions as "insight meditation," designed explicitly to cultivate those insights that lead to wisdom and thereby free ourselves and others from suffering. The Greek philosopher Heraclitus wrote, "Applicants for wisdom do what I have done: inquire within" (Hillman, 2003, p. xiii). The Buddha said, "Come and see for yourself" (*ehipassiko* in ancient Pali). For this wisdom to dawn, we need an attitude of deep acceptance toward our moment-to-moment experience and compassion toward ourselves as suffering individuals. When we use mindfulness practices to look inside in this way, we develop qualities of mind and heart—wisdom and compassion—that allow us to see clearly, to engage whatever we're feeling with tenderness and ease, and to respond effectively to emerging life circumstances.

Three Mindfulness Skills

Although mindfulness, wisdom, and compassion are *experientially* related and are cultivated by overlapping methods, they have distinct conceptual features and engage somewhat different psychological processes or skills.

The three core skills taught by most mindfulness training programs are (1) concentration (single-focus awareness), (2) mindfulness per se (open-field awareness), and (3) loving-kindness and compassion (Salzberg, 2011). Until recently, the first two psychological processes have been emphasized in mindfulness- and acceptance-based psychotherapy. Those skills are also the primary vehicles for cultivating wisdom, understood in Buddhist psychology as penetrating insight into the nature of our minds and the "self." The third skill—loving-kindness and compassion—helps to cultivate a caring attitude toward ourselves and others, especially in the midst of suffering, which, in turn, allows us to hold our moment-to-moment experience with greater mindfulness and less resistance.

Regulating Attention and Emotion

William James (1890/2007) wrote: "The faculty of voluntarily bringing back a wandering attention, over and over again, is the very root of judgment, character, and will" (p. 424). In meditation, single-focus practices such as returning attention to the breath or the soles of the feet when we're distressed serve the function of calming the mind (R. D. Siegel, 2010). Open-field awareness techniques—noticing whatever arises in our field of perception—train the mind to receive the vicissitudes of life with equanimity and insight. Taken together, learning to regulate our attention with these practices helps us regulate our emotions.

However, there are other meditation techniques, such as loving-kindness meditation (*metta*) and giving and taking meditation (*tonglen*), that have been developed over thousands of years specifically to manage difficult emotions (see Chapters 4 and 7).

The Dalai Lama notes:

> Buddhism has long argued for the tremendous potential for transformation that exists naturally in the human mind. To this end, the tradition has developed a wide range of contemplative techniques, or meditation

> practices, aimed specifically at two principal objectives—the cultivation of a compassionate heart and the cultivation of deep insights into the nature of reality, which are referred to as the union of compassion and wisdom. At the heart of these meditation practices lie two key techniques, the refinement of attention and its sustained application on the one hand, and the regulation and transformation of emotions on the other. (Society for Neuroscience, November 12, 2005)

This book explores how the theory and practice of mindfulness and compassion can blossom into wisdom and compassion in psychotherapy and beyond. We begin by examining compassion, which is a bit more familiar to clinicians and has been investigated more extensively by researchers than the more elusive and enigmatic concept of wisdom.

WHAT IS COMPASSION?

The English word *compassion* derives from the Latin and Greek roots *pati* and *pathein* ("to suffer") and the Latin root *com* ("with"), so compassion means to "suffer with" another person. The *Oxford English Dictionary* defines compassion as "sympathetic pity and concern for the sufferings and misfortunes of others" (p. 291). In 2009, thousands of religious leaders from around the world composed the Charter for Compassion in which they defined compassion as a call to "treat all others as we wish to be treated ourselves" (Armstrong, 2010, p. 6). In the hands of psychologist scholars and scientists, the quest to understand compassion becomes especially interesting and nuanced.

A shorthand, operational definition of compassion might be *the experience of suffering with the wish to alleviate it*. Similar definitions include the following:

- "Basic kindness, with deep awareness of the suffering of oneself and other living beings, coupled with the wish and effort to alleviate it" (Gilbert, 2009c, p. xiii)
- "The feeling that arises in witnessing another's suffering and that motivates a subsequent desire to help" (Goetz, Keltner, & Simon-Thomas, 2010, p. 351)
- "The wish that all sentient beings may be free from suffering" (Dalai Lama, 2003, p. 67)
- A three-part process: (1) "I feel for you" (affective), (2) "I understand you" (cognitive), and (3) "I want to help you" (motivational) (Hangartner, 2011)

Until the last decade, compassion as a distinct emotion or attitude had been relatively neglected by experimental psychologists (Davidson & Harrington, 2001; Goetz et al., 2010; Goleman, 2003; Pommier, 2010) and by psychotherapists (Gilbert, 2005, 2009a; Glaser, 2005; Ladner, 2004; Lewin, 1996). This neglect may be due, in part, to the overlap of compassion with similar constructs such as *empathy* (Batson, 1991; Hoffman, 1981), *sympathy* (Shaver, Schwartz, Kirson, & O'Connor, 1987; Trivers, 1971), *love* (Fehr, Sprecher, & Underwood, 2009; Post, 2002), *pity* (Ben Ze'ev, 2000; Fiske, Cuddy, Glick, & Xu, 2002), and *altruism* (Monroe, 2002; Oliner, 2002). How does compassion relate to these terms? A precise understanding of compassion is useful not only for developing theory, assessment tools, and applications to therapy, but also for recognizing and cultivating compassion within ourselves. (For further analysis, see Eisenberg & Miller, 1987; Goetz et al., 2010.)

Empathy

Carl Rogers (1961) defined *empathy* as an "accurate understanding of the [client's] world as seen from the inside. To sense the [client's] world as if it were your own" (p. 284). It is "having an emotional response similar to the response another person is having" (Bohart & Greenberg, 1997, p. 23). Empathy goes beyond cognitive appraisal to include a felt sense of what another person is experiencing (Feshbach, 1997; Lazarus, 1991). It is considered a common factor in psychotherapy that "accounts for as much and probably more outcome variance than does specific intervention" (Bohart, Elliott, Greenberg, & Watson, 2002, p. 96).

We can be empathic with just about any human emotion—joy, grief, excitement, boredom. Compassion, however, is a special form of empathy insofar as it is *empathy with suffering* (along with the wish to alleviate it). Suffering is a prerequisite for compassion. Since the purpose of therapy is to alleviate emotional suffering, it seems that compassion has probably been hidden under the umbrella of empathy throughout the history of psychotherapy. Systematic efforts to cultivate empathy are still relatively rare in the clinical field (Shapiro & Izett, 2007), but that may change as ancient Buddhist compassion practices are integrated into modern psychotherapy.

Sympathy

Sympathy is "an emotional reaction that is based on the apprehension of another's emotional state or condition and that involves feelings of concern and sorrow for the other person" (Eisenberg et al., 1994, p. 776).

Sympathy includes a reactive element, based on prior experience, whereas empathy is a *mirror* of another person's mental state. There appears to be more mindful awareness in empathy than in sympathy.

Love

Therapists tend to avoid the term *love*, especially with their patients, because it has multiple meanings—parental love, universal love, romantic love—that are likely to create misunderstanding. But the word *love* still retains some juiciness that helps to illuminate the meaning of compassion. Lynne Underwood (2009) prefers the term *compassionate love* to simply *compassion* because it implies more emotional engagement.

Compassion within the Buddhist context may appear to an outside observer to be detached rather than juicy (Goetz, 2010). This perception is due to the quality of *equanimity*—the ability to hold the highs and lows of our emotional lives in openhearted awareness. For example, a teenage daughter may need to temporarily reject her mother in order to develop independence before she goes out into the world. Deeply understanding this process will enable a mother to feel her own pain, fear, or anger without overreacting. Equanimity does not prevent us from jumping for joy or dissolving into tears, but it does give us the freedom to express emotion in effective ways in different situations while staying emotionally connected to others.

Loving-kindness is a "state of mind which aspires that all sentient beings may enjoy happiness," and compassion is "the wish that all sentient beings may be free from suffering" (Dalai Lama, 2003, p. 67). In the Buddhist tradition, loving-kindness practices are usually taught *before* compassion practices because compassion is more challenging. It can be rather difficult to keep our hearts open in the face of suffering—not blaming the victim or wishing that he or she would go away so that we can feel better again.

Pity

Pity is concern for the plight of others comingled with a slight sense of superiority (Fiske et al., 2002), whereas compassion is an emotion among equals. Since we all suffer, suffering is a common thread that ties us together. When we're open to suffering in a compassionate way, we feel less alone. When we block out suffering, we may feel a slight remove from others who are struggling—that is, pity. Pity can be considered a precursor to compassion—an initial opening—but it can also get in the way of the fully connected experience of compassion if it isn't recognized.

Altruism

> Compassion is not just feeling with someone, but seeking to change the situation. Frequently people think compassion and love are merely sentimental. No! They are very demanding. If you are going to be compassionate, be prepared for action!
>
> —DESMOND TUTU (Barasch, 2005)

Altruism is a quality of compassion that distinguishes it from both empathy and sympathy. Altruism can be considered either a motivation (Batson, 2002) or an action (Monroe, 2002) that "involves helping another without regard for personal gain" (Kristeller & Johnson, 2005, p. 394). Empathy and sympathy may *lead* to altruism, but they don't necessarily do so. Compassion always includes altruism.

Self-Compassion

Although compassion is generally considered an emotion or attitude toward *others*, the Buddhist definition of compassion includes all beings, *including oneself* (see Chapters 6 and 7). The Dalai Lama (2000) said:

> . . . for someone to develop genuine compassion towards others, first he or she must have a basis upon which to cultivate compassion, and that basis is the ability to connect to one's own feelings and to care for one's own welfare. . . . Caring for others requires caring for oneself.

Many people find it easier to be compassionate toward a few special beings—pets, children, loved ones—than toward themselves, so current research does not show a clear, linear relationship between self-compassion and compassion for others (Neff, Yarnell, & Pommier, 2011). It makes sense, however, that in order to be compassionate toward *all* people, we need to be accepting of the many different parts of ourselves, including our less desirable qualities (see Chapter 13). Otherwise we will have a tendency to reject in others what we don't like in ourselves.

Compassion is an inside job. Compassion can turn to *anger* if we think that the suffering individual is undeserving of help; it can turn into *distress* if we don't have the resources to help; into *schadenfreude* (pleasure at the suffering of another) if the sufferer is seen as an obstacle to one's own happiness; and sometimes even into *anger* or *shame* when the suffering individual is oneself (Goetz et al., 2010). Therefore, we need balanced (mindful) awareness of our internal world, and an attitude of self-kindness, to sustain compassion toward others.

A BRIEF HISTORY OF COMPASSION

Compassion is at the core of the world's religions. For example, Confucius was the first major teacher to put forth the Golden Rule: "Never do to others what you would not like them to do to you" (Armstrong, 2010, p. 9). The Hindu avatar Krishna said, "Out of mere compassion for them, I, abiding in their self, destroy the darkness born of ignorance" (Shankaracharya, 2004, p. 264). Jesus taught, "You shall love your neighbor as yourself" (Mark 12:31). Muhammad said, "No one is a believer unless his neighbor feels safe from harm on his account" (Taymiyyah, 1999, p. 262). In Judaism, "The kindness of the Lord is not ended, His mercies are not spent. They are renewed every morning" (Lamentations 3:22–23; see also Berlin, Brettler, & Fishbane, 2004, p. 1596). Our religious traditions all deal with the problem of human suffering. In the Buddha's teaching, suffering is the "first noble truth," and he taught compassion as a means to relieve personal pain and promote peaceful cooperation.

In the Western philosophical tradition, Aristotle was the first to consider compassion in detail (as "pity") (Cassell, 2005). Subsequent philosophers were wary of emotion, such as Kant and Nietzsche, who warned that feelings like compassion are a threat to reason and should be suppressed (Nussbaum, 1996, 2001). Other Western thinkers, however, such as Hobbes (1651/1962), Hume (1888/1978), and Schopenhauer (1844/1966), saw the value of identifying with others or imagining ourselves in their position (see Pommier, 2010).

Perhaps the close association of compassion with religion discouraged the fledgling science of psychology from exploring it more thoroughly. Nonetheless, compassion can be found embedded in familiar therapeutic concepts of empathy, the therapeutic alliance, unconditional positive regard, and acceptance.

In their historical overview of "acceptance" in psychology, John Williams and Steven Lynn (2010) identify the historical Buddha (563–483 BCE) as the first to carefully elaborate the concept. The Buddha believed that most human suffering arose from the desire for moment-to-moment experience to be other than it is (i.e., nonacceptance). To counteract this tendency, he suggested that individuals cultivate nongreed, nonhatred, mindfulness, compassion, wisdom, and a host of other mental factors to alleviate suffering (see Chapters 4 and 9).

Interest in acceptance, especially acceptance of "self" and "other," has existed in the field of psychotherapy for over a century. William James, Sigmund Freud, and B. F. Skinner all considered acceptance to be psychologically beneficial. Carl Rogers (1951) and fellow humanistic and existential therapists elevated acceptance to the status of a core change process. Interestingly, both Freud (1913/1957) and Rogers considered *self-acceptance* to be a precursor to acceptance of others, and this perspective became a focus of empirical investigation well into the 1980s. In the 1990s, research shifted focus to acceptance of *moment-to-moment experience* with the introduction of Buddhist-inspired mindfulness and acceptance-based treatments (Kabat-Zinn, 1990; Linehan, 1993a; Segal et al., 2002).

Exploring compassion, along with wisdom, appears to be the next step in the convergence of Buddhist psychology and modern psychotherapy. Familiar topics are being reexamined and new frontiers opened:

- Self-compassion is emerging as a new form of self-acceptance.
- Compassion is being explored as a type of empathy that emphasizes regulating suffering with good will.
- Compassion fatigue is being understood as what happens when we have empathy without self-compassion and equanimity.
- Compassion-oriented therapy is being developed as a focused attempt to cultivate the skill of compassion to manage emotional pain.
- Brain studies are showing that compassionate mind states include enhanced visceral sensitivity to the pain of others.

These topics and a host of others are discussed in this book.

IS COMPASSION INNATE?

It may be said that we are hardwired not only for fight and flight, but also for compassion. Our primitive, self-preservative instincts occur very quickly and automatically, but we are also naturally cooperative and altruistic (Keltner, 2009; Sussman & Cloninger, 2011). And like all mental habits, our instinct for compassion can be strengthened through practice. Evidence for innate compassion can be found in evolutionary and neurobiological arenas.

Evolution

Contrary to popular belief, Charles Darwin considered sympathy to be the strongest of our instincts, noting that "those communities, which included the greatest number of the most sympathetic members would flourish best, and rear the greatest number of offspring" (1871/2010, p. 82; Ekman, 2010). Parents need compassion to raise children to the age of reproduction, and evidence even shows that kindness is the main criterion (over financial prospects and appearance) for mate selection by both men and women (Keltner, 2009). We appear to have been naturally selected to cooperate with others even though we may never see a particular other person again (Delton, Krasnow, Cosmides, & Tody, in press).

Neurobiology

Neuroanatomically, social emotions like compassion engage regions in the brain well below the cortex, including the hypothalamus and the brain stem, that are associated with basic metabolic processes and evolutionarily old emotions such as fear (Immordino-Yang, McColl, Damasio, & Damasio, 2009; see also Chapter 8). Compassionate brain states also appear to activate the mesolimbic neural system, which may explain why compassion is intrinsically rewarding (Kim et al., 2011).

The fight–freeze–flight and competition–reward subsystems in the brain are balanced by a "safeness" subsystem (Depue & Morrone-Strupinsky, 2005; Gilbert, 2009b; see Chapter 18). The safeness system is associated with compassion—caregiving and soothing—and appears to be related to the neurotransmitters oxytocin and vasopressin. Compassionate mind states are typically calming and are characterized by decelerated heart rate (Eisenberg et al., 1988), lower skin conductance (Eisenberg, Fabes, Schaller, Carlo, & Miller, 1991), and vagus nerve activation (Oveis, Horberg, & Keltner, 2009; Porges, 1995, 2001)—the opposite of what occurs in sadness and distress (Goetz et al., 2010).

We also have mirror neurons that continually register what others are thinking and feeling (Rizzolatti & Craighero, 2004; Rizzolatti & Sinigaglia, 2010; Siegel, 2007), prompting us to relieve the suffering of others to make ourselves feel better. Finally, it appears that many individuals, especially women, have a "tend and befriend" response to stress, rather than fight and flight (Taylor et al., 2000). In sum, numerous elements in our nervous system predispose us to feel compassion.

CULTIVATION

Over the past few millennia, the efforts of countless practitioners of meditation and prayer suggest that it's possible to make compassion a habit. Long-term effects of compassion meditation on the brain are currently being explored using brain imaging and other methods (see Chapter 8). Evidence shows that we can gradually learn to use our neocortex to move from automatic fear activation of the amygdala and the "self-preservative system" to compassionate mind states and the "species-preservative system" (Wang, 2005). Only 8 weeks of mindfulness meditation, averaging

27 minutes per day, can cause changes in the structure of the brain associated with self-awareness, compassion, and introspection (Hölzel, Carmody, et al., 2011).

Mind training occurs not only on purpose with closed eyes in meditation, but also in our interactions with others from birth onward (Siegel, 2007). Childhood attachment styles can impact the capacity for compassion in adulthood (Gillath, Shaver, & Mukilincer, 2005), but even those with anxious or avoidant attachment styles can increase their compassion levels after being primed with words, memories, or stories of secure attachment (Carnelley & Rowe, 2007, 2010). Training programs designed specifically for cultivating compassion (Miller, 2009) and self-compassion (see Chapters 6 and 18) are currently under development.

COMPASSION AND WELL-BEING

Within the Buddhist tradition, love, compassion, joy, and equanimity are considered the "four immeasurable attitudes," or the abodes of the gods (see Chapter 4). The implication is that when we embody these qualities, suffering disappears.

The scientific community is beginning to explore the mental and physical health benefits of compassion (Hofmann, Grossman, & Hinton, 2011; Wachholz & Pearce, 2007). For example, individuals high in compassion are more likely to accept compassion from others and are therefore less reactive to stress (Cosley, McCoy, Saslow, & Epel, 2010). Practicing compassion can also lead to lasting improvements in happiness and self-esteem (Mongrain, Chin, & Shapira, 2011). Most of the compassion research has been conducted on correlates of compassion such as altruism, empathy, forgiveness, and other positive emotions, as well as challenges to compassion such as anger, stress, loneliness, and compassion fatigue. For example, altruism may benefit physical and emotional health by reducing stress and improving the immune response (Sternberg, 2011), and it seems to promote longevity (Brown, Nesse, Vinokur, & Smith, 2003).

The research on *self*-compassion demonstrates clear correlations to psychological well-being (see Chapter 6). At the time of this writing, there still don't appear to be any published, randomized, controlled studies on the impact of self-compassion training on mental health, but preliminary evidence indicates multiple beneficial effects (Adams & Leary, 2007; Gilbert & Irons, 2005a; Kuyken et al., 2010; Raque-Bogdan, Ericson, Jackson, Martin, & Bryan, 2011; Schanche, Stiles, McCollough, Swartberg, & Nielsen, in press; Shapira & Mongrain, 2010; Thompson & Waltz, 2008; Van Dam, Sheppard, Forsyth, & Earleywine, 2011). For example, individuals high in self-compassion who were also depressed showed significantly less depression 5 months later than those with low self-compassion, suggesting that self-compassion provides a natural buffer against emotional problems (Raes, 2011).

The question inevitably arises, "Can a mental state that embraces suffering really be good for mental health?" In practice, our focus of attention does not remain very long with suffering. We need suffering for compassion to arise, but we only need to contact it for a brief period before switching to loving feelings for the sufferer and the wish to help. Positive emotions predominate over suffering in the experience of compassion. This is the reason that compassion fatigue may actually be "empathy fatigue" (Ricard, 2010; see also Chapters 7 and 19). There is tenderness, hope, and good will in the mind of a compassionate individual—all factors that support mental and physical health.

WHAT IS WISDOM?

Almost every language has a word for "wisdom." It has been described as the highest human virtue across diverse cultures, and it figures prominently in written and oral traditions since ancient times. It's also certainly a trait most of us would like to see in a psychotherapist. And yet, until recently, modern psychologists (and even philosophers) had hardly touched the subject. In fact, they've had a very difficult time even agreeing what it is. Much like U.S. Supreme Court Justice Potter Stewart's (1964) observation that "hard core pornography is hard to define [but] I know it when I see it," a consensual definition of wisdom has been elusive, even though we recognize it when it emerges and miss it when it's absent.

The English word *wisdom* comes from the Indo-European word *wede*, meaning "to see" or "to know" (Holliday & Chandler, 1986). In English-language dictionaries, wisdom is defined variously as the "capacity of judging rightly in matters relating to life and conduct; soundness of judgment in the choice of means and ends; . . . enlightenment, learning, erudition (*Oxford English Dictionary*, 2010) or "knowledge . . . the intelligent application of learning; ability to discern inner qualities and essential relationships; insight, sagacity; . . . judgment, prudence . . . sanity" (Merriam-Webster, 2011). These overlapping definitions are multidimensional, raising the question of whether we'd be better served by seeing wisdom as a cluster of diverse human capacities rather than a single virtue. Nonetheless, the fact that people have valued "wisdom" highly across time and cultures suggests that there is something meaningful about the construct. The diverse capacities that wisdom comprises are probably interrelated, creating a whole that is greater than the sum of its component parts. As we'll see throughout this book, none of us acts very wisely when using only some components of wisdom while neglecting others.

Because the construct is so multidimensional, it may not be possible to arrive at a shorthand, operational definition of wisdom. Instead, we may need to settle for a definition that captures its essence, even if it doesn't readily lend itself to experimental design. So in the context of psychotherapy, we might think of wisdom as simply *knowing deeply how to live.* What this actually entails, however, is not so simple to describe.

One mark of a particularly hard-to-define construct is the existence of competing methods of arriving at its definition (Staudinger & Glück, 2011). Some psychologists have gone around the world asking ordinary folks to describe "wise" people, looking for patterns in their responses to identify *implicit models* of wisdom (e.g., Bluck & Glück, 2005). Other researchers have searched the world's philosophical and religious writings looking for recurring themes (e.g., Birren & Svensson, 2005; Osbeck & Robinson, 2005). Still others have tried reflecting deeply about the matter themselves, yielding a wide variety of *explicit theories* –"constructions of (supposedly) expert theorists and researchers" (Sternberg, 1998, p. 349). No consensus has emerged. The two primary psychological texts on wisdom, edited by Robert Sternberg (Sternberg, 1990a; Sternberg & Jordan, 2005), have as many definitions of wisdom as they have chapters. Luckily, however, the struggle to define wisdom is actually beginning to illuminate its nature. By elucidating its many component parts, we get hints as to how we might cultivate wisdom and use it in psychotherapy. But as you'll soon see, clinical attention has been focused even less on wisdom than on compassion.

A Top-Down Process

Modern neuroscientists differentiate between bottom-up and top-down processes. The former describe how the brain takes in basic sensory information, organizes it into perceptions, and constructs experiences of reality from these basic building blocks–as, for example, when enjoying the smell of a rose. Top-down processes involve interpreting and responding to the data continuously streaming into our brain from our sensory systems, using higher cortical faculties such as reason, judgment, and conceptual frameworks born of past experience. Thinking before acting and making balanced decisions, as we might do when choosing how to speak about a sensitive subject with a patient, are top-down processes. Wisdom, therefore, may perhaps be the highest possible top-down process. It has many components, all of which involve deliberation, emotional regulation, and perspective taking. Like many other top-down processes, it is integrative–involving communication among the body, head, and heart.

Although theorists disagree about its particulars, almost all agree that wisdom is the opposite of acting impulsively out of instinct, habit, or unmodulated passion (Sternberg, 2005a; see also Chapter 11).

One reason that wisdom has received so little attention until recently from either academic or clinical psychology is that it is such a complex top-down process. Since its beginnings in the late 1800s, academic psychology has focused on more elemental psychological processes—phenomena that could readily be defined operationally and experimented upon, such as perception or behavioral conditioning (Birren & Svensson, 2005). Psychotherapists have also shied away from examining wisdom, perhaps seeing it as more rightly the province of philosophy or religion. Even modern philosophers have ignored it, noting its historical interest but not wanting to spend much time with a construct that is so multidimensional (Smith, 1998). Yet this was not always the case among the world's deepest thinkers.

A BRIEF HISTORY OF WISDOM, WEST AND EAST

Some of the earliest existing wisdom writings are found on fragments of clay tablets in Mesopotamia dating back 5,000 years. Here we find such sage advice as, "If we are doomed to die—let us spend"; and "He who possesses much silver, may be happy; he who possesses much barley, may be happy; but he who has nothing at all, can sleep" (Hooker & Hooker, 2004), along with admonitions for "good" and "effective" behavior (Baltes, 2004, p. 45). Ancient Egyptian wisdom writings from 2000 BCE foreshadow many later conceptions of wisdom, including the inadvisability of thinking of oneself as wise: "Be not puffed up with thy knowledge, and be not proud because thou are wise" (Readers Digest Association, 1973).

Yet it was the ancient Greek philosophers, "lovers of wisdom," who established the intellectual framework for this quality that dominated Western thinking in subsequent centuries. From Socrates (470–399 BCE) to Plato (428–322 BCE) to Aristotle (384–322 BCE), the idea of wisdom or *sophia* evolved and was eventually distinguished from knowledge, craftsmanship, and other capacities. Socrates described "the narrow intelligence flashing from the keen eye of a clever rogue" as distinct from wisdom, and repeatedly underscored the importance of knowing one's limitations (Osbeck & Robinson, 2005, p. 65). His pupil, Plato, emphasized that the cultivation of wisdom is a "daily discipline" that we should undertake "with all earnestness" by developing "reason" to control our spirit and appetites. Aristotle entertained the notion of the "Golden Mean"—finding balance in the degree to which we express various aspects of our character

(Center for Ethical Deliberation, 2011). All of these ancient themes have made their way into modern definitions of wisdom.

In later Hebrew and Christian texts, wisdom became revelation of truth from God (Birren & Svensson, 2005). Adherence to faith was the path to wisdom, and, as can be seen in Job's Old Testament struggle, wisdom included knowing our place in the world, accepting that much is beyond our capacity to understand, and remaining faithful to God (Rad, 1972). Later, in the teachings of St. Augustine (354–430 CE), wisdom became moral perfection without sin (Birren & Svensson, 2005). Not surprisingly, these more theological notions have not been widely adopted by modern psychologists studying wisdom.

Great thinkers in the West have typically emphasized some combination of the importance of reason (Frances Bacon, 1561–1626 CE; Descartes, 1596–1650; Plato), knowing God (Locke, 1632–1704), and just action (Kant, 1724–1804; Montaigne, 1533–1592) in describing wisdom (Birren & Svensson, 2005). It was generally seen as a set of cognitive capacities involving both the acquisition of knowledge and the development of the skill to utilize it effectively in the world.

Asian wisdom traditions typically have a different flavor. They emphasize the *transformative* power of wisdom in positively affecting our cognitive, intuitive, affective, and interpersonal experience (Takahashi & Overton, 2005). Our earliest written records of Asian wisdom teachings are the *Upanishads*, recorded between 800 and 500 BCE (Durant, 1935). Here the collected stories of saints and sages describe wisdom that was not only distinct from factual knowledge, but included transcendent spiritual experiences beyond those of our familiar sensory world. Around 600 BCE the diverse collection of teachings we call Taoism emerged in China. In this tradition, intuition, compassion, and, above all, living a balanced life in harmony with natural laws are seen as the essence of wisdom. Logical thought, reason, and customs are seen as suspect—too easily influenced by narrow self-interest and alienating us from the totality of nature (Birren & Svensson, 2005). Soon after, also in China, Confucius (551–479 BCE) taught that living a moral life and maintaining the social order were hallmarks of wisdom (Baltes, 2004; Birren & Svensson, 2005).

Influential as these wisdom traditions have been in shaping Asian culture, it is the teachings of the Buddha (563–483 BCE) that are currently having the most direct impact on Western psychological thought and practice—primarily through the adoption of mindfulness-based treatments. As we'll see shortly, in Buddhist teachings wisdom is seen as insight into both the patterns of the natural world and the ways in which our conventional mental habits create suffering. As in the Taoist tradition, reason and accumulated knowledge are seen as less important than intuitive insight, and insight is seen as radically transforming of both our experience and behavior.

WISDOM IN WESTERN PSYCHOLOGY

Given the importance of wisdom in Western thought, the foundational theorists of both academic psychology and psychotherapy traditions have had surprisingly little to say about it. This absence is particularly striking considering that "wise" people were the mental health professionals of old—people routinely sought their counsel when upset by life's difficulties.

Traditional compendia of psychological knowledge, such as the *Handbook of General Psychology* (Wolman, 1973) or *An Intellectual History of Psychology* (Robinson, 1995), make no mention of the topic. Despite being philosophically oriented, William James didn't discuss wisdom in *The Principles of Psychology* (1890/2007) nor even in *The Varieties of Religious Experience* (1902/2010), in which he quotes numerous religious texts that use the word, but never explores the construct himself. Sigmund Freud, despite being counted by many as a wise master, hardly mentions the word throughout his voluminous writings.[1] Carl Jung, also appreciated for his wisdom, describes transcendent experiences and discusses dream and mythical images of the "wise old man" and "wise old woman," but doesn't describe wisdom per se nor how to develop it.

Among foundational theorists, Erik Erikson (1950) was the first to address wisdom in any detail. He described it as the outcome of successfully negotiating the eighth and final stage of human development: "ego integrity vs. despair." In later writings, he provided a bit more detail, describing wisdom as "an informed and detached concern with life itself" or "truly involved disinvolvement" (Erikson & Erikson, 1982/1998, p. 61). Related to Erikson's idea that wisdom involves successfully navigating developmental challenges, George Vaillant, who conducted the Harvard Study of Adult Development, came to the conclusion that "maturity of defenses," reflected in people's behavior rather than in their words, is the best measure of wisdom (2003, p. 255). Mature defenses, such as humor, sublimation, and altruism, tend to bring well-being to oneself and others, while less mature defenses such as projection, hypochondriasis, and passive–aggressive behavior tend to cause grief.

Of major psychological theorists, Abraham Maslow has probably contributed most to our understanding of wisdom, though he, too, didn't discuss the term in great detail. The "self-actualizing" individuals he studied

[1]Based on an online search of Freud's writings using the keyword *wisdom*.

to develop his hierarchy of needs embrace reality and facts rather than denying truth, are spontaneous, focus on problems outside themselves, can accept their own human nature with all its shortcomings, are accepting of others, and lack prejudice (Maslow & Lowry, 1973). As we'll see, these are all widely recognized as important components of wisdom.

Despite historical neglect by Western psychology, a more recent growing interest in lifespan development and, subsequently, in positive psychology (the study of happiness) has inspired a small but dedicated group of theorists and researchers to study wisdom explicitly (Hall, 2007; Sternberg, 1990a; Sternberg & Jordan, 2005).

Empirical Research

Empirical research in this area began with a doctoral dissertation in 1976 by Vivian Clayton, who set out to investigate what wisdom might be and whether it's affected by age (Hall, 2007). Studying ancient Western texts in an effort to define it, she came to the conclusion that wisdom generally involved acquiring knowledge, applying it to human social situations, reflecting upon it, and using judgment to make decisions influenced by compassion. She then tried to measure wisdom using existing psychological tests and came to the conclusion that, unlike many other cognitive abilities, wisdom resisted erosion over time and could actually increase with age (Hall, 2007).

In the early 1980s, Paul B. Baltes, a pioneer in lifespan developmental psychology, founded the Berlin Wisdom Project, which became the largest program to date studying wisdom in the laboratory. He and his colleagues defined wisdom as "highly valued and outstanding expertise in dealing with fundamental . . . problems related to the meaning and conduct of life" (Kunzmann & Baltes, 2005, p. 117). They studied wisdom by presenting subjects with open-ended, hypothetical situations and inviting them to "think aloud" about how they might respond. They found that, compared to others, those whose responses demonstrated aspects of wisdom such as rich factual and procedural knowledge, perspective, tolerance, and acceptance of uncertainty, tended to be less "self-centric" and have less interest in pursuing a pleasurable and comfortable life. These "wise" individuals focused instead on personal growth and insight, and other-oriented values related to "environmental protection, societal engagement, and the well-being of friends" (Kunzmann & Baltes, 2005, p. 126). Wise people also prefer cooperative approaches to conflict management, rather than those that reflect either a one-sided concern with one's own interests (dominance) or others' interests (submission), or no concern at all (Kunzmann & Baltes, 2005, p. 126). The Berlin group found that wisdom is rare and doesn't necessarily increase with age (findings repeatedly replicated by many researchers; e.g., Baltes & Staudinger, 2000; Jordan, 2005; Staudinger, 1999), though training and practice in trying to understand oneself and others seem to help (Kunzmann & Baltes, 2005). Interestingly, they also came to see wisdom as a socially interactive product (Staudinger & Baltes, 1996) that can't really be located in individuals but rather is shared by communities.

Although the Berlin project has produced the largest body of empirical research on wisdom, it has its critics. The most often cited concerns are that this research (1) measures how people think, rather than how they act, and (2) neglects emotion. Beginning in 1997, Monika Ardelt, a sociologist, recruited senior citizens to help develop a "three-dimensional" wisdom scale that measures *cognitive, reflective*, and *emotional* domains. In her framework the emotional sphere involves feeling compassion toward others and being able to deal constructively with adversity. Ardelt argues that including compassion reveals what really constitutes a wise person—not just one who can demonstrate intellectual skills. Quoting the philosopher John Kekes, she notes that "a fool can learn to say all the things a wise man says, and to say them on the same occasions" (Ardelt, 2004, p. 262), but this isn't real wisdom. In support of her model, she points out that Jesus, Buddha, Muhammad, Gandhi, Christian saints, and Zen masters all perceive a deeper truth that eludes others, are able to transcend their subjectivity and projections and look at events objectively from multiple perspectives, and have compassion for others (Ardelt, 2004, p. 279).

Another major contributor to empirical wisdom studies is Robert Sternberg (see Chapter 11). In his model, a wise person works toward a common good "through *balance* among a) intrapersonal, (b) interpersonal, and (c) extrapersonal interests to achieve a balance among (a) adaptation to existing environments, (b) shaping of existing environments, and (c) selection of new environments, over the long term as well as the short term" (Sternberg & Lubart, 2001, p. 507; Chapter 11). Foolishness is what erupts when we're out of balance—relying only on some of our faculties, considering only some interests, or focusing exclusively on either short- or long-term consequences (Sternberg, 2005a; Chapter 11).

Seeking Consensus

So how might we sift through these many perspectives to arrive at an understanding of wisdom that is useful to psychotherapists? Several writers have tried to identify common themes in historical accounts and modern models. Neurobiologists Thomas Meeks and Dilip Jeste (2009; Chapter 14) identified six key components of wisdom: (1) prosocial attitudes/behavior, (2) social decision making/pragmatic knowledge of life, (3) emotional homeostasis, (4) reflection/self-understanding, (5) value relativism/tolerance, and (6) acknowledgment of and dealing effectively with uncertainty/ambiguity. Judith Glück (2008; of the Berlin Project) and Susan Bluck also surveyed existing definitions and identified four components of wisdom, summarized by the acronym *MORE*: mastery, openness to experience, a reflective attitude, and emotion regulation skills. Although we still don't have a consensus definition, at a 2010 meeting of philosophers and psychologists exploring the topic, the simplified MORE framework gained some support as a way to encompass diverse perspectives (Tiberius, 2010).

Neurobiology

Not surprisingly, given our difficulty even defining wisdom, our understanding of its neurobiology is currently limited. Meeks and Jeste (2009) have tried to describe what may be happening in different brain regions when various components of wisdom are active, though they caution that the map is speculative because we don't have a consensus definition of wisdom, and because brain imaging research has not focused specifically on the neurobiology of wisdom. Despite these and other limitations, we can get a clearer idea of the dynamics of wisdom by exploring what sorts of brain activity are associated with each of its subcomponents (see Chapter 14).

Clinical Explorations

The psychological construct of wisdom has been largely ignored in the clinical field. Many books and articles discuss "clinical wisdom," the "wisdom of the body," and the "wisdom of the unconscious," but relatively few have grappled with what wisdom might be and how it might inform psychotherapy.[2]

The most in-depth clinical explorations of wisdom in the context of psychotherapy are found in the realm of transpersonal psychology. This discipline, which initially grew out of research with psychedelic drugs in the 1960s and subsequent countercultural interest in Asian meditation and yoga practices, is "concerned with the study of humanity's highest potential, and with the recognition, understanding, and realization of intuitive, spiritual, and transcendent states of consciousness" (Lajoie & Shapiro, 1992, p. 91). Its goal is to "integrate timeless wisdom with modern Western psychology and translate spiritual principles into scientifically grounded, contemporary language" (Caplan, 2009, p. 231). In addition to Maslow's work on "self-actualizing" individuals, Stanislav Grof's

[2]Based on a search of PsycINFO in February 2011 using the keyword *wisdom*.

(1975, 1998) studies of the consciousness-expanding effects of LSD helped to launch the field. Probably because the field grew out of a countercultural milieu, borrows liberally from esoteric spiritual traditions, and is particularly interested in mystical experiences, it has not received a lot of attention from mainstream clinicians.

As far as we can determine, there has only been one systematic attempt to apply the findings of academic wisdom research in the clinical arena. Michael Linden, a German psychiatrist practicing in Berlin, has developed a treatment he calls "wisdom therapy." It uses a modification of the Berlin Wisdom Project's research protocol to cultivate wisdom in clients. These individuals are asked to consider difficult life situations from multiple perspectives, with the aim of developing several components of wisdom, including flexibility of view, empathy, acceptance of emotions, value relativism, acceptance of uncertainty, and a long-range perspective (Linden, 2008).

When we began planning this book, we thought of wisdom simply as having a deep understanding of how to live. While this definition still captures its essence, we've since learned that wisdom is a high-level, multidimensional human capacity that manifests differently under different circumstances. It involves balance among, and integration of, many faculties, and has taken varying forms across cultural and historical contexts. Developing targeted interventions or clinical training models to cultivate such a multidimensional virtue therefore will be a challenge indeed.

WISDOM FOR THE PSYCHOTHERAPIST

We conducted an informal survey of experienced clinicians, asking them what constitutes a "wise" therapist (see Chapter 10). Based on their responses, combined with the historical and modern models just discussed, we identified the following attributes of wisdom that may be useful to consider—both to work more wisely as therapists and to cultivate wisdom in our patients:

- Factual knowledge relevant to the problem at hand
- Reasoning and problem-solving ability
- Capacity for common sense as well as expert judgment
- Ability to hold multiple perspectives and competing values simultaneously
- Awareness of the limits of our knowledge
- Comfort making decisions amidst ambiguity and uncertainty
- Awareness that all thoughts are constructed

- Intuitive grasp of the interdependent, ever-changing nature of all phenomena and how the mind constructs a conventional "reality" of separate, stable objects
- Ability to appreciate absolute (transcendent, transpersonal, interdependent) reality along with conventional reality
- Ability to observe, reflect on, and understand our own cultural, familial, and personal conditioning and psychological dynamics
- Interest in personal growth and learning from experience
- Openness to experience
- Concern for the effects of actions on the near and wider world in the long and short term
- Ability to tolerate and reflect upon affects and urges without necessarily acting on them
- An understanding of human nature as it changes through physical, psychological, and spiritual developmental stages
- Understanding the causes of human suffering and its alleviation
- Social or emotional intelligence—the ability to understand and communicate with others
- Compassion for self and others

It's a long list that may seem like a tall order. But these capacities tend to be interrelated, and by developing one we tend to strengthen others.

CULTIVATING WISDOM

Although numerous investigations have come to the conclusion that wisdom is a rare development and doesn't necessarily increase with age, occasionally it does (Baltes & Staudinger, 2000; Jordan, 2005; Staudinger, 1999; Vaillant, 2003). But can we deliberately cultivate it? A study by the Berlin school indicates that clinical psychologists demonstrate more wisdom than the population at large, at least when describing solutions to complex human problems (Smith, Staudinger, & Baltes, 1994; Staudinger, Smith, & Baltes, 1992). This finding suggests that training can help, although therapists may be a self-selected sample. It's nonetheless likely that holding the intention to understand others and develop other aspects of wisdom over the course of a lifetime is one factor supporting its development (Jordan, 2005). Traditional conceptions of wisdom are in line with this view. Plato suggested that developing wisdom requires a "daily discipline," and in early Buddhist traditions, wisdom is developed by following the eightfold path requiring, among other things, persistent "right effort."

The Role of Mindfulness

Most wisdom traditions suggest that deliberately engaging in meditative or contemplative practices can help us become wiser. In the Buddhist tradition, mindful awareness practices were developed explicitly as a means of cultivating wisdom—"seeing things as they are, rather than as we'd like them to be" (Surya Das, 2011, p. 1). How might this work? Let's look at some of the components of mindfulness practices, and how each may in turn develop various components of wisdom.

Stepping Out of the Thought Stream

By returning our attention repeatedly to moment-to-moment sensory experience (e.g., the sensations of the breath), rather than remaining embroiled in thoughts, we begin to gain perspective on our thought processes. This practice allows us to see how thoughts are conditioned by family and culture, and how they change with moods and circumstances (R. D. Siegel, 2010). We also get to see our intellectual defenses at work—the resistance that arises in response to unsettling thoughts, and our urges to maintain comforting ideas or interpretations. Seeing these mental processes in action helps us develop a central feature of wisdom found across many definitions: the ability to entertain multiple perspectives. In the Buddhist tradition, this "perspective taking" goes even further, to gain firsthand insight into how the mind constructs a seemingly stable reality out of the ever-changing flux of experience (see Chapter 9).

Being with Discomfort

By turning our attention toward, and opening to, uncomfortable emotions and physical sensations, mindfulness practice helps us tolerate and accept physical and emotional discomfort (Germer et al., 2005; R. D. Siegel, 2010). Many definitions of wisdom point to the capacity to step back, resist the urge for immediate personal comfort, and act in the interest of the greater good. This is possible only if we can get beyond our instinctual habit of seeking personal comfort and avoiding pain. Much as our muscles become stronger by lifting weights at the gym, we become better able to endure pain by practicing mindfulness. This endurance is cultivated both by observing that our pain, like all things, changes on its own, and by not identifying with the discomfort as being about "me" (more on this shortly).

Disengaging from Automatic Responses

When we're not mindful, many of our reactions are impulsive. They're either instinctual or conditioned through reward and punishment, modeling, and/or classical conditioning. Mindfulness practice teaches us to observe stimulus-response processes in microscopic detail, so that we can experience the arising of a sensation, thought, or feeling, followed by the urge to act in response to it, finally followed by overt behavior. Instead of automatically enacting the sequence, with practice we can develop the ability to pause, take a breath, and evaluate whether or not the action would actually lead to desirable results. In this way mindfulness practice can help us develop the capacity for emotional regulation—restraint from acting automatically on affects or urges—which figures prominently in most definitions of wisdom.

Transpersonal Insight

A key purpose of mindfulness within the ancient Buddhist mind-training tradition is to yield direct insight into *anatta* (see Chapters 9 and 13)—the lack of a separate, enduring self or identity. This insight is closely related to insight into what later Buddhist traditions refer to as *shunyata*, or *emptiness*: the observation that all perceived phenomena arise interdependently with all other phenomena, and their apparent separate nature is an invention of our conceptual minds. Mindfulness practices help us see this interdependence by revealing that all experience is in constant flux, with our minds relentlessly generating words to organize this flux into what we take as conventional reality. We notice that we are, as neuroscientist Wolf Singer (2005) puts it, "an orchestra without a conductor." This awareness not only helps develop wisdom in the Buddhist sense—insight into the way things really are—but also dissolves the barrier between "me" and "mine" and "you" and "yours," leading to compassion, another cornerstone of wisdom.

Moment-to-Moment Observation of the Mind's Antics

While mindfulness practice can lead to a radical reappraisal of who we think we are, along the way it usually illuminates what psychodynamic traditions call *defenses*. Noticing what the mind is doing in each moment, we see how we often project onto others and have difficulty seeing them clearly as they are. We notice our minds stereotyping, judging, jealously competing, idealizing, denigrating, and doing all the other not-so-noble things that are part of human nature. Seeing this mental busyness enables us to reflect on our reactions to things, increasing the possibility that we'll develop the introspective attitude and self-understanding that is another important component of wisdom.

Seeing How the Mind Creates Suffering

Mindfulness practices were also developed to help practitioners see how the mind creates suffering for itself, and how this suffering can be alleviated (R. D. Siegel, 2010). Like Goldilocks and the Three Bears, the mind is forever making comparisons and judgments, struggling to get things "just right" and then keep them from changing. Our attempts to cling to pleasant moments and avoid or push away unpleasant ones inevitably fail, causing endless distress. One moment we're winning, but the next moment we're losing. Insight into these processes, which arises spontaneously during mindfulness practice, gives us a rich understanding of human nature—a dimension of wisdom particularly relevant to psychotherapy practice.

Embracing Opposites

When we step out of the thought stream and observe the moment-to-moment activity of the mind, we see that our dearly held views of reality—"I'm smart," "I'm stupid," "I'm kind," "I'm mean"—are merely mental constructions. That understanding helps us tolerate the views of others and find cooperative solutions to conflicts—both of which are frequently mentioned dimensions of wisdom.

Mindfulness can also help us embrace different levels of reality simultaneously. We can be aware of what Buddhist psychology describes as *absolute reality*: emptiness and *anatta* (the interdependence of all phenomena and lack of any separate, enduring "self"), *anicca* or impermanence (the fact that all phenomena are in constant flux), and *dukka* or suffering (how the mind creates suffering by clinging to pleasant and rejecting unpleasant experience). At the same time, we can be aware of conventional or *relative reality*: the fact that we naturally want to protect ourselves and our loved ones; we want to be healthy, safe, secure, and loved; we fear the unknown; we have natural sexual and aggressive urges; as well as all the other tendencies that make us human. As we'll see throughout this volume, being able to embrace both of these levels is particularly important to acting wisely as a therapist, since sometimes our patients need us just to understand their ordinary emotional experience, whereas other times they need us to see the bigger picture and understand how the mind creates suffering by not perceiving absolute reality.

Developing Compassion

Several definitions of wisdom include compassion toward others (Ardelt, 2004; Clayton, 1982; Meeks & Jeste, 2009). Conversely, effective compassionate action must include wisdom, lest we inadvertently harm those we're trying to help. As we discussed earlier, mindfulness practice can be a great support for cultivating compassion, in part by showing how interconnected we all are. When we have the ability to abide peaceably in the midst of our own suffering, we see that everyone else also suffers, and we spontaneously feel like helping others, much as the right hand assists the left hand when it's injured. Experiencing interdependence and feeling compassion are fundamentally inseparable. As the 10th-century Indian sage Atisha put it: "The supreme goal of the teachings is the emptiness whose nature is compassion" (Harderwijk, 2011).

Other Paths to Wisdom

One aspect of wisdom does not naturally arise from mindfulness practice: acquiring the knowledge and experience needed to solve concrete worldly problems. We're unlikely to learn to fix an automobile, speak a foreign language, or perform surgery wisely by just sitting on a meditation cushion. These aspects of wisdom are probably best learned through conventional methods, such as self-study, schooling, and apprenticeships.

Many practices designed to cultivate wisdom are associated with theological frameworks that require belief in a divinity and/or otherwise require faith. Mindfulness practices, in contrast, have been refined in Buddhist traditions with an attitude expressed by the Pali word *ehipasiko*—meaning, come and see for yourself—which fits nicely with modern psychological attitudes that value observed experience over doctrine. This is not to suggest, however, that other means of cultivating wisdom, including those drawn from Western and other Eastern religious traditions, might not also be important to psychotherapy (see Chapter 22). It's easy to imagine how many different forms of contemplative practice, as well as many different types of therapy, could support the development of the attitudes and capacities that we've been discussing.

Wisdom is also contagious. Throughout history people have sought contact with great teachers and sages for precisely this reason. And many wise figures point to the tutelage of their mentors as important developmental influences. In fact, one reason why having a wise therapist is important is that wisdom will be transmitted in the therapy process. This seems particularly likely in light of studies showing that clients' values tend, over time, to become increasingly like those of their therapists (Williams & Levitt, 2007).

To some extent, wisdom can also be acquired through books. But it appears that most aspects of wisdom—seeing how the mind constructs reality, learning to tolerate personal discomfort, developing emotional regulation, experiencing care and compassion, seeing the interdependence of things, developing self-understanding, and deeply appreciating human nature—all require personal, introspective discipline.

TWO WINGS OF A BIRD

In Tibetan Buddhism, wisdom and compassion are considered to be "two wings of a bird" (Dalai Lama, 2003, p. 56; see also Chapter 4). The bird cannot fly with only one wing, nor when one wing is significantly weaker than the other. In psychotherapy, if we feel compassionately toward a patient but have no wisdom, we are liable to lose our compassion, become overwhelmed with emotion, lose the path through suffering, and conclude that the treatment is hopeless. Conversely, if we can wisely comprehend the multidetermined nature of a patient's problem but are out of touch with the patient's despair, our supposedly wise therapeutic suggestions will fall on deaf ears. Our patients need both; they need to "feel felt" (Siegel, 2009), and they need a realistic path through their suffering.

At an absolute level, wisdom and compassion are inseparable. Shortly before his death, Thomas Merton (2008) said, "The whole idea of compassion . . . is based on a keen awareness of the interdependence of all these living beings, which are all part of one another, and all involved in one another" (p. 30). A Buddhist friend echoed this vision: "Wisdom is concerned with penetrating and abiding in the ultimate truth, while compassion is the movement of the heart from this deep understanding to relate to the ups and downs and struggles of life as it unfolds" (Chodon, personal communication).

We hope that this introduction to wisdom and compassion in psychotherapy has kindled your interest and tempted you to read on. It's usually easiest to learn or refine a skill when we have some understanding of its component parts and the methods others have used to develop it before us. In the pages ahead, you'll find diverse perspectives on compassion and wisdom, varied ways to cultivate them, and concrete applications we can use as therapists and offer to our patients. By looking together at the many facets of these highest of human potentials, may we all find ways to live more wisely and compassionately, so that we, our patients, and everyone else can live happier, healthier, more meaningful lives.

CHAPTER 2

Mindful Presence

A Foundation for Compassion and Wisdom

Tara Brach

Do you pay regular visits to *yourself*?
—RUMI (Barks, 1995, p. 80)

I was bringing a daylong meditation workshop to a close when Pam, a woman in her late 60s, drew me aside. She and her husband Jerry were at the end of an ordeal that had begun 3 years earlier. Now near death from lymphoma, Jerry had asked Pam to be his primary caregiver, the person guiding and supporting him in his passing. "Tara," she implored, "I really need some help."

Pam was desperate to do anything she could for Jerry, who was enduring intense pain, nausea, and exhaustion. "I wanted so much to save him," she told me. "I looked into ayurvedic medicine, acupuncture, Chinese herbs, every alternative treatment I could find, tracked every test result . . . we were going to beat this thing." She slumped wearily in her chair. "And now, I'm keeping in touch with everyone, giving updates . . . coordinating hospice care. If he's not napping I try to make him comfortable, read to him . . . "

I responded gently, "It sounds like you've been trying really hard to take good care of Jerry . . . and it's been *very busy*." At these words, she gave me a smile of recognition. "Hmm, *busy*. That sounds crazy, doesn't

---

This chapter is adapted from *True Refuge* (Brach, 2012). Copyright 2012 by Tara Brach. Adapted by permission.

it?" She paused, "As far back as I can remember I've really been busy. But now . . . well, I just can't let him go without a fight."

Pam was silent for a few moments and then looked at me anxiously. "He could die any day now, Tara. Isn't there some Buddhist practice or ritual that I should learn? Is there something I should be reading? What about *The Tibetan Book of the Dead*? . . . How can I help him with this . . . with dying?"

Hearing the urgency behind her questions, I asked her to listen inwardly and to let me know what she was feeling. "I love him so much, and I'm terrified that I'm going to let him down." She began weeping. After some time, she spoke again. "All my life I've been afraid of falling short–I guess I've always been on overdrive. Now I'm afraid I'm going to fail at the thing that matters most. He'll die and I'll feel *really* alone because I failed him. I just don't trust that I can handle this."

"Pam," I said, "You've already done so much . . . but the time for all that kind of activity is over. At this point, you don't have to make anything happen, you don't need to *do* anything." I waited a moment and then added, "Just *be* with him. Let him know your love through the fullness of your presence."

At this difficult time I was calling on a simple teaching that is central to my work with both my meditation students and therapy clients: *It is through realizing and trusting our capacity for a wise and loving presence, through* being *that presence, that we discover freedom from suffering. In the face of life's greatest challenges, this timeless presence brings healing and peace to our own hearts and to the hearts of others.* The deepest transformations in therapy arise out of a person's capacity to hold his or her own inner life with a loving, wise awareness. This awareness is cultivated by paying attention with unconditional presence: seeing clearly what is–right now–with compassion. When therapists offer such fullness of presence to their clients, they model how that person can attune to him- or herself; they also directly offer the healing balm of undivided attention. Such presence, offered to ourselves or others, is not passive. Rather it is an engaged, receptive state that is the very ground for wise action.

Pam had nodded when I spoke of "the fullness of presence." She and Jerry were Catholic, she told me, and they'd found that the mindfulness practice they'd learned in my weekly class had helped them experience their faith more deeply. But in this crisis, any reserves of trust–in herself, in others, in God–seemed out of reach: "I know the hospice aides are doing everything they can to help, but I just feel like this shouldn't be happening. . . . No one should have to go through something like this–it's just plain wrong." For Pam, as for so many people, sickness, with its sometimes relentless discomfort and pain, was an unfair and cruel enemy. At times she felt betrayed and angry at life, and at other times, she sank into a sense of personal failure. Trapped in fear and aloneness, Pam was living in what I call a "trance" (Brach, 2003), identified as a deficient, isolated, and threatened self.

"In those most difficult moments," I suggested, "You might pause and recognize what you are feeling—the fear or anger or grief—and then inwardly whisper the phrase 'I consent.'" I had recently heard this phrase from Father Thomas Keating, and I thought that, as a Catholic, Pam might find it particularly valuable. Saying "I consent," or, as I more frequently teach, "yes," relaxes our armoring against the present moment and allows us to see more clearly what is happening within and around us.

Pam was nodding again, but she had an intent, worried look. "I want to do this, Tara, but when I'm most upset, my mind speeds up. I start talking to myself . . . I talk to him . . . how will I *remember* to pause?" It was a good question, one that I'm often asked. "You probably will forget, at least some of the time," I responded, "and that's totally natural. All you can do is have the intention to pause, the intention to feel what is going on and 'let be.'" Pam's face softened with understanding. "That I can do. I can intend, with all my heart, to be there for Jerry."

MINDFULNESS: THE GROUND OF COMPASSION AND WISDOM

In the simplest terms, mindfulness is the intentional process of paying attention, without judgment, to the unfolding of moment-to-moment experience. It is the opposite of *trance*, a word I use to describe all the ways in which we—therapists and clients alike—live inside a limiting story about life. The Buddha often referred to this virtual reality of incessant thinking and emotional reactivity as a dream, and he taught that mindfulness wakes us up (Gunaratana, 1991). For example, if you get lost in worries about paying bills, mindfulness notices the worry thoughts and the accompanying feelings of anxiety. If you get lost in rehearsing how you will explain a mistake to your supervisor, mindfulness notices the inner dialogue and the feelings of excitement or fear. If you are hunched over, gazing intently into your computer screen composing a response to an annoying e-mail, mindfulness notices the irritation, the mental tightness, and the sensations of your frozen and strained physical posture. Mindfulness recognizes and allows, without any resistance, all these thoughts, sensations, and feelings as they come and go.

Here is an image that is helpful in introducing mindfulness (Siegel, 2010b): Imagine your awareness as a great wheel. At the hub of the wheel is mindful presence, and from this hub, an infinite number of spokes extend out to the rim. Your attention is conditioned to react to whatever arises—whether within you or outside you—by grasping after pleasant experience, avoiding what is unpleasant, and being inattentive if it is neutral. This means that the mind habitually leaves the hub, moves out along the spokes, and affixes itself to one part of the rim after another. Plans for dinner segue into a disturbing conversation, a self-judgment, a mental note about making a phone call, irritation at the volume of the radio, anxiety about a persistent backache. Or, as Pam found, attention can get lost in obsessive thinking, circling endlessly around stories and feelings about what is wrong. While attention naturally moves in and out of presence, the problem is that it is easy to get stuck on the rim. If you are not connected to the hub, if your attention is trapped out on the rim, you are cut off from your wholeness and living in trance. You have lost contact with your physical aliveness, your feelings, and your heart. Mindfulness is a pathway home.

The Buddhist tradition offers simple but powerful techniques to cultivate present-centered, lucid, and compassionate attention (Goldstein & Kornfield, 1987). Meditation practice, designed to cultivate mindfulness, often begins with preselecting a home base or anchor, such as the in and out of the breath, the sounds in the room, or moment-to-moment bodily sensations. Because the mind is so habituated to moving into the future and the past, to creating stories about what is happening, it rarely stays focused on the anchor for long. Although it is possible to train attention to become deeply stable and concentrated on a single object, this is not the purpose of an anchor in mindfulness training. Rather, the purpose is to help us recognize when the mind has wandered and become lost on the rim, and to guide us back to the hub. "*Coming back*" is necessary if we are to connect with the reality that is here and now. Once we're back at the hub, the anchor also helps us to quiet and calm the mind. No matter how often our attention flies out to some problem or fantasy or memory on the rim, we gently pause, return to the hub, and ground ourselves, once again, in presence.

Whether in formal meditation or in the midst of daily life, a key skill for cultivating mindful presence is remembering to pause (Brach, 2003). When we're in trance, we're often tumbling forward through time—"on our way" somewhere, trying to get through the day, reacting to one thing, then another. I sometimes refer to "the sacred pause," because if we can remember to pause, we begin to contact the healing space of presence. We can see we've been circling on the rim and choose to come back. My students and clients often report that, perhaps more than any other meditative guideline, the sacred pause has enabled them to wake up from habitual patterns of obsessive thinking. Just a taste of pausing and experiencing a little space around the compelling stream of worries and plans can be tremendously freeing.

As our attention becomes more settled, we will sense that the boundaries of the hub are softening and opening. This is the phase of training in mindfulness that might be called "*being here*." We continue to be in touch with the movement of our breath (or with another anchor), but at the same time we are aware of the sound of a dog barking, the pain in our knee, a thought about how long we'll continue to meditate. In this state, we're neither fixating on these experiences nor pushing them away. We "recognize and allow" the thoughts, feelings, and sensations that come to our attention; they are free to come and go. If the emotions are strong, as was the case for Pam, the allowing can be deepened by saying "yes," or "I consent." Naturally the mind will still sometimes lose itself in reactivity, and at these times, when we notice, we again gently return to the hub—"coming back" and "being here" are fluid facets of practice.

The more we inhabit the alert stillness at the center of the wheel and include in awareness whatever is happening, the more the hub of mindful presence becomes edgeless, warm, and bright. In the moments when there is no controlling of experience—when there is effortless mindfulness—we enter fully into natural presence. This timeless presence is filled with infinite possibilities. The hub, spokes, and rim are all floating in our luminous open awareness—we are home. In these moments, our minds are sourced in an unobstructed view of reality—wisdom—and our hearts, in unconditioned love or compassion.

CULTIVATING COMPASSION AND WISDOM IN DIFFICULT WEATHER

Sustaining presence with our intra- and interpersonal lives is much easier said than done. Each of us knows what it is like when someone criticizes us, challenges our sense of competency, brings out our feelings of guilt or shame. We know what it is like when we are with a client and reacting with a sense of personal failure ("I'm not helping") or judgment ("You're not trying to help yourself"). And we know what it is like when we, like Pam, face a major life crisis—perhaps a sense of betrayal in a relationship, financial insecurity, a life-threatening illness. Rather than staying grounded in a mindful presence, we become lost in our spinning thoughts, in our urgent efforts to control what is happening, in addictive behaviors, in our habitual judgments and defenses. We become simultaneously less clear-minded and less open-hearted. How do we strengthen mindfulness at those moments when we are most inclined to go into trance?

Some years ago, a number of Buddhist teachers began to share a new mindfulness tool based on the acronym *RAIN*. This training in presence is "in-the-trenches" support for working with intense and difficult states of mind—for awakening wisdom and compassion when we're most inclined to become confused or self-absorbed. While it is most effective when combined with ongoing practice in mindfulness meditation, it provides an accessible approach to mindfulness even for clients who might resist anything they thought was "meditation." I have now taught RAIN to thousands of students, clients, and mental health professionals, adapting and expanding it into the version you'll find in this chapter. I've also made it a core practice in my own life. When, like Pam, we are caught up and suffering in the trance of fear and separation, RAIN can help bring us home to full mindfulness by directing our attention in a clear, systematic way.

R-A-I-N

R	***R**ecognize* what is happening.
A	***A**llow* life to be just as it is.
I	***I**nvestigate* inner experience with kindness.
N	***N**onidentification;* rest in ***N**atural awareness.*

Recognize What Is Happening

Recognition starts when you focus your attention on whatever thoughts, emotions, feelings, or sensations are arising in the present moment. Recognition is seeing what is true in your inner life. You can awaken recognition simply by asking yourself: "What is happening inside me right now?" Call on your natural curiosity as you focus inward. Try to let go of any preconceived ideas about what is happening and, instead, listen in a kind, receptive way to your body and heart.

Allow Life to Be Just as It Is

Allowing means "letting be" whatever thoughts, emotions, feelings, or sensations you discover. It can be helpful to ask yourself, when difficult experiences arise, "Can I be with this?" or "Can I let this be, just as it is?" You may feel a natural sense of aversion, of wishing that unpleasant feelings would go away, or find yourself filled with thoughts of blame or shame. But as you become more willing to be present with "what is," a different quality of attention will emerge. Learning to *be with* difficult experiences in this way is necessary for wise action, since without it we will react automatically, rather than thoughtfully, to difficulties. It is also necessary to cultivate compassion because if we cannot tolerate our own pain, we will not be able to tolerate others' pain (see Chapter 1).

The realization that allowing is intrinsic to understanding and healing can give rise to a conscious intention to "let be." Many clients and students I work with support their resolve to accept what is happening by mentally whispering an encouraging word or phrase. For instance, they might feel the grip of fear and whisper "let be," or experience the swelling of deep grief and whisper "yes." They might use the words, "this too," or, as I suggested to Pam, "I consent." At first many feel a sense of tentatively "putting up" with unpleasant emotions or sensations. Or they might say "yes" to fear, hoping that saying "yes" will make the fear magically disappear.

In reality, we have to consent again and again and sometimes recognize even the subtlest ways in which we are tensing against fear or pain. Yet even the first gesture of allowing–simply whispering a phrase such as "yes" or "I consent"–begins to create a space that softens the harsh edges of your pain. Your entire being is not so rallied in resistance. Offer the phrase gently and patiently, and in time your receptivity will deepen. Your defenses relax and you may feel a physical sense of yielding or opening to waves of experience.

Sometimes, however, just the notion of allowing brings up vehement resistance. "What do you mean!" someone might say. "Am I supposed to accept that he betrayed me?" "Am I supposed to say 'yes' to feeling self-loathing?" "To this awful anxiety?" In these situations it is important to point out that we are agreeing only to the experience–in our body, heart, mind–*in the present moment*. We're not being asked to accept the situation itself or another person's behavior, just the felt experience, here and now. In fact, when resistance arises, our first step is to accept the experience of resisting. We recognize and allow the disgust, the tension in the body, the blaming thoughts, the aversion. As I often teach it, "You are saying 'yes' to your 'no'!"[1]

Investigate with Kindness

At times, simply working through the first two steps of RAIN–the basic components of mindfulness–is enough to provide relief and reconnect

[1] It is also important to note that for someone who has experienced trauma, RAIN may initially be contraindicated and potentially retraumatizing. We need to feel a degree of safety and trust to say "yes" and open to raw feelings. When there is very intense fear or terror lurking, it may be wise to honor the "no" of our protective defenses and first to cultivate the inner and outer resources of safety and compassion that provide a groundwork for practicing RAIN.

you with presence. In other cases, however, the simple intention to recognize and allow is not enough. For instance, if you are in the thick of a divorce, about to lose a job, or dealing with the distress of a loved one, you may be easily overwhelmed by intense feelings. Because these feelings are triggered over and over—you get a phone call from your soon-to-be ex, your bank statement comes, you wake up to pain in the morning—your reactions can become very entrenched. In such situations, you may need to further awaken and strengthen mindful awareness with the *I* component of RAIN.

Investigation means calling on your natural interest—the desire to know truth—and directing a more focused attention to your present experience (Goldstein & Kornfield, 1987). Simply pausing to ask "What is happening inside me?" might initiate recognition, but with investigation you engage in a more active and pointed kind of inquiry. You might ask yourself: "How am I experiencing this in my body?" or "What does this feeling want from me?" or "What am I believing about myself?" "About others?" The impetus for such inquiry arises out of our innate intelligence. We discern that we need to open ourselves to a deeper understanding of our situation.

The investigation phase of RAIN is especially suited for the therapeutic relationship. Although we might sense that we need to look more closely at what is happening inside us, we often don't ask ourselves the very questions that might most unhook us from an unconscious identification with our thoughts and feelings. For instance, if a client is possessed by feelings of fear and hurt, suggesting that he or she inquire "What am I believing right now?" may uncover the stories of personal failure or mistrust that have been fueling the feelings. Consciously naming the belief can weaken its grip, opening the way to ask "Is that really true?" On the other hand, if a client is lost in obsessive thinking, he or she might not remember to ask "What am I feeling in my body?" This question helps us to step out of the intellectualization, judgments, and mental commentary that obscure genuine insight into "things as they are," and to directly contact the felt sense of vulnerability or woundedness that can give rise to authentic self-compassion.

Wisdom begins to unfold as we include in mindful awareness whatever we have habitually avoided or covered over. As you investigate, you might contact sensations of hollowness or shakiness, and then tap into a story you've told yourself for years about always being pushed away by those to whom you most want to be close. This might lead to a memory of rejection, and then to feelings of shame, hurt, or loneliness. Buried in these responses you might feel a yearning for acceptance, for connection. Unless these parts of your psyche are consciously contacted, they will control your experience and perpetuate the identification with a threatened, deficient self. Only when we shine the light of awareness on previously hidden experiences does the assumed identification start to loosen. We begin to see that our being is more than an insecure, limited self, and this realization enables us to respond wisely to our situation rather than react out of emotional pain.

However, such inquiry alone is not enough to arouse full mindful presence. In order for investigation to be healing and freeing, we need to approach our experience with a kind quality of attention. This means contacting a sense of care and warmth and offering a gentle welcome to whatever arises. Without this heart energy, investigation cannot penetrate and awaken our natural wisdom; there is not enough safety and openness for real contact: Self-compassion is an inherent ingredient in a mindful presence.

Imagine that your child has been bullied at school and comes home in tears. What is needed is both understanding (investigation) and compassion. In order to find out what happened and how your child is feeling, you have to offer a kind, receptive, gentle attention. In a similar way, when a client arrives at a session wildly upset, our caring and acceptance create a safe and healing space for the emotions to be felt, examined, and transformed. In RAIN, this intimate attention is offered to our inner life. It softens the armoring of the heart and makes inquiry, and ultimately insight and healing, possible.

Because so many clients suffer from shame and self-aversion, they have little or no experience of self-compassion. As therapists, our own compassionate attention begins to transform this emotional patterning. Then building on this, training in mindfulness gradually cultivates the client's capacity to hold difficult inner experience with kindness. The seeds of this shift in relating to one's inner life are planted in the initial phase of RAIN—recognizing a painful emotional state and allowing it to be as it is. Research done with brain imaging has shown that mindful attention itself activates parts of the brain associated with compassion and empathy (Cahn & Polich, 2006; Hölzel et al., 2011). The *I* of RAIN—investigating and intentionally offering a kind attention—both strengthens and deepens mindfulness, giving rise to a full and authentically compassionate presence. In this way, compassion, like wisdom, can be understood to be an intrinsic component of mindful presence, and also a precious fruit.

Realize Nonidentification; Rest in Natural Awareness

The lucid, open, and kind presence evoked in the *R*, *A*, and *I* of RAIN leads to the *N*: the freedom of *nonidentification* and the realization of *natural awareness* or natural presence. Nonidentification means that your self-sense is not fused with, or defined by, any limited set of emotions, sensations, or stories about who you are. This realization that you are "no-thing"—that there is not a static, solid self—is the ultimate expression of wisdom and the essence of freedom (Rahula, 1974; see also Chapters 9 and 13). Identification keeps us locked into the "small self," the self of trance. When identification with the small self is loosened, when we are no-thing, we begin to intuit and live from the aliveness, openness, and love that express our natural awareness. As Indian teacher Nisargadatta Mahraraj (1973) describes it:

> Love says, "I am everything."
> Wisdom says, "I am nothing."
> Between these two my life flows. (p. 269)

This awakening of wisdom and love (or compassion) affects us in a very immediate way: We find that we have more choices about how to respond to life—new possibilities open up, fresh ways of relating with ourselves, with loved ones and colleagues—and we are filled with more gratitude, greater ease.

The first three steps of RAIN require intentional activity. In contrast, the *N* of RAIN expresses the result of mindfulness: a liberating realization of natural awareness. Although for some people, this kind of awakening might uproot the suffering of trance once and for all, for most of us, freedom from emotional suffering unfolds more gradually. We might find ourselves moving through many rounds of getting lost in the old stories of what is wrong with us, wrong with others, wrong with our lives—and then remembering to arrive once again in mindful presence. Because there is a persistent "forgetting," it often takes faith in ourselves—and in our clients—to allow this process to unfold. Yet with each round, the understanding that we are not the isolated, deficient, endangered self depicted in our stories deepens; and with each round the realization of our true potential—awakened, loving presence—blossoms more fully.

COMING HOME TO LOVING PRESENCE

This is how it happened for Pam. A month after my meeting with her, she called to let me know that Jerry had died. Then she told me what had happened the evening after she and I had talked. When she arrived back at their apartment, she had invited Jerry to join her in silent prayer. "When we were done," she told me, "we shared our prayers. I let him know how much I wanted him to feel my love." Pam was quiet a moment, then her voice choked up. "He had been praying for the same . . . in reverse. We just hugged and cried."

Even in those final weeks, Pam acknowledged, she had continued to struggle with the urge to be busy, to find ways to feel useful. But she had gained the all-important skill of noticing her reactivity, recognizing when she had contracted away from mindful presence. One afternoon, Jerry began talking about having only a short time left, and about not being afraid of dying. She bent over, gave him a kiss, and said quickly, "Oh dear . . . today's been a good day, you seemed to have more energy . . . let me make you some herbal tea." He fell silent, and the quietness shook her. "It became so clear to me in those moments that anything other than listening to what was really going on—anything other than being fully present—actually separated us. I hadn't wanted us to admit his dying out loud, that just made it too real. So I avoided reality by suggesting a cup of tea. But the attempt to steer away from the truth of what was happening took me away from him, and that was heartbreaking."

While Pam boiled water for tea, she prayed, asking that her heart be fully present with Jerry. This prayer guided her in the days that followed: "Over those last few weeks I had to keep letting go of all my ideas of how his dying should be and what else I should be doing, and just remind myself to say 'I consent.' At first I was mechanically repeating the words, but after a few days I felt as if my heart actually started consenting." She described how she would pause when she recognized she was gripped by strong feelings, and then investigate to see what was going on. When her gut tightened with clutches of fear and feelings of helplessness, she'd stay with the feelings, consenting to the depth of her vulnerability, intending to be kind. When the restless urge to "do something" arose, she'd notice that and be still, letting it come and go. When the great waves of grief rolled through, she'd again say "I consent," opening herself to the huge aching weight of loss. And as the days went by, she realized that her tone in saying "I consent" was becoming increasingly tender.

This intimate, mindful presence with her inner experience allowed Pam to attend fully to Jerry, and to act from her inner wisdom. As she put it, "When all of me was truly consenting to the fear and pain, I knew how to take care of him. I sensed when to whisper words of encouragement or just listen, ways to reassure him with touch . . . how to sing to him, be quiet with him, *be* with him." Before she ended the call, Pam shared with me what she considered to be the gift of her last days with Jerry, the answer to her prayers: "In the silence I could see past a sense of 'him' and 'me' . . . it became clear that we were a field of loving—total openness, warmth, light. He's gone, but that field of loving is always with me. My heart knows that I came home . . . truly I came home to love."

TRUSTING YOUR HEART AND AWARENESS

For Pam, a mindful presence awakened her intuition and her heart. She moved from her fear of failing herself and Jerry, her painful isolation and anger, into realizing the truth of belonging, an ever-present love that could sustain her even after he died. This wisdom of nonseparation is the gift of mindfulness.

As a Buddhist teacher, I would say that mindfulness is our gateway to realizing the vibrant aliveness, love, and luminous wakefulness that is our essential nature. From a therapeutic perspective, I would say that mindfulness loosens the grip of preconditioned, engrained tendencies created by temperament and personal history. The liberating "mechanism" in mindfulness is expressed in the *N* of RAIN: nonidentification. In cultivating a full presence, we begin dissolving our identification with our habitual defensive patterns and reactions. Released from the trance that constricts and limits us, we open to a vaster and more lucid awareness. This open awareness allows our innate capacities for intelligence and compassion to unfold spontaneously, along with fresh perceptions, creativity, and learning. Whether we are relating with our clients, our partners, our children, or our inner life, we are living from a space of wisdom and kindness that is no longer clouded over by trance.

At my first meditation retreat one of our teachers conveyed a story about a conference in India with the Dalai Lama. A group of Western Buddhist teachers had asked him for the most important message they could bring back home to their meditation students. After a few thoughtful moments the Dalai Lama nodded and smiled broadly. "Tell them that they can trust their hearts and awareness to awaken in the midst of all circumstances." This has stayed with me ever since.

We long to trust that in the face of difficulty, we can find our way home to our inner wisdom and compassion. Mindfulness training cultivates this trust, but not necessarily right away! I've seen how, for many people, the single most challenging deterrent to sustaining a mindfulness practice is the sense of doubt: "I'm not doing this right. I'm not getting it. This isn't working." Therapists whom I've trained in mindfulness, as well as my clients and students, tell me that they are regularly lost in obsessive thinking, that they are not able to maintain any experience of "being here" in mindful presence. They wonder why meditating is so hard.

Training our attention *is* hard. As other contributors to this volume will discuss, it takes time and repeated practice to reshape the brain structures that embody our mental and emotional "default" settings. When we train our attention, we're also going against the grain of our culture, with its incessant distractions and multitasking. And more importantly, we're going against the grain of countless hours lost in thoughts and unconsciously driven by wants and fears. It's as though we'd spent our lives on a bicycle, peddling hard to get away from the present moment. We peddle to resist what is happening, we peddle to try to make something happen, we peddle to try to get somewhere else. The more we feel like something is missing, or something is wrong, the faster we peddle. Even in the midst of a meditation we might realize we are peddling–straining to be with the breath, chasing after a fantasy, trying to figure something out. Training in mindfulness is a setup for feeling deficient unless we respectfully acknowledge the strength of our conditioning to race away from presence. *It's not our fault!* (see Chapter 18). Given this conditioning, how can we follow the Dalai Lama's advice and trust our heart and awareness?

The key elements in cultivating trust are *intention* and *attention*. As Zen master S. Suzuki Roshi (2007) said, "The most important thing is to find out what is the most important thing" (p. 79). If we have the sincere intention to become more present in every part of our lives, that will open the door. And if we remember to pause and offer our attention whenever we realize we've been lost in trance–even for a few moments!–we are on our way home.

This homecoming can happen in any situation. We might be in the middle of an argument with our partner, and instead of saying the next thing to prove our point, we pause. In that pause we can allow ourselves to contact the insecurity or hurt that lies under our defensiveness, which in turn may open the door to honest communication and more mutual understanding. We might be harshly self-critical for having overconsumed food, or for a session that went poorly. But when we remember to pause, to sense the pain, yet again, of being at war with ourselves, the space of self-compassion can open up (see Chapters 6 and 7). We might be listening to a client and simultaneously planning an intervention, and in pausing recognize our own restlessness and fear of falling short. Mindfully contacting and acknowledging our own experience allows us to listen more deeply to our client.

Pausing and arriving in the space of mindful presence makes room for our natural intuitive intelligence and care to emerge. Our life becomes full with possibility and more clearly interconnected with all life everywhere. In time, mindful presence reveals the power of our heart and awareness and allows us to trust and embody our innate compassion and wisdom. By extension, we come to recognize that this same basic goodness shines through our clients and all those whom we meet.

CHAPTER 3

Building Lives of Compassion and Wisdom

Barbara L. Fredrickson

> Love, compassion, and tolerance are necessities, not luxuries. Without them, humanity cannot survive.
>
> —TENZIN GYATSO, the 14th Dalai Lama (1999, p. 3)

Someone cuts you off in traffic.
Your boss overlooks your many contributions to a team effort while lauding others.
Your partner snaps at you and tells you to back off.

These and other upsets can ignite anger, dismay, downward spirals, and a whole host of related painful experiences and destructive behaviors. We're only human, after all.

Yet, as humans, we have enormous choice in how we respond to the slings and arrows of daily life. What would it take to experience these and other upsets *without* inner turmoil or outer destructiveness? Is it possible?

Indeed it is possible. What it takes are healthy doses of compassion and wisdom, the central characters of this volume: compassion to accept and even love others *as they are*, even when they present you with unexpected and challenging behavior; wisdom to realize that their behavior often arises out of their own suffering and their own deeply rooted conditioning from past experiences.

People enter psychotherapy because they are suffering, either from unwanted painful emotions or destructive behavioral patterns. Clients and therapists alike often hold out happiness as the end goal, seeing the process of psychotherapy as one of alleviating suffering and cultivating the conditions for happiness. This understanding of the therapeutic process, while both noble and accurate, nonetheless conceals the important role of *positive* emotions. More than a decade of empirical work on the broaden-and-build theory of positive emotions (Fredrickson, 1998, 2001; see Fredrickson, 2009, for a review) casts positive emotions as key engines of personal growth and resilience, not simply the products of them. Put differently, emotions such as joy, serenity, gratitude, love, and compassion, along with attitudes such as equanimity, are important tools within the psychotherapeutic toolkit, and not just the yardsticks by which to measure success.

In this chapter, I describe how positive emotions can widen one's perspective on life and build personal skills such as mindfulness and the ability to connect with others. Then I show how momentary states of compassion and wisdom can grow into more stable personality traits. Finally, I offer two exercises that can help therapists and their clients experience positive emotions—love, kindness, gratitude, joy—more frequently in daily life.

POSITIVE EMOTIONS AS MEANS, NOT ENDS

Positive Emotions Open Minds

The first tenet of the broaden-and-build theory is that positive emotions expand people's awareness, temporarily allowing them to take in more of their surrounding contextual information than they do during neutral or negative states (Fredrickson, 1998, 2001). This momentary cognitive effect of positive emotions has been demonstrated in a wide range of tightly controlled experiments carried out in multiple laboratories. For instance, experimentally induced positive emotions have been shown to broaden the scope of people's visual attention in behavior tests (Fredrickson & Branigan, 2005), including tests that measure fine-grained behavioral responses using milliseconds of reaction times (Rowe, Hirsh, & Anderson, 2007) and eye-tracking technology (Wadlinger & Isaacowitz, 2006). Moreover, experiments with brain imaging (e.g., functional magnetic resonance imaging) reveal that positive emotions expand people's field of view at very early perceptual encoding stages (Schmitz, De Rosa, & Anderson, 2009; see also Soto et al., 2009). Positive emotions, then, quite literally widen people's outlook on the world around them.

Although the expansion of awareness that comes with positive emotions is as subtle and short-lived as the emotion itself, it accounts for positivity-related increases in creativity (Rowe et al., 2007), and may well account for the documented benefits of positive emotions for autobiographical memory (Talarico, Berntsen, & Rubin, 2009), integrative decision making (Estrada, Isen, & Young, 1997), test and work performance (Bryan & Bryan, 1991; Staw & Barsade, 1993), coping and resilience (Fredrickson, Mancuso, Branigan, & Tugade, 2000; Tugade & Fredrickson, 2004), interpersonal trust (Dunn & Schweitzer, 2005), social connection (Johnson & Fredrickson, 2005; Waugh & Fredrickson, 2006), teamwork (Sy, Cote, & Saavedra, 2005), and negotiation ability (Kopelman, Rosette, & Thompson, 2006). In short, open and flexible awareness is a core attribute of positive emotional states.

Positive Emotions Transform Lives

The second tenet of the broaden-and-build theory is that, over time, the momentary states of expanded awareness sparked by positive emotions accumulate and compound to build durable personal and social resources that ultimately reshape people's lives for the better (Fredrickson, 1998, 2001, 2009). In the context of psychotherapy, this means that teaching clients specific skills for self-generating positive emotions—which in turn allow them to increase their daily diets of positive emotions—builds resources and resilience that help to minimize future suffering and cultivate well-being. Recent randomized controlled trials have tested the effects of teaching people loving-kindness meditation (LKM) as a means to self-generate positive emotions more frequently. Results indicate that LKM practice reliably raises a wide range of self-reported positive emotions. The durability and pervasiveness of these effects suggest that enduring upward shifts in positive feelings are indeed possible, especially among those who invest more time in their meditation practice (Cohn & Fredrickson, 2010; Fredrickson, Cohn, Coffey, Pek, & Finkel, 2008).

Most importantly, however, the upward shift in positive emotions evident in people practicing LKM also increased their personal resources, including their mindfulness, their environmental mastery, their positive relations with others, and their self-reported health. In turn, these increased resources accounted for reduced depressive symptoms and improved life satisfaction (Fredrickson et al., 2008). As LKM increases daily positive emotions, it has also been shown to increase cardiac vagal tone (Kok et al., 2010), a marker of both physical health and behavioral flexibility (Thayer & Sternberg, 2006). This nascent research on the long-range health and psychological benefits of cultivating positive emotional states provides a compelling rationale to consider the value of positive emotions in psychotherapy.

UPWARD SPIRALS COUNTER DOWNWARD SPIRALS

Because both positive and negative emotions alter people's attention, thinking, motivation, and behavior, they also trigger self-perpetuating dynamics—or spirals—that can either drag people down or buoy them up. To illustrate, the negative emotions of anger, stress, or sadness each narrows people's attention and reinforces emotion-consistent appraisal patterns (e.g., blame, threat, or loss, respectively) that initiate further bouts of anger, stress, or sadness, with attendant social friction or isolation. These cycles perpetuate themselves to produce the downward spirals all too familiar to therapists.

The broaden-and-build theory holds that positive emotions create opposing upward spiral dynamics, in which the broadened awareness that accompanies positive emotions allows people to step back or "decenter" from stressful circumstances and appraise them in a more positive light, which in turn can trigger further experiences of positive emotions. As this upward spiral unfolds, it creates resilience, well-being, and greater opportunities for social connection. A number of prospective studies have now documented this upward spiral dynamic (Burns et al., 2008; Cohn, Fredrickson, Brown, Mikels, & Conway, 2009; Fredrickson & Joiner, 2002; Kok & Fredrickson, 2010), and my collaborators and I have recently outlined how upward spirals might drive neuroplasticity in ways that can be applied productively within psychotherapy (Garland et al., 2010).

CLINICAL APPLICATIONS OF THE BROADEN-AND-BUILD THEORY

The broaden-and-build theory originated to explain how positive emotions were shaped by the forces of natural selection. The key is that, over time and through repeated experiences, these fleeting pleasant states augmented our human ancestors' resources for survival. Although the theory has been tested primarily in healthy populations with typical life stressors, more recently, clinical scientists have created clinical applications of the theory, targeting a range of psychological disorders characterized by emotion dysfunctions and deficits, such as depression, anxiety, and schizophrenia (for a review, see Garland et al., 2010). For instance, promising results have emerged from a pilot test that used LKM to unlock more frequent self-generated positive emotions as a means to treat the negative symptoms of schizophrenia, which include anhedonia (diminished pleasure), avolition (diminished motivation), asociality (diminished desire for interpersonal relationships), alogia (diminished speech), and blunted affect (diminished expression of emotion) (Johnson et al., 2011; see also Johnson et al., 2009). Likewise, initial evidence suggests that depression and anxiety disorders can be successfully treated using adaptations of cognitive-behavioral therapy that more explicitly cultivate positive emotions, either through mental imagery (Rudd, Joiner, & Rajab, 2001; Tarrier, 2010) or positive reappraisals (Garland, Gaylor, & Park, 2009). In light of these promising early returns, it would be particularly interesting to explore whether positive states of compassion and wisdom could be considered mechanisms of action in clinical applications.

COMPASSION AND WISDOM THROUGH THE LENS OF BROADEN-AND-BUILD

A key process illuminated by the broaden-and-build theory is that even short-lived positive emotions and mind states can spark dynamic upward spirals that facilitate personal growth and transformation, ultimately reshaping a person's enduring traits and habits of mind. From this perspective, compassion and wisdom can each be viewed as both momentary *states* and as enduring personality *traits*. The following sections unpack this perspective further.

Compassion and Wisdom as States

The 10 positive emotions I have targeted in my research over the last decade include joy, gratitude, serenity, interest, hope, pride, amusement, inspiration, awe, and love. With one exception, I typically list these emotions in their order of their relative frequency, starting with the positive emotions people feel most frequently. The exception is love. Feeling love, closeness, or trust appears to be the positive emotion people feel most frequently—at least among the adults I've tested. This makes sense when considering that, like poets, artists, and songwriters before them, emotion theorists have viewed love as a many-splendored thing (Fredrickson, 2009; Izard, 1977). That is, momentary states of love are actually comprised of the other nine positive emotions: joy, gratitude, serenity, and so on.

The context of these other positive emotions is what recasts them as love. Love is experienced in contexts of safe, often close, relationships. In the early stages of a relationship, for instance, tied up with initial attraction, people are deeply *interested* in anything and everything this new person says and does. They share *amusement* and laugh together, often as a result of the awkwardness of coming together for the first time. As a relationship builds and perhaps surpasses expectations, it brings great *joy*. People begin to share their *hopes* and dreams for their future together. As the relationship becomes more solid, they may sink back into the cozy *serenity* that comes with the security of mutual love. At this stage, people in loving relationships often feel *grateful* for the joys their beloved brings into their life, as *proud* of their achievements as they are of their own, *inspired* by their good qualities, and perhaps in *awe* of the forces of the universe that brought and keep them together.

Each of these pleasant momentary states might equally be described as love. Viewing love in this way also sharpens our ability to see love as a temporary state that ebbs and flows, and not simply a description of a stable relationship. In its most basic form, love is the positive emotion that arises from trusting connections with others. When we become aware of interconnection and delight in it, we experience love. Open acceptance is key here, and it shows up in the characteristic nonverbal displays of love—the leaning toward, the affirming head nods. It creates the urge to be kind, friendly, to show care and concern. This is not a conditional love that says "*I love you if . . . when* . . . or . . . *as long as. . . .* " Those conditions describe a way of clinging to a certain fixed way of viewing the other person or the relationship, a rigidity that defies the openness inherent within truly open and heartfelt moments of love.

Such open and accepting states of love are tightly interwoven with states of compassion. Indeed, compassion can be viewed as a key variant of love: Whenever the other person (or being) with whom we connect is suffering, love and compassion become one and the same (see Chapter 1). Given the ubiquity of suffering, the appropriateness of compassion is widespread. Moreover, when we connect with those who suffer, with kindness, clear eyes, and open acceptance, we are naturally drawn to care, help, or give. The feeling itself inspires us to do what we can to relieve the other person's suffering. Compassion motivates action.

To the extent that positive emotions such as love and compassion expand people's momentary awareness, they may also increase people's momentary wisdom. One way that psychologists have defined wisdom is as "expertise in the fundamental pragmatics of life," with particular emphasis on the ability to see holistically and integrate seemingly contradictory perspectives to achieve balance and well-being (Baltes, Glück, & Kunzmann, 2002; see also Sternberg, 1998, and Chapter 1). Broadened awareness—being able to "see the big picture"—can thus be viewed as a core facet of wisdom. Recognizing that the scope of awareness changes dynamically over time—it narrows with negative emotions and broadens with positive ones—moments of compassion and moments of wisdom may go hand in hand.

The term *equanimity* might be reasonably used to describe wisdom in this state form. In the context of love and compassion, equanimity refers to the awareness that, despite our best wishes and efforts, we and our loved ones will still suffer from time to time, and that our suffering is often tied to our entrenched habits of mind. This broadened awareness of equanimity is what supports openness and acceptance within moments of compassion. It creates a willingness to accept whatever comes next, without attaching contingencies on our provision of care and concern for the other—for instance, a contingency that our helping efforts do indeed alleviate suffering (see Chapter 6).

Compassion and Wisdom as Traits

According to the broaden-and-build theory, teaching clients and ourselves to self-generate moments of love and compassion—and endorsing the value of doing so frequently—generates concomitant moments of expanded awareness, a mental state that supports wisdom and equanimity. Over time, such moments accumulate and compound to reshape people's enduring traits, which in turn hold potential to create abiding new resources of compassion and wisdom, thereby promoting wellness and health. Compassion and wisdom become traits when they become automatic and habitual. Put differently, when people's thresholds for experiencing a particular emotional or mental state are low and evidenced in multiple and varied circumstances, that frequent state can be reframed as a trait—a description of enduring character more generally, not just of responsiveness in one moment or one circumstance.

Personality is thus, to some degree, plastic, subject to change over time based on people's habitual emotions and mind states. By increasing our daily diets of love, compassion, and other positive emotions, then, we nourish character development and psychological growth. If we wish to build more compassionate and wise communities, we can start by turning our attention to "micromoments" of loving social connection and cultivating these micromoments more frequently.

EXERCISES TO SELF-GENERATE POSITIVE EMOTIONS

Loving-Kindness Meditation

My own recent empirical tests of the hypothesis that positive emotions build consequential personal resources draw on an ancient Buddhist mind-training practice we've already encountered: loving-kindness meditation (LKM; Germer, 2009; Salzberg, 1997). Whereas most Western science on meditation has centered on mindfulness meditation, I chose to study the effects of LKM because it more directly aims to evoke positive emotions, especially within relationships. LKM is a technique used to condition one's habitual responses to increase good will and feelings of warmth and caring for self and others. Like other meditation practices, it involves quiet contemplation in a seated posture, often with eyes closed and an initial focus on the breath and the heart region. Beginners might do this for 10 minutes or so. As the practice becomes more familiar and comfortable, people can experiment with longer meditation times, aiming for 25 minutes of daily practice when possible. Randomized controlled trials reveal a wide array of benefits of such practice after just 2–3 months (Fredrickson et al., 2008).

LKM is a bit like guided imagery, although the practice targets feelings of love and compassion more than visual images per se. To some, LKM may at first blush seem saccharin or unrealistic. This reaction can be countered by balancing the practice with the wisdom of equanimity. You might do this by lightly bringing your awareness not only to the reality and inevitability of suffering and the conditions that create suffering, but also to the vast interconnections between people and the fundamental similarity of all humans. It is into this context that we put forth the wishes for happiness and well-being that are central to LKM.

LOVING-KINDNESS MEDITATION

- Bring your awareness to the sensations of your own heart in this quiet moment and reflect on a person for whom you already feel warm, tender, and compassionate feelings. This could be your child, spouse, even a pet—someone whom the mere thought of makes you smile. Your goal is to rouse warm and tender feelings naturally, by visualizing how connecting with this loved one makes you feel.
- Once these tender feelings of love and compassion have taken hold, creating genuine warmth and kindness in you, gently let go of the image of that particular loved one and simply hold the feeling in your heart region.
- Now, extend that warm feeling to yourself. Cherish yourself as deeply and as purely as you would cherish your own newborn child. For many—especially Westerners—this is a large hurdle. We're not accustomed to directing our love inward. It takes patience and practice to make it genuine. At first, you might spend the entire time directing love to yourself before this happens.
- Traditional LKM comes with a set of statements that you repeat silently to yourself. The words themselves are not as critical as the sentiments and

emotions they evoke. Rephrase the statements in ways that stir your heart most. The traditional statements go something like this: *"May this one* (or *I, we, he, she*, or *they*) *feel safe. May they feel happy. May they feel healthy. May they live with ease."* Repeat these phrases slowly and silently to yourself. Let them cultivate genuine warmth and tenderness as you move your attention from yourself to an ever-widening circle of others.

- Next, radiate your warm, tender, and compassionate feelings to others, first to a person you know well, then gradually calling to mind all your friends and family, and then all people with whom you have a connection—even remote connections, like the service person you reached on your last call for tech support.
- Ultimately, extend your feelings of love and kindness to all people and creatures of the earth. To do this you might visualize your city, your region of the country, your continent, and finally the whole planet.
- As you end your meditation, gently remind yourself that the purpose of your practice is to condition your own heart and emotions so that you can generate these feelings of kindness and warmth more readily any time you wish.

Empirical evidence suggests that regular LKM practice indeed makes it easier to find the joy in day-to-day interactions with others (Fredrickson et al., 2008).

Positivity Portfolio

LKM is not the only way to increase one's daily diet of positive mind states, such as compassion and wisdom. I describe more than a dozen evidence-based techniques for doing so in my book *Positivity* (Fredrickson, 2009). I wrote this book for a general audience, with the intent that it might be a resource for people–including clients in psychotherapy–who wish to learn more about how the new science of positive psychology can help them to flourish in life, becoming happier and more resilient. One additional technique I describe in *Positivity* is the process of building and using portfolios of pictures, quotes, objects and other mementos to evoke each of the 10 positive emotions. These positivity portfolios, whether they are physical folders or digitized assemblies, help to personalize each individual's ability to rekindle specific positive emotions when they are needed most. When malaise or mushrooming negative emotions threaten to pull us on a downward spiral, a positivity portfolio can be a game changer, a breath of life that inspires us to find our way back to the nourishing upward spiral of positivity.

POSITIVITY PORTFOLIO

One particularly effective kind of positivity portfolio focuses on love. To build your own, start by answering the following questions:

- *When do you feel the warmth of love well up between you and another?*
- *When do you feel close, safe, secure, and trusting?*
- *When does a relationship of yours spark one of the other forms of positivity—joy, gratitude, serenity, interest, hope, pride, amusement, inspiration, or awe?*
- *When do you find yourself leaning in toward your beloved, affirming his or her uniqueness?*
- *When do you have the urge just to be with and enjoy your beloved's companionship, to cherish him or her or to bask in his or her reflected glory?*

Next, go on a treasure hunt. Find photos or other mementos that carry the capacity to reignite feelings of love in you. Don't rush through the process of assembling your love portfolio—savor and enjoy it. Resonate with the feelings of love created by building a portfolio that truly moves you. The idea is to create a personalized shrine to love that reflects the inner workings of your own heart. Whereas nutritionists ask their clients to pay attention to how certain foods make them feel, the goal here is to pay attention to how certain activities, circumstances, and lines of thinking make you feel. As you become more familiar with what uplifts and enlivens you, you gain both insight into and control over your daily emotional experiences, which can carry over to your day-to-day interactions and experiences.

I regularly assign students enrolled in my positive psychology course to create a portfolio focused on a specific positive emotion (e.g., joy, love, gratitude) in one week, and then in the following week to be alert to the downward tug of negativity and, in that context, to engage with their positivity portfolio, reflecting on its contents with the intent of lightly and sincerely rekindling that positive feeling.

One of my former first-year students, Patty, gave me permission to share her experience using her portfolio this way, which she had described in her learning journal for my course. The first week she wrote that building her portfolio was a joyful and relaxing experience and that she continued to collect mementos for it, not because it was homework, but because it was fun. The next week, she wrote that she became frustrated and angry because she felt that her best friend (who was a first-year student at another university) was ignoring her. That was her cue to take out her portfolio. As she mindfully engaged with it, she felt her anger fade away. She felt better and more open. Her openness allowed her to see the situation from her friend's perspective and to be more forgiving. She admitted to herself that she'd actually be worried for her friend's well-being were her friend not keeping busy, making new friends, and enjoying her new college life. So instead of staying angry and letting the friendship die—which Patty admitted she'd done with other friends in the past—she wrote her friend an honest, compassionate letter describing her feelings and included a small gift (a "best friend" charm). After her friend received her letter, she called Patty in tears, and they had their best bonding moment ever. When I touched base with Patty more than a year later, she reported that this friendship continued to thrive, which she credited to her timely use of her positivity portfolio.

When people come to understand how positive emotions such as love and compassion work—how they open minds, transform futures, and create uplifting upward spiral dynamics—they are more likely to see the wisdom of cultivating these heartfelt momentary experiences more frequently. Seen from the perspective of the broaden-and-build theory, unlocking more momentary experiences of love and compassion is not simply the end goal of the therapeutic process, but rather, doing so is an important vehicle for reshaping people's abiding levels of compassion and wisdom as well as a host of other resources and personality traits that make life more satisfying and meaningful.

PART II

The Meaning of Compassion

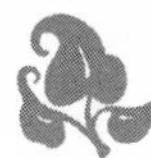

Suffering is unavoidable, yet suffering is precisely what brings people into therapy. How do clinicians endure, even thrive, in the presence of so much sorrow? Compassion seems to help–a positive attitude that feels more like love than misery. Compassion also allows therapists to stay emotionally connected with their clients during difficult periods, such as when we feel afraid, helpless, or inadequate to the task.

Chapter 4 reviews how the three main psychological traditions of Buddhism understand compassion, sometimes even as our fundamental, unconditioned nature. Chapter 5 shows how compassion is a way of knowing, an eye through which we may still see the fullness of another human being when the person is buried in suffering or we're incapable of altering the course of a tragic life. In Chapter 6, the author reminds us to include ourselves in our circle of compassion. She describes exactly what self-compassion means, and how it may positively affect our lives and work. Chapter 7 expands on the theme of self-compassion as a goal of therapy and offers numerous exercises and suggestions for how to cultivate a compassionate attitude in the context of psychotherapy. Finally, we see in Chapter 8 how training the mind in compassion can alter brain function, whether by practicing for relatively short periods or throughout a lifetime.

CHAPTER 4

Compassion in Buddhist Psychology

John Makransky

> Thus we can reject everything else: religion, ideology, all received wisdom. But we cannot escape the necessity of love and compassion.
>
> —TENZIN GYATSO, the 14th Dalai Lama (2001a, p. 234)

In Buddhist psychology, compassion is a form of empathy. We sense others' suffering as like our own and naturally wish them deep freedom from it. A compassionate mind, as opposed to a cruel and angry one, is understood to be much more closely attuned to our actual condition. Thus, compassion is informed by the wisdom that understands our basic situation: the inner causes of our suffering and our potential for freedom and goodness. From a Buddhist perspective, compassion with wisdom is the foundation of emotional healing and inner freedom.

Compassion is also characterized as a mental capacity that, when cultivated and strengthened, empowers all positive states of mind as we awaken to our fullest human potential. In Buddhist psychology, the patterns of our experience unfold based on our habits of intention and reaction. "All phenomena of experience have mind as their forerunner, mind as chief, and they are mind-made" (*Dhammapada*, Chapter 1, vss. 1, 2). Thus, a loving, compassionate state of mind supports our own happiness and well-being and helps bring out this potential in others, whereas cruel, malicious, and envious states of mind do the opposite. In Buddhist meditation systems, compassion is also closely connected with love, sympathetic joy, and equanimity—called the "four immeasurable attitudes"—as bases for powerful meditative insight. In sum, compassion is viewed as a power for purifying the mind of confusion, for inner healing, and for protection of self and others.

Compassion has been taught and practiced for millennia in three main Buddhist traditions: Theravada, Mahayana, and Vajrayana. These approaches to the alleviation of suffering could be viewed as more akin to psychology and philosophy than religion insofar as they do not require belief in a higher power to reap their benefits. As clinical scientists and psychotherapists begin to systematically explore the concept of compassion, it may be helpful to consider the nuances in understanding that have emerged within these traditions in different parts of the world.

COMPASSION IN EARLY BUDDHISM AND THERAVADA TRADITION

Because compassion in Buddhist psychology involves a wish for beings to be deeply free of their sufferings, Buddhists' understandings of "suffering" (in Pali, *dukkha*) are crucial to their understanding of compassion. Theravada traditions of Southeast Asia, which systematized the early teachings of the Buddha, describe three levels of suffering: (1) obvious suffering, (2) the suffering of transience, and (3) the suffering of self-centered conditioning (Harvey, 1990; Nyanamoli, 1964). *Obvious suffering* includes all physical and mental forms of misery that we normally associate with the word *suffering*: the miseries of illness and physical injury, of old age and dying, of grief, mental anguish, and distress. The *suffering of transience* stems from the futile attempt to get, have, and hold onto pleasant things as if they could be a stable source of security and well-being. The passing things to which our minds cling for happiness and security transform into conditions of suffering as we lose them throughout life and inexorably approach death.

The *suffering of self-centered conditioning* underlies the prior two. This form of suffering is inherent in the mind's subconscious attempt to create from the impermanent flow of its experience the impression of a substantial, unchanging, and separate sense of self surrounded by a stable world. The mind's ongoing attempt to fabricate such a reified, unchanging impression of self and world, in turn, conditions numerous anxious patterns of thought and reaction: clinging to whatever seems to affirm a fixed, unchanging self and its world, fearing or hating whatever seems to threaten it (see Chapters 9 and 13). To oscillate uncontrollably through such feelings in reaction to our mental constructs of self and others is the suffering of self-centered conditioning (Makransky, 2007).

The sufferings of transience and self-centered conditioning are not fully conscious to most of us, but the Buddha's process of awakening, it is taught, made him vividly aware of them. The Buddha's compassion, in wishing persons to be free from suffering, focused on *all three* levels, the last two of which are present even when obvious sufferings are not. For this reason, the Buddha's compassion extended to all beings equally. It is this impartial, unconditional, and all-inclusive compassion that the Buddha imparted to his followers.

Mindfulness

In the path of awakening explained by the Buddha, mindfulness is key. To cultivate mindfulness is to cultivate conscious awareness of present experience without judgment (see Chapter 2). As noted, the sufferings of transience and self-centered conditioning are mediated by unconscious habits of reification—the mind's attempt to generate and cling to a sense of permanence in self and world that the mind projects onto its impermanent experience. As our tendencies to cling to illusions of permanence are illuminated by mindful awareness, we become newly conscious of how much anxiety and unease our clinging has generated. We can then start to recognize the same subconscious layers of suffering operating in all others. Thus sympathy and compassion for self and others emerge with increasing power as we gain insight into impermanence and the constructed nature of self. Such sympathy and compassion in relation to our selves inform the gentle, accepting quality of mindful attention, giving our mind permission to open to further insight. And this, in turn, helps empower an increasingly compassionate and discerning awareness of others in their conscious and subconscious sufferings.

The inmost causes of suffering diagnosed by the Buddha—the illusion of a reified fixed, unchanging self and the deluded reactions of attachment and aversion that constellate around it—are progressively weakened by such deepening insight or wisdom. Cutting through the mind's construct of separateness, this insight allows us to experience others as fundamentally like ourselves, thereby strengthening our sympathy for them (Fulton, 2005). When an individual is fully released from inner causes of suffering by such insight, it is taught, nirvana is attained—inmost freedom from the sufferings of self-grasping. As such insight progressively deepens in its realization of nirvana, it also recognizes the commonality of self and others in their underlying potential for such inner freedom. The compassion that emerges from that liberating insight is therefore not discouraged or depressed by the layers of suffering it senses in beings, but instead holds in mind their potential for deep freedom from suffering. Such compassion does not just uphold others in their underlying potential, but also challenges aspects of their thought and action that hide their potential (Aronson, 1986; Makransky, 2007).

The Eightfold Path

Compassion is thus implicitly associated with the whole process of awakening that unfolds through deepening mindfulness and insight, which are referred to as *right mindfulness* and *right understanding* in the Buddha's *eightfold path* of liberation. Compassion is also implicitly related to the other six factors cultivated within the *eightfold path*: *right thought, speech, action, livelihood, effort*, and *concentration. Right thought*, informed by insight into selflessness, is thought directed away from grasping, cruelty, and ill will and toward compassion and love (Harvey, 2000). Such thought is the power of intent that motivates right speech, right action, and right livelihood (Harvey, 2000; Rahula, 1974). And such compassionate thought and activity inform the sort of *effort* that is needed to complete this path—the compassionately gentle, caring focus of disciplined energy in mind and body that helps us nurture and sustain wholesome states of mind. *Right concentration* is the cultivation of deep tranquility through focused attention to a meditation object. To accomplish such concentration, besides other objects of meditation, the Buddha frequently taught intensive meditations on love (in Pali, *metta*), compassion (*karuna*), sympathetic joy (*mudita*), and equanimity (*upekkha*) (Aronson, 1986, note 6). When those states of mind are cultivated impartially and all-inclusively in meditative concentration, they become the *four immeasurable attitudes* that are said to give the mind tremendous power to overcome obstacles, to live with happiness and ease, to support one's progress in all aspects of the path, and to elicit the potential in others for similar states of mind (Aronson, 1986; Harvey, 2000).

The Four Immeasurable Attitudes

Given such benefits, Theravada Buddhism has emphasized the cultivation of the four immeasurable attitudes, which are explained systematically in Buddhaghosa's classic text *The Path of Purification* (Nyanamoli, 1964). Here, *love* (or loving-kindness) is the open-hearted wish for beings to experience happiness and well-being. It is not to be confused with self-centered attachment or possessiveness. Love undercuts tendencies toward ill will and fear and is thus characterized as a protective power for oneself and a protective influence on others.

Love

In the meditative cultivation of love that Buddhaghosa describes, the wish of love is directed first toward ourselves since deep self-acceptance is crucial to the deep acceptance of others, all of whom are like us in their layers of suffering and their wish to be happy. First, we generate positive wishes and feelings of love and acceptance for our self by repeating phrases such as: "May I have well-being and happiness; may I be free from enmity and danger" (see Chapter 3). When the wish and feeling of love become established in regard to the self, then in recognizing that others also wish to be happy, it feels natural to extend the same wish to others. We begin extending the wish to someone who strongly elicits it, such as an especially inspiring teacher or mentor. The wish and feeling of love are next extended to a dear friend. As the power of love for such dear beings emerges, it can be harnessed and directed to less obvious beings: first to a neutral person (someone previously viewed as a stranger who now becomes the object of the same loving wish and feeling), then to someone who has been hostile. Increasingly, we recognize every kind of living being as like us—worthy recipients of love, no matter how they superficially appear—and the wish of love is progressively extended until it literally includes all beings everywhere. This focus draws our mind into a state of deep absorption, with a sense of immeasurable inclusiveness, stability, tranquility, and joy (Aronson, 1980; Harvey, 2000; Nyanamoli, 1964; Salzberg, 1997). This kind of concentration can then be deepened into further levels of meditative absorption. Buddhaghosa was the first to fully articulate and systematize this practice, described in Chapter 3 (along with detailed instructions) as "loving-kindness meditation."

Compassion

Based on this cultivation of love, we are ready to cultivate *compassion*, the empathic wish for beings to be free from suffering. As a mental power, compassion undercuts tendencies toward cruelty. It is not to be confused with sadness about suffering, since what it wishes for beings—inner freedom from suffering—is seen as a real possibility within the Buddha's path of awakening. Sensing all beings as dear through the practice of love, and reflecting on the sufferings they undergo, compassion for them naturally arises. Because the initial cultivation of love began with love for self, compassionate self-acceptance is also now assumed. Buddhaghosa instructs us to focus first on someone experiencing intense misery because such an image easily and strongly evokes our compassionate wish for him or her to be free from that suffering. We then direct our mind with the same empathic feeling and wish of compassion to a friend, then a neutral person, then someone who has been hostile. Finally, as with immeasurable love, the wish of compassion is extended to all beings everywhere, becoming all-inclusive, stable, and joyful as it deepens into increasingly subtle levels of meditative absorption. We can focus compassion on all sentient beings, including those who are not presently experiencing obvious misery, by recalling their ever-present sufferings of transience and self-centered conditioning (Harvey, 2000; Nyanamoli, 1964).

Sympathetic Joy

Love and compassion for living beings naturally evoke our joy in their happiness and good fortune, so the next cultivation is that of *sympathetic joy*. The quality of sympathetic joy, which takes quiet joy in the happiness of others (rather than becoming overexcited or giddy), undercuts tendencies toward jealousy and aversion when others may be doing better than we are. In practice, we reflect first on the happiness and success of a dear friend, taking joy in the friend's happiness with thoughts such as "How wonderful! How fine!" We then turn our mind to the happiness of a neutral person, then to one who has been hostile, and finally to all beings everywhere.

Equanimity

Equanimity is a peaceful calmness in the face of the ups and downs that all beings undergo, a recognition that their potential for happiness and suffering is conditioned by their own patterns of intention and reaction to experiences (Harvey, 2000). Equanimity also includes the power of impartiality that senses all beings as essentially the same in their layers of suffering and their wish and potential for freedom from distress. This quality thus supports the impartial extension of love, compassion, and sympathetic joy to all. Although equanimity undercuts partiality, it is not to be confused with apathy. The cultivation of equanimity focuses first on a neutral person, then a dear one, a deeply revered friend, a hostile person, and finally all beings everywhere. Such immeasurable equanimity, Buddhaghosa says, is established on the highest level of meditative absorption, based on previous levels of absorption that were attained in the prior three meditations (Nyanamoli, 1964).

The blending of equanimity with the other "immeasurable attitudes" helps to maintain their purity. For example, equanimity protects love from degrading into unnecessary clinging to the object of affection, it protects compassion from turning into a sense of superiority or pity, and it protects sympathetic joy from devolving into an ungrounded giddiness. And as mentioned in Chapter 3, equanimity as a state of mind is also associated with wisdom.

The four immeasurable attitudes of love, compassion, joy, and equanimity, cultivated in this way, are also referred to as the "four divine abodes," states of mind akin to those of a god in ancient Indian lore. Thus, in early Buddhist and Theravada understanding, compassion is most fully realized when cultivated in close connection with the related attitudes of love, joy, and equanimity. Together, they constitute an ancient and high-minded "positive psychology"—the happiness of the gods.

COMPASSION IN MAHAYANA BUDDHISM

The Theravada path of awakening noted above is modeled on practices of accomplished disciples of the Buddha known as *arhats*, those who are said to have attained nirvana: inner liberation from suffering. Although, as noted above, compassion in Theravada Buddhism is implicitly related to each part of the path, it was not given the same central importance as wisdom, the insight that explicitly liberates from suffering (see Chapter 9). Because insight or wisdom recognizes the *impermanent, selfless* nature of experience, it alone releases the mind from its tendencies to reify and cling to its constructed sense of self, freeing us from inmost causes of suffering. Therefore, insight, rather than compassion per se, is upheld as the core liberating principle of the Theravada path of the *arhats* (Aronson, 1980).

Other movements in the development of Indian Buddhism emerged from the first century BCE that constellated under the term *Mahayana*, meaning "Great Vehicle." Mahayana traditions gave compassion a greater centrality because they placed a fresh emphasis on the kind of awakening that the Buddha had realized that set him apart from other *arhats*. The Buddha's realization gave him the power to skillfully *communicate* the insight of his awakening in ways that benefited countless people over many generations. Indeed, the Buddha's power to beneficially affect others through his presence and speech, exceeding other *arhats*, was taken as an indication that the Buddha's wisdom also far exceeded theirs. For his wisdom not only freed himself from the root causes of suffering but enabled him to point so many others to the same essential freedom. The Buddha's long prior training in impartial compassion was viewed as the means by which he deepened his wisdom to the point that he could know others so profoundly and teach them so skillfully. Compassion is thus raised up in Mahayana traditions as ultimately inseparable from wisdom within the fullest form of awakening (Harvey, 2000). Those who choose to follow the Buddha's own distinctive path of awakening—to realize and communicate the inseparability of wisdom and compassion for the sake of the world—are called *bodhisattvas* in this tradition.

Compassion and Emptiness

The wisdom taught in Mahayana traditions opens us to others in compassionate intimacy not only through insight into their condition but also through recognition of the ultimately undivided nature of all that exists. According to Mahayana teachings, not only are phenomena found to be impermanent and beyond reification into "me" or "mine" (as in Theravada), but upon further investigation, no independently existent phenomenon of any kind, impermanent or otherwise, is even findable. So, for example, a wooden table initially appears to us as an intrinsically unified entity that seems to exist of itself, independently, as though unrelated to prior causes, conditions, or parts, and as if it had nothing to do with the constructive activity of the observer's mind. But upon investigation, Mahayana texts assert, no such independently existent table can be found. Instead, the table can be analyzed into innumerable causes, conditions, and parts that have been cognitively organized into the *appearance* of a separate, self-existent "table" through the conceptual construction of the observing mind (see Chapter 9).

On the level of appearances, this means that the wooden table cannot be separated from all the causes and conditions that contribute to its existence: a carpenter, trees, atmosphere, sunlight, soil, water, earthworms, insects, etc., each of which exists in dependence upon further innumerable causes and conditions that finally relate each thing to all other things, and each sentient being to all other beings. On the level of deep insight, no independent, separate thing can be found anywhere—every seemingly separate "thing" is *empty* (Sanskrit: *sunya*) of the sort of isolated self-existence that it appeared to have prior to such deep investigation.

In Mahayana Buddhist understanding, the insight that thus recognizes phenomena to be *empty* of self-existence cuts even more deeply into the inner causes of suffering than the insight into impermanence—more fully deconstructing the tendency to reify and cling to experiences, since the wisdom of emptiness doesn't find any independent thing to which even impermanence can be ascribed. To thus realize the empty nature of phenomena is to go beyond even the reified conceptual construct of a separate "observer" and "observed," to relax into a nonconceptual, nondual awareness that recognizes the entire world and its beings as ultimately like undivided space (Conze, 1973). This is not a form of nihilism, for things continue to appear through the force of their interdependently generated modes of existence, and beings continue to suffer by reifying, clinging, and reacting to things and to each other as if they were all inherently separate and self-existent—as if they were not empty. Rather, the nondual wisdom of emptiness recognizes *all beings* as *undivided from oneself in the empty, interdependent ground of all things* (Sanskrit: *dharmadhatu*), which supports an all-embracing, unconditional *compassion* for all creatures.

To realize the emptiness of the world in this way is to realize that nirvana, the empty essence of experiences, is undivided from the world of interdependent, changing appearances in the same way in which space is undivided from all the forms that it pervades. To realize emptiness thus gives one the freedom to *participate* in the world without clinging to it, with *unconditional compassion* for all who suffer by clinging and reacting to their own concretized projections of self and other as self-existent. As one scholar notes, "[This] means, for example, that a bodhisattva can rub shoulders with wrong-doers, to reach them and draw them toward the good, as he knows that their bad characteristics are not inherent realities" (Harvey, 1990, p. 125). Such radical compassion is also essential when practicing psychotherapy—especially with those who cause harm to others.

To have nonconceptual insight into emptiness (Sanskrit: *sunyata*) then, beyond all reification and grasping (and thus beyond the inner causes of suffering), is to feel tremendous compassion for *all* persons who continue to be caught in causes of suffering and who are sensed as ultimately undivided from oneself. That profound insight, as the basis for such all-inclusive compassion, is called the *perfection of wisdom* (Sanskrit: *prajna-paramita*).

The Six Perfections

In early Mahayana texts, the four immeasurable attitudes of love, compassion, joy, and equanimity are freshly articulated in line with these teachings. Deepest equanimity is now identified with the perfection of wisdom itself—which is intrinsically stable, tranquil, and free of expectation or partiality because it is grounded in the unconditioned, undivided, empty nature of things beyond discrimination (Conze, 1973, 1979). The love, compassion, and sympathetic joy that radiate from such wisdom, aware of how beings suffer by clinging to their experiences, motivate actions to meet each level of their need and ultimately to point them to complete freedom. Such activity is described as "generous, disciplined, patient, indefatigable, and deeply grounded" (Conze, 1973, p. 199). Those five paradigmatic aspects of other-directed activity, together with the perfection of wisdom that informs them, are the *six perfections* that comprise the *bodhisattva* path of awakening.

Cultivating Wisdom and Compassion Together

As mentioned in Chapter 1, Buddhist traditions see wisdom and compassion as interrelated—two wings of a bird. Although we all have the potential to realize the perfection of wisdom, our entrenched tendencies to cling to things as intrinsically separate and self-existent make it difficult for us to move beyond a merely conceptual understanding of such teachings to a nonconceptual, nondual realization of their meaning that can profoundly transform our responses to others. Since all-inclusive compassion is the primary response of nondual wisdom to the world, to train in such compassion *before* we have directly realized that wisdom is to harmonize the mind with its potential *for* that wisdom. In other words, to cultivate universal compassion helps release the mind from the narrow confines of its clinging to self and to dualism, giving it the courage and power to release its frames of reference into the boundless emptiness of nonconceptual wisdom. To cultivate the wisdom of boundless, undivided emptiness, in turn, further empowers an analogously boundless, impartial compassion (Harvey, 1990; Makransky, 2007). So, in Mahayana traditions from India, practitioners train extensively in meditations of compassion to empower their minds to realize nonconceptual wisdom, and as nonconceptual wisdom emerges, it is harnessed to strengthen compassion.

The systematic cultivation of compassion and wisdom is explained in a group of texts called *The Stages of Meditation* (Beyer, 1974b) by the eighth-century Indian Mahayana teacher Kamalasila. He gives instruction on cultivating compassion for dear, neutral, and hostile persons, culminating in compassion for all beings everywhere. At each stage, we reflect on the sameness of self and others in their three levels of suffering and in their wish to be free of misery. We also reflect on our relation to all others through interdependent connection, and we endeavor to learn to view everyone equally, as part of our own suffering family.

As you may notice, this meditation is similar to Theravada cultivation of compassion, but in the Mahayana tradition the force of compassion is immediately channeled into a strong aspiration to attain a buddha's awakening, the kind of enlightenment that possesses the skillful means to help all others find freedom from suffering. This aspiration is called the spirit of enlightenment (*bodhicitta*) and is reinforced by the *bodhisattva* vow to fully realize the skillful means of compassion and wisdom for the sake of all (Beyer, 1974b). Empowered by that solemn vow, the *bodhisattva* enters stages of meditative concentration that give the mind enough stability to investigate the insubstantial nature of all aspects of experience until nonconceptual wisdom dawns. This dawning *wisdom* of emptiness strengthens the *bodhisattva*'s *compassion* for all who suffer by clinging to what is empty (Beyer, 1974b, p. 110), which empowers his or her mind to release itself further into the wisdom. This synergy of compassion and wisdom is worked out through the *bodhisattva*'s practice of the six perfections on the path to buddhahood–at each stage compassionately offering his or her time, energy, patience, resources, and power of presence in whatever ways may help ease and release the suffering of beings, while recognizing the empty nature of all such activity.

In Tibetan Mahayana training systems that draw on such Indian systems of praxis, compassion is cultivated by recalling one's mother as a source of loving-kindness, eliciting one's natural response of love in return. This loving response is then transferred to all beings as past mothers, whose suffering in all three levels becomes the object of one's all-inclusive compassion. Such compassion evokes one's aspiration to help beings find freedom from suffering by helping them fully realize their potential (Harvey, 2000; Makransky, 2007).

Exchanging Self and Other

Another renowned eighth-century Indian teacher, Santideva, by pointing out the constructed nature of concepts of self and other, shows us how to reemploy those concepts to reconfigure our world into an expression of compassion and wisdom, thereby placing us on the *bodhisattva* path. *Self* and *other* are merely relative, contextual terms, Santideva argues, like *this bank* and *the other bank* of a river. Neither side of a river is intrinsically an "other bank" (Harvey, 2000). Similarly, it is a cognitive error to think of other beings as intrinsically "other." For all are "self" from their own perspectives; all are like oneself in their deepest potential, desire for happiness, and deluded patterning; and all are undivided from oneself in the empty, interdependent ground of all things (Wallace & Wallace, 1997). By reflecting on the sameness of self and others in such ways, and the tremendous benefit to our mind that would come by reversing the usual constructs of self, other and associated feelings, we explore viewing others as our very self while sensing our self as a neutral other. Through such practice, we discover, the great burden and suffering of clinging to ourselves over others is relieved, and we can increasingly give rise to the compassion and wisdom that feel and recognize all beings as like ourselves (Wallace & Wallace, 1997).

In Tibet this practice of "exchanging self and other" is commonly given the form of *tong-len* meditation, in which we exchange self for other by imagining that we take others' sufferings into the empty ground of our being while freely offering others all of our own virtue, well-being, and resources (see Chapter 7 for instructions). This imaginative pattern helps conform our mind to the wisdom of emptiness that recognizes others as ultimately undivided from ourselves, and gives that wisdom its most fundamental compassionate expression (Chödrön, 2001a). Part of the power of *tonglen* is the way it is also applied to recontextualize and transform our own experiences of suffering. When we undergo difficulties, we sense right through our own suffering the analogous suffering that many others undergo, then imagine joyfully relieving those others of their suffering by undergoing our own on *their* behalf. People tend to experience the grief of loss, for example, as isolating them from others. But in this practice, *through our own feelings* of loss and grief, we sense what many others feel, making a strong empathic connection to them. And this connection helps our mind to further release its grip on its isolated sense of self, to relax into the empty essence of experience, to sense the ultimate undividedness of self and other, and thus to become more fully present to others in relationship and service. By familiarizing with applied *tonglen* in this way, we can gradually learn to take all of our own suffering into the path of compassion and wisdom even unto death (Chödrön, 2001b; Makransky, 2007).

COMPASSION IN VAJRAYANA (TANTRIC) BUDDHISM

Further traditions of Buddhism emerged in India from the eighth century CE that came to be called *Vajrayana* ("diamond vehicle"), which became central within the spread of Buddhism to Tibet and other Himalayan regions of Asia. Based in part on the teachings above, some Mahayana schools had posited that a tremendous capacity for compassion and wisdom, and for all associated qualities of awakening, is innate—already given in the deepest, unconditioned nature of our minds. Vajrayana traditions put special emphasis on this teaching of *Buddha nature,* in relation to which the foundational teachings of suffering and its causes were reframed.

Our Buddha Nature

Our fundamental awareness, Vajrayana asserts, prior to all patterns of self-centered clinging, is essentially unconditioned, pure and undefiled. Our basic awareness is a limitless expanse of emptiness and cognizance, like boundless space pervaded by sunlight, already endowed with all-encompassing wisdom and compassion. Individual and socially conditioned habits of reification and grasping have hidden much of this underlying potential. To cultivate compassion and wisdom, therefore, is not to generate new states of mind and make them grow stronger (as was understood in Theravada and some earlier Mahayana traditions), but rather to help the mind relinquish its deluded tendencies so that its innate, unconditioned power of boundless compassion and wisdom, its *Buddha nature,* can spontaneously manifest. Holding this vision in awareness, a psychotherapist can nourish and support a patient's deepest nature, regardless of the prevailing emotional struggle.

The deep primordial nature of mind, Vajrayana thus asserts, contains all positive energies and qualities of awakening in potential. When a person's attention is habitually caught in patterns of self-centered thought and reaction, those innate energies become patterned into deluded emotions such as fear, possessiveness, and aversion—into inner causes of suffering (Bokar Rinpoche, 1991). Vajrayana practice is designed to transform and liberate these confused patterns of emotion by letting one's innate, primordial awareness recognize all experiences as expressions of its own empty cognizance, beyond reification or clinging. When one's innate awareness recognizes thoughts and emotions as patterns of its own cognizant emptiness, emotions spontaneously self-release within their own unconditioned emptiness, like writing on water dissolving back into its own unchanging wateriness. Then the innate energies that had fueled deluded emotions are freed from their distorted patterning to manifest as energies of all-inclusive compassion, wisdom, and presence to others (Dilgo Khyentse Rinpoche, 1992; Makransky, 2007; Ray, 2001; Sogyal Rinpoche, 2002). Compassion is thus understood as an intrinsic capacity of fundamental awareness—an innate quality of primordial mind that is unleashed automatically when the mind is freed from its habitual patterns of self-centered conceptualization and reaction.

Because all persons share this same innate capacity for spontaneous awakening, the compassion of a Vajrayana practitioner knows other beings not only in their suffering but also in their immeasurable dignity, primordial purity, and innate potential. Someone who has actualized his or her Buddha nature, then, communes with the *un*actualized Buddha nature in other persons, mirroring their deepest potential back at them and thereby helping to evoke it in them (Makransky, 2007). Awakening to one's own innate potential becomes infectious.

Tibetan Vajrayana meditation practice embodies this infectiousness. We bring to mind a host of awakened benefactors, in human or symbolic form, whom we regard as embodiments of deepest compassion and wisdom, of actualized Buddha nature. We commune deeply with these compassionate figures, ritually offering all of our outer and inner experiences to the Buddha nature that they represent. Held within their pervasive compassion and wisdom, our own layers of suffering can now be experienced with a sense of deep acceptance and safety, helping us to release the grip of our emotional patterning, finally to merge with our benefactors in the ground of their pervasive compassion, Buddha nature, the limitless expanse of emptiness and cognizance (Thondup, 1995). From that place, our own innate capacity can now be unleashed—our compassion for all others in their analogous layers of suffering and underlying potential can spontaneously unfold. As we learn in this gentle way to come into recognition of our Buddha nature and to extend its compassionate energy to all others, we learn to take our own place among awakened benefactors and become an extension of their activity for beings (Bokar Rinpoche, 1991; Dilgo Khyentse Rinpoche, 1992; Makransky, 2007).

In summary, compassion and wisdom are interrelated in varying ways in three leading Buddhist traditions. In early and Theravada Buddhism, compassion is seen as a power for deep mental purification, protection, and healing that can support inner freedom. In Mahayana Buddhism, compassion becomes the primary means to empower and communicate a nonconceptual wisdom in which self and others are experienced as undivided. In Vajrayana Buddhism, unconditional compassion radiates forth all-inclusively as a spontaneous expression of the mind's deepest unconditioned nature.

Systematic ways of cultivating wise compassion have been developed within each tradition. In our modern global culture, clinicians have the opportunity to explore which approach may best inform and nourish themselves or their psychotherapy clients. In consultation with experienced teachers of these meditation traditions, clinicians can also explore how existing concepts and techniques may be adapted to their settings. May this book foster and facilitate that noble effort.

CHAPTER 5

The Compassionate Therapist

Elissa Ely

People aren't solved.
—DIANA TRILLING (1982, p. 339)

Editors' note: Most therapists consider themselves compassionate, and indeed they are. Yet we all face limits to what we can do. The following story illustrates the challenge of remaining compassionate in the face of the world's limitless, untold suffering.

Two nights a week, I visit a homeless shelter. Many of the patients there hear voices, and sometimes they believe they are being punished for crimes they never committed. They live in terror of horrific events that will not happen to them, and sometimes they can't forget horrific events that *have* happened to them.

I prescribe meditations, hold their hands metaphorically, admire their strengths, and imply that if they just hold on—if they take their meds, come to see their therapists regularly, stay away from substances—their symptoms will diminish and their lives will improve.

But I know this is not always so.

This is a story about a shelter patient. It begins with a newspaper piece I wrote about him. His Full Scale IQ was under 70. He didn't drink or use drugs, but he did have a hard time controlling his urge for lottery tickets. When his numbers came up, he would treat the many sudden friends around him to Chinese dinner and sometimes a movie in the Cineplex.

He was waiting for services from the state. Each morning he walked across the bridge to a local arboretum. He wandered all day, doing isometric exercises, watching birds, and then he walked back to the homeless shelter. Nature delighted him. The shelter agitated and intimidated him. His hands were huge and his arms were like pipes from all the push-ups he did. Walls and garbage cans suffered.

Afterwards, he was full of remorse. "I never want to take these hands outta my pants and hit someone again, ma'am," he said after each misdeed. Willingly, he took medication for his anger.

Social services had been slow in coming. The Department of Mental Health wasn't interested in someone without a history of hospitalizations, suicide attempts, or psychosis. On the basis of his mildly low IQ, we thought he might be better served by an agency for mental retardation.

Weeks passed after the application was submitted—and then it was rejected without explanation. An administrator's voice somewhere told us that the patient was entitled to write a detailed letter of rebuttal on behalf of himself, which would serve as an appeal. It seemed a contradiction to write a highly sophisticated document defending one's own incapacity, but one cannot argue with the administrative mysteries of the state.

He continued to do his push-ups, take his anger pills, and walk outside except on frigid winter days. He was trying to treat himself. But he began to slide backwards, shoving garbage cans, threatening bunkmates. He took his large hands out of his pants often.

One night we brought him into the office. We needed to tell him that the rebuttal we had helped him write had also been rejected, that he had still not been accepted for housing or treatment programs, and that no change was anticipated. We had interrupted him in the middle of dinner. He carried a Hoodsie ice cream cup with him and sat, eating it slowly. To prolong the telling of bad news, we asked about his day.

"I was in the park," he said. "I do my push-ups there. I like to smell the trees in the morning, and watch the bugs. There's a hawk nest I found. One of the hawk's red-tailed, that's the woman. The white-tailed, that's the guy, he's a titch bigger."

He was full of proud knowledge.

"You know what, ma'am? I seen the same white-tailed hawk right here at dinnertime," he said. "He flies across the bridge to this place, looking for pigeons. That's a steak dinner to them birds. You get nothing but feathers when they're done."

Standing up, he directed our gaze with an ice cream spoon out the window. "You gotta watch that tree at dinner time," he said. "It's beautiful. It makes me feel lucky."

He stretched out his pipe arms.

"Oh yes, ma'am," he said, remembering. "I feel lucky."

I wrote that profile about him for the local paper. The piece was a poem (not in execution, but in subject), and the response was uplifting.

Readers felt they were taking part in a redemptive moment. They were left with an irresistible image: peaceful nature savant, gesturing with his plastic spoon at the hawks. Briefly, he enjoyed a state of semifame; it was like coming up all numbers in the lottery.

That was the end of the story I wrote.

But it wasn't the end of the story he lived.

A few weeks later, a woman in the shelter accused him of fondling her breast. No one witnessed it. She had made numerous similar accusations before about other men. But these are times when allegations carry heavy weight, and he was barred from the shelter.

He was unable to comprehend what it meant to be barred. The concept made no sense to him. Our shelter was the home he knew, and for the first few days, he slept on the bench outside the front door, begging staff to let him back in. Eventually he made his way to the city hospital emergency room and begged them to send him back to us. All he wanted was to take his anger pills, do his push-ups in the park, wander with avian knowledge.

Finally, he disappeared. We hoped he had found his way to another shelter, but we never heard. We grew busy with a hundred other homeless men.

About a year later, I got a call from a nurse practitioner. She was consulting to a nursing home behavioral unit. Our patient had been admitted in a nearly catatonic state. He gave the shelter as his home address.

The nurse described the fit, lucky man we had known as stiff, sedated, and hostile. He was also—deadliest of chart terms—behaviorally inappropriate, masturbating in the hallways. This behavior was all the staff had to know him by. He was overcome by imprisonment, inarticulation, and anxiety, and his simple-minded panic had chosen exactly the wrong expression. As it happened, the nurse practitioner had read the piece I wrote about him. She would never have recognized that poetic man in this one.

She called several times over the next months, bless her, to consult. His behaviors had not lessened, and he was wearing an ankle bracelet that beeped when he wandered through the ward door. He was not allowed outside the building, onto open land, or near the birds that were his best treatment.

When the nursing home was scheduled for closure, she called one last time. He had not been reassigned yet, and she did not know where he would be transferred. "It's a shame people don't know what happens next in these stories," she said one day. "You ought to write that, too."

After the shelter barred him, he had disappeared from our view, then emerged briefly (just long enough to be sighted and misunderstood), then disappeared again. Yet all this time, in and out of our sight and our awareness, he was still alive, growing more forsaken and less understood. His life, beyond our view, continued.

And then, the nurse disappeared, too.

Four years after he first described his luckiness to us, a letter arrived from a neurology clinic in another part of the state. The envelope ought to have been thrown out, the name on it was so old, but by good luck someone at the front desk had recognized it and passed it onto us. Apparently he was still giving the shelter as his home address.

The consultation inside chilled the spirit. It had been written as if there were no person left in this patient–there was not a single quotation, not even a physical description of him. You got the feeling the neurologist was a little at the end of his own rope. He wrote that without any history on this man–and he had no history whatsoever–there was no way to understand his downward trajectory. The only conclusion that could be drawn, and drawn by observation alone, was that his target behaviors had worsened. The plan, therefore, would be to increase the medications.

We called the neurologist. Our patient is living in a group home now. He is a complete cipher, incomprehensible, identified only by his ongoing problem behaviors. No one wants to take a chance on lowering his medication. No one would dream of letting him walk outside. The published and admired lucky man, the bird-loving him, is unrecognizable. That person may have ceased to exist.

We sent our records to the clinic, all the ones we had, so that they could know the patient now as we had known him then. We also sent a copy of the old newspaper piece, hoping it would inspire them to treat him with tenderness, exert a VIP effect, humanize him. We had lost sight of him again–but again, *his* life had continued. We lose sight of patients, but their lives go on. Even this is not the end of his story. It is only the end of the story I am writing.

Sometimes what we do is as simple as listening. Sometimes what we do should be even simpler: reminding others of who the unrecognizable patient is. Patients, therapists, neighbors, family, we are snapshots, unknown to each other in our fullness. Most of us endure lives of partial recognition because survival does not hinge on it. But now and then, it does.

CHAPTER 6

The Science of Self-Compassion

Kristin D. Neff

> When you begin to touch your heart or let your heart be touched, you begin to discover that it's bottomless, that it doesn't have any resolution, that this heart is huge, vast, and limitless. You begin to discover how much warmth and gentleness is there, as well as how much space.
>
> —PEMA CHÖDRÖN (2001a, p. 128)

To understand what is meant by the term *self-compassion*, it is useful to first consider what it means to feel compassion more generally. When we experience compassion, we notice and are moved by the suffering of others. Rather than rushing past a homeless man begging for change on your way to work, for example, you might actually stop to consider how difficult his life must be. The moment you see the man as an actual human being who is suffering, your heart connects with him (compassion literally means "to suffer with"; see Chapter 1). Instead of ignoring him, you find that you're moved by his pain and feel the urge to help in some way. And importantly, if what you feel is true compassion rather than simply pity, you may say to yourself, "There but for the grace of God go I. If I'd been born in different circumstances, or maybe had just been unlucky, I might also be struggling to survive. We're all vulnerable."

Compassion, therefore, presupposes the recognition and clear seeing of suffering. It entails feelings of kindness, care, and understanding for people who are in pain, so that the desire to ameliorate suffering naturally emerges. Finally, compassion involves recognizing the shared human condition, fragile and imperfect as it is.

Self-compassion has exactly the same qualities—it's just compassion turned inward. In this chapter, I describe what self-compassion is and isn't, how self-compassion is related to well-being, and how it contributes to healing in psychotherapy.

WHAT IS SELF-COMPASSION?

Drawing on the writings of various Buddhist teachers (e.g., Bennett-Goleman, 2001; Brach, 2003; Goldstein & Kornfield, 1987; Salzberg, 1997), I have defined self-compassion as composed of three main components: self-kindness, a sense of common humanity, and mindfulness (Neff, 2003b).

Self-Kindness

Self-compassion entails being warm and understanding toward ourselves when we suffer, fail, or feel inadequate, rather than flagellating ourselves with self-criticism. It recognizes that being imperfect and experiencing life difficulties are inevitable, so we soothe and nurture ourselves when confronting our pain rather than getting angry when life falls short of our ideals. We clearly acknowledge our problems and shortcomings without judgment, so that we can do what's necessary to help ourselves. We can't always get what we want. We can't always *be* who we want to be. When this reality is denied or resisted, suffering arises in the form of stress, frustration, and self-criticism. When this reality is accepted with benevolence, however, we generate positive emotions of kindness and care that help us cope.

Common Humanity

One of the biggest problems with harsh self-judgment is that it tends to make us feel isolated. When we notice something about ourselves we don't like, we irrationally feel like everyone else is perfect and it's only *me* who is inadequate. This isn't a logical process, but a kind of distorted self-centeredness: focusing on our inadequacies gives us tunnel vision so that we can't see anything else but our own feeble, worthless self (see Chapter 3). Similarly, when things go wrong in our external lives, we feel that somehow other people are having an easier time of it, that our own situation is abnormal or unfair. When our experiences are interpreted from the perspective of a separate self, we have trouble remembering the similar experiences of our fellow humans (like the dying 84-year-old man whose final words were "Why me?"). Self-compassion recognizes that life challenges and personal failures are part of being human, an experience we all share. In this way, it helps us to feel less desolate and isolated when we are in pain.

Mindfulness

Mindfulness is a nonjudgmental, receptive mind-state in which thoughts and feelings are observed as they are, without suppressing or denying them (see Chapter 2). You can't ignore your pain and feel compassion for it at the same time. Of course, you may think that suffering is blindingly obvious. But how many of us, when we look in a mirror and don't like what see, remember that this a moment of suffering worthy of a compassionate response? Similarly, when life goes awry, we often go into problem-solving mode immediately without recognizing the need to comfort ourselves for the difficulties we're facing. Conversely, mindfulness requires that we not overly identify with negative thoughts or feelings, so that we are caught up and swept away by our aversive reactions (Bishop et al., 2004). This type of rumination narrows our focus and exaggerates implications for self-worth (Nolen-Hoeksema, 1991). The mental space provided by taking a mindful approach to our difficult feelings, however, allows for greater clarity, perspective, and emotional equanimity (Baer, 2003; Shapiro, Carlson, Astin, & Freedman, 2006).

SELF-COMPASSION PHRASES

When you're feeling stress or emotional pain—perhaps you are caught in a traffic jam, are arguing with a loved one, or are feeling inadequate in some way—it's helpful to have a set of phrases memorized to help you remember to be more compassionate toward yourself in the moment. You can take a deep breath, put your hand over your heart, or gently hug yourself (if you feel comfortable doing so), and repeat the following phrases:

This is a moment of suffering.
Suffering is a part of life.
May I be kind to myself.
May I give myself the compassion I need.

These phrases capture the essence of the three components of self-compassion. The first phrase helps to mindfully open you to the sting of emotional pain. (You could also say "This is really hard right now" or "This hurts.") The second phrase reminds us that suffering unites all living beings, and it reduces the tendency to feel ashamed and isolated when things go wrong in our lives. The third phrase begins the process of responding with self-kindness rather than self-criticism. The final phrase reinforces the idea that you both need and deserve compassion in difficult moments. Be experimental with the phrases. Other phrases that may feel more authentic in a given situation are "May I accept myself as I am," "May I forgive myself," or "May I learn to accept what I cannot change." As you may have noticed, this practice is similar to the loving-kindness meditation introduced in Chapter 3.

WHAT SELF-COMPASSION IS NOT

Self-Pity

People often avoid taking a compassionate stance toward themselves because they confuse self-compassion with self-pity. Western culture has a strong "stiff-upper-lip" tradition in which we're taught that we should just carry on without complaint. Self-compassion is very different from self-pity, however. When individuals feel self-pity, they become immersed in their own problems and forget that others have similar problems. They ignore their interconnections with others and act as if they are the only ones in the world suffering. Self-pity emphasizes egocentric feelings of separation and exaggerates the extent of personal distress. Self-compassion, however, allows us to see the related experiences of self and other without distortion or disconnection. When we acknowledge how hard it is for us in the moment, the rest of humanity is automatically included in our concerned attention. Moreover, when we think about what others are going through, we are often able to put our own situation into greater perspective.

Self-Indulgence

An even greater block to self-compassion is the belief that it's self-indulgent to be kind to oneself. Many people think that self-criticism is necessary to motivate themselves, and that if they're too self-compassionate they'll just sit around all day watching TV and eating ice cream. But is this true? A good analogy can be found in how parents motivate their children. When a mother cares about her son and desires his well-being, does she indulge him by letting him do whatever he wants (like sitting around all day watching TV and eating ice cream)? No. She'll make sure he does things like eat well, go to school, finish his homework, brush his teeth, and go to bed early—even if he doesn't want to—because it's necessary for him to grow and be healthy. Her child will also be more motivated to reach his goals in life when he can count on his mother's encouragement and support even when he fails.

On the other hand, if a mother ruthlessly criticizes her son when he messes up, telling him he's a good-for-nothing failure who'll never amount to anything, how is that going to make him feel? Inspired, motivated, ready to take on the world? Of course not. Constant criticism makes us feel worthless and depressed—not exactly a get-up-and-go mindset. And yet, isn't that how most of us act toward ourselves? We somehow have the notion that self-criticism is a more effective motivator than giving ourselves nurturance, support, and encouragement.

You might say that the motivation of self-compassion arises from love, whereas the motivation of self-criticism arises from fear. To the extent that self-criticism *does* work as a motivator, it's because we're driven by the desire to avoid self-judgment when we fail. But if we know that failure will be met with a barrage of self-criticism, sometimes it can be too frightening to even try. This is why self-criticism is associated with underachievement and self-handicapping strategies such as procrastination (Powers, Koestner, & Zuroff, 2007).

Self-criticism is also used as a means of shaming oneself into action when confronting personal weaknesses. However, this approach backfires if weaknesses remain unacknowledged in an unconscious attempt to avoid self-censure (Horney, 1950). For instance, if you have an anger problem but continually blame things on your partner because you can't face up to the truth about yourself, how are you ever going to achieve a more harmonious relationship? With self-compassion, however, we strive to achieve for a very different reason—because we *care*. If we truly want to be kind to ourselves, we'll do things to help ourselves be happy, such as taking on challenging new projects or learning new skills. And because self-compassion gives us the safety needed to acknowledge our weaknesses, we're in a better position to change them for the better.

Self-Esteem

It's also important to distinguish self-compassion from self-esteem. *Self-esteem* refers to the degree to which we evaluate ourselves positively. It represents how much we like or value ourselves, and is often based on comparisons with others (Coopersmith, 1967; Harter, 1999). In American culture, having high self-esteem means standing out in a crowd—being special and above average (Heine, Lehman, Markus, & Kitayama, 1999). In contrast, self-compassion is not based on positive judgments or evaluations—it is a way of *relating* to ourselves. People feel self-compassion because they are human beings, not because they are special or above average. It emphasizes interconnection rather than separateness. This means that with self-compassion, you don't have to feel better than others to feel good about yourself. It also offers more emotional stability than self-esteem because it is always there for you—when you're on top of the world *and* when you fall flat on your face.

EMPIRICAL DATA

OK, but what does the research show? So far, the majority of studies on self-compassion have been correlational and have used the Self-Compassion Scale (Neff, 2003a)—a 26-item self-report measure. (You can take this scale online at *www.Self-Compassion.org.*) However, more recent research has started to examine self-compassion using experimental manipulations or interventions.

Self-Compassion and Emotional Well-Being

One of the most consistent findings in the research literature is that greater self-compassion is linked to less anxiety and depression (see Neff, 2009, for a review). Of course, a key feature of self-compassion is the lack of self-criticism, and self-criticism is known to be an important predictor of anxiety and depression (Blatt, 1995). However, self-compassion still offers protection against anxiety and depression when controlling for self-criticism and negative affect (Neff, 2003a; Neff, Kirkpatrick, & Rude, 2007). Thus, self-compassion is not merely a matter of looking on the bright side of things or avoiding negative feelings. Self-compassionate people recognize when they are suffering, but are kind toward themselves in these moments, acknowledging their connectedness with the rest of humanity.

In support of this idea, my colleagues and I conducted a study involving a mock interview task in which participants were asked to write an answer to the infamous question, "Please describe your greatest weakness" (Neff, Kirkpatrick, & Rude, 2007). Not only did self-compassionate people experience less anxiety after the task, they also tended to use more connected and less isolating language when writing about their weaknesses. Similarly, Leary and colleagues (Leary, Tate, Adams, Allen, & Hancock, 2007) investigated the way that self-compassionate people deal with negative life events by asking participants to report about problems experienced over a 20-day period. Individuals with higher levels of self-compassion had more perspective on their problems and were less likely to feel isolated by them. They also experienced less anxiety and self-consciousness when thinking about their difficulties.

Self-compassion is associated with greater wisdom and emotional intelligence (Neff, 2003a; Neff, Rude, & Kirkpatrick, 2007), suggesting that self-compassion represents a wise way of dealing with difficult emotions. For instance, self-compassionate people engage in rumination and thought suppression less often than those low in self-compassion (Neff, 2003a; Neff, Kirkpatrick, & Rude, 2007). They also report greater emotional coping skills, including more clarity about their feelings and greater ability to repair negative emotional states (Neely, Schallert, Mohammed, Roberts, & Chen, 2009; Neff, 2003a; Neff, Hseih, & Dejitthirat, 2005).

Self-compassion appears to bolster positive states of being as well. For example, self-compassion is associated with feelings of social connectedness and life satisfaction—important elements of a meaningful life (Neff, 2003a; Neff, Pisitsungkagarn, & Hseih, 2008). It is also linked to feelings of autonomy, competence, and relatedness (Neff, 2003a), suggesting that self-compassion helps meet the basic psychological needs that Deci and Ryan (1995) argue are fundamental to well-being. Self-compassionate people tend to experience more happiness, optimism, curiosity, and positive affect than those who lack self-compassion (Neff, Rude, & Kirkpatrick, 2007). By wrapping one's pain in the warm embrace of self-compassion, positive feelings are generated that help balance the negative ones.

Self-Compassion, Motivation, and Health

Research supports the idea that self-compassion enhances motivation rather than self-indulgence. For instance, while self-compassion is negatively related to perfectionism, it has no association with the level of performance standards adopted for the self (Neff, 2003a). Self-compassionate people aim just as high, but also recognize and accept that they can't always reach their goals. Self-compassion is also linked to greater personal initiative—the desire to reach one's full potential (Neff, Rude, & Kirkpatrick, 2007). Self-compassionate people have been found to have less motivational anxiety and engage in fewer self-handicapping behaviors such as procrastination than those who lack self-compassion (Williams, Stark, & Foster, 2008). In addition, my colleagues and I (Neff et al., 2005) found that self-compassion was positively associated with mastery goals—the intrinsic motivation to learn and grow—and negatively associated with performance goals—the desire to enhance one's self-image (Dweck, 1986). This relationship was mediated by the lesser fear of failure and perceived self-efficacy of self-compassionate individuals. Thus, self-compassionate people are motivated to achieve, but for intrinsic reasons, not because they want to garner social approval.

Self-compassion also promotes health-related behaviors. For instance, a study by Adams and Leary (2007) demonstrated that self-compassion can help people stick to their diets. Dieters often display a paradoxical tendency—if they break their diet and eat high-calorie foods, they tend to eat more afterward as a way to reduce bad feelings associated with their lapse (Heatherton & Polivy, 1990; see abstinence violation effect, Chapter 16,). This study demonstrated that helping women to feel compassionately about blowing their diet attenuated this tendency. Similarly, Kelly, Zuroff, Foa, and Gilbert (2009) examined whether self-compassion could help people stop or reduce smoking. Individuals trained to feel compassionate about the difficulties of giving up smoking reduced their smoking to a greater extent than those trained to reflect upon and monitor their smoking. The self-compassion intervention was especially effective among those who were highly self-critical or resistant to change. Similarly, a study of women's goals for exercising found that self-compassionate women had intrinsic rather than extrinsic motivation to exercise, and their goals for exercising were less related to ego concerns (Magnus, Kowalski, & McHugh, 2010; Mosewich, Kowalski, Sabiston, Sedgwick, & Tracy, 2011). They also reported feeling more comfortable with their bodies and had less anxiety regarding social evaluations of their physique. Thus, self-compassion appears to enhance both physical and mental well-being.

Self-Compassion and Interpersonal Functioning

While there is evidence that self-compassion psychologically benefits the individual, there is also evidence that self-compassion benefits interpersonal relationships. In a study of heterosexual couples (Neff & Beretvas, in press), self-compassionate individuals were described by their partners as being more emotionally connected, accepting, and supportive of autonomy while being less detached, controlling, and verbally or physically aggressive than those lacking self-compassion. Self-compassion was also associated with greater relationship satisfaction and attachment security. Because self-compassionate people give themselves care and support, they appear to have more emotional resources available to give to their partners.

Another study (Yarnell & Neff, in press) found that self-compassionate college students were more likely to compromise in conflict situations with mothers, fathers, and romantic partners, whereas those lacking self-compassion tended to subordinate their needs to partners. This pattern makes sense given that people with high levels of self-compassion say they tend to be equally kind to themselves as others, but people with low levels of self-compassion say they tend to be kinder to others than themselves (Neff, 2003a). The study also showed that self-compassionate people felt more authentic and experienced less turmoil when resolving relationship conflicts, and reported a greater sense of well-being in their relationships.

An interesting question concerns whether self-compassionate people are more compassionate toward others in general. Cultivating an openhearted stance toward oneself that recognized human interconnectedness should theoretically facilitate being kind, forgiving, and empathetic towards other. While there needs to be more research on this topic, preliminary findings suggest that self-compassion is linked to other-focused concern, but this link differs somewhat according to age and life experiences.

Neff and Pommier (in press) examined this question among college undergraduates, an older community sample, and individuals practicing Buddhist meditation. Self-compassion was significantly linked to compassion, empathetic concern for others, and altruism among the community and Buddhist samples, but not the undergraduates. It may be that the sense of interconnectedness facilitating an association between kindness toward self and others does not develop until later in life. Among all three groups, however, self-compassionate people were more likely to forgive others who had harmed them. They also showed enhanced perspective-taking skills, an important component of wisdom (see Chapter 1).

Similarly, Richie Davidson and colleagues conducted a study with a group of participants who were trained in loving-kindness meditation (which intentionally cultivates compassion for the self and others) and found that the training increased self-compassion levels (Davidson, 2007; see also Weibel, 2007). Brain scans were then conductedt on participants while showing them images of suffering (e.g., a child with an eye tumor). Participants who had larger increases in self-compassion experienced greater empathy (as evidenced by increased activity in the insula, a brain area also associated with perspective taking). This body of research suggests that self-compassion helps engender compassion toward others.

Self-Compassion versus Self-Esteem

The psychological benefits of high self-esteem (e.g., lessened depression and anxiety) have been touted for decades (McKay & Fanning, 1987). However, psychologists are now starting to question whether self-esteem is all it's made out to be (for reviews, see Blaine & Crocker, 1993; Crocker & Park, 2004). For instance, people with high self-esteem often engage in downward social comparisons with others, meaning they put others down and puff themselves up as a way to feel better about themselves (Tesser, 1999). Self-esteem is also associated with narcissism (Twenge & Campbell, 2009), inflated and unrealistic self-views (Sedikides, 1993), prejudice

(Aberson, Healy, & Romero, 2000), ego-defensive aggression (Baumeister, Smart, & Boden, 1996), and bullying (Salmivalli, Kaukiainen, Kaistaniemi, & Lagerspetz, 1999). The motivation to protect feelings of self-worth can also lead to increased "need for cognitive closure" (Taris, 2000), in which alternative viewpoints are not tolerated. Self-esteem thus seems to work against the development of wisdom. And self-esteem often fluctuates because self-evaluations are continually changing. As the Hollywood saying goes, you're only as good as your latest success (at least when viewing the world through the lens of self-esteem). This type of instability undermines emotional well-being (Kernis, Cornell, Sun, Berry, & Harlow, 1993). Self-compassion, on the other hand, appears to offer many of the benefits of high self-esteem with fewer downsides (Neff, 2011a).

Research indicates that self-compassion is moderately associated with trait levels of self-esteem (Leary et al., 2007; Neff, 2003a; Neff, Kirkpatrick, & Rude, 2007), as one would expect, given that both represent positive attitudes toward the self. However, self-compassion still predicts greater happiness and optimism as well as less depression and anxiety when controlling for self-esteem (Neff, 2003a). Moreover, the two constructs differ in terms of their impact on well-being.

In a survey I conducted with Roos Vonk (Neff & Vonk, 2009) involving a large community sample in the Netherlands, self-compassion was shown to be a stronger predictor of healthy functioning than self-esteem. For one thing, self-compassion was associated with more stability in state feelings of self-worth over an 8-month period (assessed 12 different times) than trait self-esteem. This finding may be related to the fact that self-compassion was also found to be less contingent on things such as physical attractiveness or successful performances than self-esteem. Results indicated that self-compassion was associated with lower levels of social comparison, public self-consciousness, self-rumination, anger, and need for cognitive closure, than self-esteem. Also, self-esteem had a robust association with narcissism, whereas self-compassion had no association with narcissism. These findings suggest that in contrast to those with high self-esteem, self-compassionate people are less focused on evaluating themselves, feeling superior to others, worrying about whether or not others are evaluating them, defending their viewpoints, or angrily reacting against those who disagree with them.

Leary and colleagues (2007) compared self-compassion and self-esteem using a mood induction method. Participants were instructed to recall a previous failure, rejection, or loss that made them feel badly about themselves and were then asked a series of questions that assessed their feelings about the event. In the self-compassion condition, participants responded in writing to prompts designed to lead them to think about the event in ways that tapped into the three components of self-compassion:

self-kindness, common humanity, and mindful acceptance. In the self-esteem condition, participants responded to prompts designed to protect or bolster their self-esteem. Participants who received the self-compassion induction reported less negative emotions when thinking about the past event than those in the self-esteem condition. Moreover, those in the self-compassion condition took more personal responsibility for the event than those in the self-esteem condition, suggesting that self-compassion does not lead to "letting oneself off the hook."

Gilbert and Irons (2005b) suggest that self-compassion enhances well-being because it helps people feel a greater sense of interpersonal connection. They propose that self-compassion deactivates the threat system (associated with feelings of insecure attachment, defensiveness, and autonomic arousal) and activates the self-soothing system (associated with feelings of secure attachment, safeness, and the oxytocin–opiate system) (see Chapter 18). In contrast, self-esteem is thought to be an evaluation of superiority–inferiority that helps to establish social rank stability and is related to alerting, energizing impulses and dopamine activation. Whereas self-compassion enhances feelings of safety and interconnectedness, self-esteem positions the self in competition with others and amplifies feelings of distinctness and separation.

Self-Compassion in Therapeutic Settings

An exciting area of research concerns the implications of self-compassion for clinical practice (Baer, 2010b). People who lack self-compassion are more likely to have critical mothers, come from dysfunctional families, and display insecure attachment patterns than are self-compassionate people (Neff & McGeehee, 2010). Given that therapy clients often have problems related to their family backgrounds, they may be especially likely to benefit from developing greater self-compassion.

It is an interesting empirical question whether self-compassion is implicitly generated in psychotherapy and is one of the factors underlying effective treatment. This certainly seems to be the case, and may have important implications for understanding the therapeutic process.

My colleagues and I conducted a study that tracked changes in self-compassion experienced by therapy clients over a 1-month interval (Neff, Kirkpatrick, & Rude, 2007). Therapists used a Gestalt two-chair technique designed to help clients lessen self-criticism and have greater compassion for themselves (Greenberg, 1983; Safran, 1998). Results indicated that increased self-compassion levels over the month-long period (assessed under the guise of an unrelated study) were linked to fewer experiences of self-criticism, depression, rumination, thought suppression, and anxiety.

Paul Gilbert (2009c) has developed a group-based therapy intervention called compassionate mind training (CMT) that is designed to help people develop skills of self-compassion, especially when their more habitual form of self-to-self relating involves self-attack. In a pilot study of CMT involving hospital day patients with intense shame and self-criticism issues, significant decreases in depression, self-attacking, shame, and feelings of inferiority were reported after participation in the CMT program (Gilbert & Procter, 2006). Moreover, almost all of the participants felt ready to be discharged from their hospital program at the end of the study. (For more on Gilbert's CMT and compassion-focused therapy [CFT], see Chapters 7 and 18.)

Therapeutic approaches that rely on mindfulness, such as Jon Kabat-Zinn's (1990) mindfulness-based stress reduction (MBSR) program, may also be an effective way for people to develop self-compassion. Mindfulness teaches people to notice the difficult thoughts and emotions that arise in present-moment awareness, so that they can be experienced with kindness, acceptance, and nonjudgment. MBSR courses are commonly taught by therapists and other health professionals to help people deal with stress, depression, and other forms of mental suffering. Research has demonstrated that MBSR significantly increases self-compassion (Shapiro, Astin, Bishop, & Cordova, 2005; Shapiro, Brown, & Biegel, 2007). Research also shows that people who regularly practice mindfulness meditation are more self-compassionate than those who are less experienced (Lykins, & Baer, 2009; Neff, 2003a; Orzech, Shapiro, Brown, & McKay, 2009).

Chris Germer, an editor of this book who specializes in mindfulness- and acceptance-based psychotherapy, views therapy through the lens of mindful self-compassion. As he notes in his book *The Mindful Path to Self-Compassion* (2009), self-compassion adds another dimension to mindful acceptance: "Whereas acceptance usually refers to *what's happening to us*—accepting a feeling or a thought—self-compassion is acceptance of *the person to whom it's happening*. It's acceptance of ourselves while we're in pain" (p. 33). This is a key insight. When we are soothed and comforted by self-compassion, it becomes easier to relate to painful feelings in a mindful way. Thus, training that explicitly teaches self-compassion in addition to mindfulness skills may be especially useful in therapy.

To this end, Chris and I are currently developing an 8-week training program in mindful self-compassion (MSC), which is designed to explicitly integrate self-compassion and mindfulness training. The program has structural elements similar to Kabat-Zinn's MBSR course (eight sessions, plus a retreat day; formal and informal meditation) and will hopefully provide a useful complement to it. On the first day of the program we mainly focus on defining self-compassion and explaining how it differs from self-esteem, self-pity, and self-indulgence. During the following weeks, we teach a variety of mindfulness and self-compassion practices for dealing with difficult emotions and challenging relationships in daily life.

An exercise from the MSC program—writing a compassionate letter to oneself (see also Shapira & Mongrain, 2010)—follows. For more examples of exercises and meditations provided in the MSC program, visit *www.Self-Compassion.org* or *www.MindfulSelfCompassion.org*.

SELF-COMPASSIONATE LETTER

- Candidly describe a problem that tends to make you feel bad about yourself, such as a physical flaw, a relationship problem, or a failure at work or school. Note what emotions come up—shame, anger, sadness, fear—as you write.
- Next, think of an imaginary friend who is unconditionally accepting and compassionate; someone who knows all your strengths and weaknesses, understands your life history, your current circumstances, and understands the limits of human nature.
- Finally, write a letter to yourself from that perspective. What would your friend say about your perceived problem? What words would he or she use to convey deep compassion? How would your friend remind you that you're only human? If your friend were to make any suggestions, how would they reflect unconditional understanding?
- When you're done writing, put the letter down for a while and come back to it later. Then read the letter again, letting the words sink in, allowing yourself to be soothed and comforted.

We recently conducted a randomized controlled study of the MSC program, comparing outcomes for the treatment group to those in a wait-list control group. Results indicated that participation in the workshop significantly increased self-compassion, mindfulness, compassion for others, and life satisfaction, while significantly decreasing depression, anxiety, stress, and the impact of trauma. The degree to which participants' self-compassion level increased was significantly linked to how much informal and formal self-compassion practice they did over the course of the program. We also explored whether enhanced well-being was primarily explained by increases in self-compassion, or if it was also explained by increased mindfulness. We found that while most of the gains in well-being were explained by increased self-compassion, mindfulness explained variance in terms of happiness, stress, and the impact of trauma. This suggests that both self-compassion and mindfulness are key benefits of the MSC program.

Whereas clients may learn to relate to their troubles in a healthier way through a relationship with a compassionate therapist, self-compassion practice can help people be their own therapists *between* sessions. Therapists also need self-compassion, of course, especially for the compassion fatigue that can result when outcomes are not necessarily as expected (see next chapter). Not only is self-compassion associated with less compassion fatigue among counselors (Ringenbach, 2009), it is also linked to greater "compassion satisfaction"—the positive feelings experienced from one's work such as feeling energized, happy, and grateful for being able to make a difference in the world.

In *Toward a Psychology of Being*, Maslow (1968) argued that emotional maturity entails nonjudgmental, forgiving, loving acceptance of oneself. Self-compassion epitomizes this way of being and may help mental health professionals understand and foster this type of emotional wisdom within themselves and in others.

CHAPTER 7

Cultivating Compassion in Psychotherapy

Christopher K. Germer

> If you want others to be happy practice compassion; and if you want yourself to be happy practice compassion.
> —TENZIN GYATSO, the 14th Dalai Lama (Dalai Lama & Cutler, 2009, p. x)

Therapists can get a bad name for wallowing in pain. Yet it's precisely because life is heartbreaking that our profession has persisted, even thrived, over the past century. Therapists have an uncanny ability, or at least a strange willingness, to bear emotional pain. How do they do it?

Compassion is a quality of mind that can transform the experience of pain, even making it worthwhile. When we open to pain in a compassionate way, there is a feeling of freedom—of nonresistance, noncontraction—and a deep sense of connection to others—of expanding beyond ourselves. In the words of Tsoknyi Rinpoche (2004), a Tibetan meditation teacher:

> What is the experience of true compassion? . . . there's some sense of being wide awake and free . . . at the same time, there's some tenderness that arises without any cause or condition. There is a deep-felt sense of being tender. . . . Not sad in a depressed in a hurting way, but tender, and somewhat delighted at the same time. There's a mixture. . . . It's slightly joyful and slightly sad. There's no sadness for oneself . . . nor is there sadness for anyone in particular either. It's like being saturated with juice, just like an apple is full of juice. (p. 159)

Indeed, many therapists return home after a full day at the office feeling buoyant and content, despite having listened to almost unbearable sorrow.

The previous chapter made the empirical case for self-compassion as a foundation for emotional well-being and satisfying interpersonal relationships. This chapter explores how to help our patients cultivate compassion for themselves when they need it the most, and how to promote that process by modeling a compassionate response to suffering. It also explores what supports and hinders a therapist's compassion in the consultation room, and offers two simple strategies for managing compassion fatigue.

COMPASSION AND SORROW

Ethan was a very depressed, middle-age man who returned after a yearlong hiatus from therapy. He was going through a divorce and was temporarily living in a dumpy apartment with a friend. In addition, Ethan's business was drying up due to the economy, and he was about to lose the house he'd built because he couldn't make monthly payments. He couldn't sleep, was losing weight because he had no appetite, and his antidepressant and antianxiety medications weren't working. Ethan was experiencing the full catastrophe. He had suicidal thoughts, but no plan. It was as Nietzsche (1923/2010) said: "The thought of suicide is a great consolation: by means of it one gets successfully through many a bad night" (p. 48).

I had known Ethan for almost 10 years and had never seen him in such a state. Our previous pattern had been to brainstorm together about his life problems. But this time I became frustrated because each question I raised was met with a web of problems that rendered it meaningless. Eventually Ethan stopped me and asked if I had grown tired of him. He added plaintively, "I know we've known each other for almost a decade, but have you stopped liking me?"

That's when I slowed down and took the time to just *be* with Ethan—and to be with myself. I gave up the rush to fix him and prevent a possible suicide, to avert foreclosure on the home his wife was living in, or to keep him from becoming emotionally disabled. I said to myself, "This is the only moment of our lives, no matter how painful it may be. It's just Ethan and me." I allowed myself to enter Ethan's reality and let his pain become my own.

When I did that, I began to realize how overwhelmed *I* was feeling and how incapable of helping Ethan I felt. I suspected that Ethan was feeling exactly the same way. Our conversation became much simpler:

ETHAN: I don't know what to do.

CKG: Neither do I. Certainly not now.

ETHAN: I'm really alone here—no wife, no job, nobody.

CKG: It's pretty bad, I know.

ETHAN: I'm just so overwrought. I wake up in terror.

CKG: Terror?

ETHAN: Mostly about money, how I'll survive.

CKG: Can you feel the terror in your body?

ETHAN: Definitely . . . here in my belly. I wake up with a knot in my stomach almost every morning.

I had suspected that Ethan felt fear in his belly because I was feeling the same sensation at the time. As Ethan spoke about his experience, I waited for the muscles in my abdomen to relax—to stop resisting—before I felt ready to return to the subject of how Ethan could safely get through the day. Ethan beat me to it. He stopped calling himself a "complete failure" and wanted to discuss how to stay out of the hospital by nourishing himself with regular meals and going to bed when he felt tired instead of sitting up all night ruminating. When Ethan made me stop and pay attention to my own experience in this way, the therapy began to move forward again, this time with much less effort.

Compassion is a skill that allows us to open to sorrow. When we resist the sorrow that arises in our own lives, or fight the pain we feel for others who are suffering, we cannot be compassionate. In the case of Ethan, I was grieving that his life was falling apart, I was afraid he would commit suicide under my watch, and I was vainly trying to recreate the happier times we'd had together in the past. I simply wasn't willing to feel fear and sorrow, both his and mine. It's often the clinician's resistance to what's occurring in the therapy room that hampers progress in treatment the most.

But sorrow is not such a bad thing. It's only a problem if it interferes with our ability to function. Seasoned meditators actually welcome sorrow as a sign of progress on the path. It means that our eyes and hearts are open to the inevitable pain in life. Over time, we learn that our personal struggles and failures—not knowing enough, not owning enough, not being happy, healthy, or successful enough—are part of the human condition. It's the nature of the mind to paint our lives as "not quite right" (see Chapters 9 and 10). As Buddhist scholar Mu Soeng (2007) puts it, "An upwelling of sadness toward one's mistakes in life and the cumulative mistakes of all humanity helps serve as a backdrop to the arising of compassion" (p. 65).

The fruit of meditation—of sitting with oneself for extended periods of time (and perhaps sitting with our patients over the years)—includes insight into the universality of suffering and the discovery that compassion is a uniquely healthy and intelligent response to it. Compassion alleviates suffering. The opposite reaction—resistance to emotional discomfort—simply adds insult to injury, layering more stress upon an already difficult situation. There is a Hasidic saying, "He who feels no compassion will become insane."

WARMING UP THE CONVERSATION

When things go wrong in our lives, as they inevitably will, we typically engage in an unholy trinity of reactions: self-criticism, self-isolation, and self-absorption (Germer, 2009; Chapter 6). These reactions seem to be manifestations of our fight–flight–freeze response to threat. We may attack and criticize ourselves for what went wrong ("I'm an idiot!"), flee from ourselves (into work, alcohol, food, etc.), and/or get stuck in our heads ("Why me?"). Self-compassion, in contrast, consists of self-kindness, a sense of common humanity, and mindfulness (see Neff, 2003b; Chapter 6). Compassion changes the *tone* of the inner conversation—it "warms it up" (P. Gilbert, personal communication; see Chapter 18).

Feeling connected to others goes a long way toward reducing human sorrow. Regardless of where it is directed, our compassion helps us recognize that we are all human beings, full of personal inadequacies and vulnerable to sickness, aging, social pain, and death. Most of what goes on in our lives is determined by an infinite number of factors (where and when we were born, to whom, and with what genetic loading), not just our personal choices. When we see the background to our lives, there is less blame. This expanded, less self-centered view reduces shame and gives us strength to address our problems. When our patients feel less alone in their suffering, as Ethan did in the story above, they too can find the courage to turn toward the broken places in their lives with greater energy and curiosity. The conversation becomes more encouraging for everyone.

COMPASSION-ORIENTED PSYCHOTHERAPY

All psychotherapy models suggest that treatment should be conducted in a compassionate manner. Research evidence is accumulating that self-compassion is an underlying mechanism of change in psychotherapy (Baer, 2010a; Birnie, Speca, & Carlson, 2010; Hofmann, Grossman, & Hinton, 2011; Hollis-Walker & Colosimo, 2011; Kuyken et al., 2010; Raes,

2010; Raque-Bogdan, Ericson, Jackson, Martin, & Bryan, 2011; Schanche, Stiles, McCollough, Swartberg, & Nielsen, in press; Van Dam, Sheppard, Forsyth, & Earleywine, 2011). This finding suggests that treatments could be rendered more effective if they were specifically geared toward the cultivation of compassionate mind states—what might be called "compassion-oriented therapy." How is this accomplished? Under the umbrella of compassion-oriented therapy, patients can develop compassion either by learning and practicing compassion exercises ("compassion-*based* psychotherapy") or through the therapy relationship ("compassion-*informed* psychotherapy"). These two approaches to incorporating compassion into the therapy process are considered later on in this chapter.

Self-compassion is the goal of most compassion-oriented psychotherapy. When we suffer from intense and disturbing emotions, often we first need to calm and soothe ourselves before we can be emotionally available to others. On occasion, however, the best way to care for ourselves is to practice compassion for others because doing so tends to improve interpersonal relationships and enhance personal well-being (Cosley et al., 2010; Crocker & Canevello, 2008; Dunn, Aknin, & Norton, 2008; Mongrain, Chin, & Shapira, in press).

The Compassion-Focused Therapy Model

A new, empirically supported, compassion-oriented approach to psychotherapy is "compassion-focused therapy" (CFT), developed by Paul Gilbert (2005, 2009a, 2009b, 2010a, 2010b, 2010c; see also Chapter 18) and colleagues. Gilbert's model integrates evolutionary psychology (Bell, 2001; Gilbert & Bailey, 2000), attachment theory, and the neurobiology of affiliative emotions (Carter, 1998). CFT is based on the current evidence that there are at least three interacting affect regulation systems that have different functions and evolved for different reasons: (1) threat, linked to detecting danger and protection; (2) drive, linked to securing and enjoying resources; and (3) contentment and soothing, linked to feeling safe and secure in relationship (Depue & Morrone-Strupinsky, 2005). The contentment and soothing system has been especially important in the evolution of attachment behavior insofar as affiliation and attachment can downregulate the other two emotion systems—for example, kindness can calm us down when we feel scared.

All three emotion regulation systems are necessary for survival, have evolved over millions of years, and function best when they are in balance. Nowadays, however, our threat and drive systems are often disproportionately triggered in our competitive, individualistic culture. Also, many individuals have not been sufficiently comforted as children to activate the soothing system as adults when they are emotionally overwhelmed, or they may not have inherited the inclination to do so. The goal of CFT is to teach patients how to evoke compassionate mind states. Although the threat system is hardwired by evolution to respond instantaneously to danger, we are also hardwired, and therefore eminently predisposed, to comfort ourselves in the absence of clear and present peril.

CFT was especially developed to address the self-criticism and shame that arises when we suffer intensely or persistently over time (Gilbert, 2010b; Gilbert & Bailey, 2000; Gilbert & Irons, 2005a). When our lives fall apart, we tend not only to *feel* bad; we believe we *are* bad. The sense of self gets engulfed in suffering, and we don't know where the pain ends and our self begins. We may think, "I'm defective," "I'm weak," "I'm unlovable," or a host of other negative, threatening beliefs (Young, Klosko, & Weishaar, 2003). These self-statements trigger the threat system. By activating the soothing system with self-compassion, the self-critical inner conversation loses its grip, enabling us to reestablish perspective and make necessary changes in our lives.

It's common for clients in traditional cognitive-behavior therapy to say that they are *aware* of their negative self-talk and can repeat positive alternatives, but they still feel bad (Stott, 2007). Why is that? As children, our caregivers hopefully rescued us from major distress and protected us from the difficulties of life. This kind of comfort through affiliation activates the soothing system and helps make it an emotional habit when we are under stress as adults. CFT argues that, for some people, particularly those from difficult or emotionally neglectful backgrounds, changing the *content* of our internal dialogue is not sufficient to change our mood. Rather, we need to change the emotional *tone* of the conversation. This means validating ourselves ("That hurts!"), expressing empathy ("Of course, you feel sad right now"), encouraging ourselves ("You *can* do it"), and whatever else is needed to feel whole and secure again. Luckily, soothing ourselves, making ourselves feel safer, and caring for ourselves when we need it the most are skills that can be learned (see Chapters 6 and 18; also Germer, 2009; Gilbert, 2010c; Lee, 2005; Neff, 2011b).

Childhood Factors

Some individuals seem to have an easier time experiencing self-compassion than others. The ability to be self-compassionate may depend on how secure we felt as children in relationship to our primary caregivers (Neff & McGeehee, 2010). We all have "internal working models" of attachment figures that we carry into adulthood (Bowlby, 1969, 1973). Mary Ainsworth (Ainsworth, Blehar, Waters, & Wall, 1978) and other theorists identified different adult "attachment patterns" that shape how we behave in relationship to others (Collins, 1996; Collins & Feeney, 2000; Mulkiner &

Shaver, 2007). For example, a person with a "secure" attachment pattern was probably raised by parents who validated his or her needs and adequately responded to them. Securely attached adults feel relatively safe in relationship, expecting the best and forgiving minor transgressions. They are likely to express their views, share, and listen. In contrast, it is thought than an insecurely attached person with an "anxious-ambivalent" attachment pattern might have had parents who were more self-focused and inconsistent, leading the adult to be distrusting of relationships and to need a lot of reassurance. An insecure person with an "avoidant" attachment style might have had parents who were dismissive or critical, leading the adult to minimize his or her needs and avoid close relationships so as not to be disappointed (Cassidy & Shaver, 2010; Wallin, 2007; Zayas, Mischel, Shoda, & Aber, 2011).

Self-compassion training, in particular, is a way of relearning how to soothe ourselves and feel more secure in relationship. Paul Gilbert describes nonsecure attachment patterns as symptomatic of overactivation of the threat system in early childhood that probably continues into adulthood and interferes with giving and receiving compassion.

It's also necessary to learn self-compassion because, as adults, the days are long gone when we can reliably expect another person to know what we're feeling at a particular moment and to respond in just the right way. Furthermore, the tendency to blame ourselves when things go wrong springs eternal. To live our lives happily, not only do we need to repair our childhood wounds, but we need a compassionate relationship with ourselves in general. When things go wrong, how do you motivate yourself to improve? For example, after going off your diet, do you motivate yourself by examining yourself in the mirror, noting your physical flaws and reminding yourself how hopeless you are? Or can you say to yourself, "I know you feel badly about eating a second piece of chocolate cake. It was awfully tasty. It's not a crime to blow your diet, but why not give yourself a really delicious, nutritious meal the next time you sit down for dinner?" (Adams & Leary, 2007; Fain, 2011; Goss & Allen, 2010).

COMPASSION-BASED PSYCHOTHERAPY

In compassion-based psychotherapy, patients are taught specific exercises to evoke a compassionate state of mind, and the possibilities are endless. Although formal meditation is rarely practiced more than 1 hour per day, we can direct our intentions, thoughts, emotions, and behavior toward compassion throughout our waking hours. The principle behind this practice was beautifully expressed by poet Mary Oliver (1986): "You only have to let the soft animal of your body love what it loves" (p. 14).

FIVE PATHWAYS TO SELF-COMPASSION

- *Physical*: Soften the body; stop tightening up (e.g., breathe deeply; take a warm bath; pet the dog; soften the belly; exercise; have sex; take a nap).
- *Mental*: Allow thoughts to come and go; stop fighting them (e.g., do concentration or mindfulness meditation; prioritize, think of death; pray, "Thy will be done").
- *Emotional*: Befriend feelings; stop avoiding them (e.g., do loving-kindness meditation; put your hand on your heart; practice forgiveness of self and other; listen to soothing music; ask, "What would your best friend say now?").
- *Relational*: Connect safely with others; stop isolating (e.g., do compassionate image meditation; share lunch; express gratitude to an old friend; make amends; volunteer).
- *Spiritual*: Commit to larger values; stop "selfing" (e.g., engage in prayer/meditation; share your faith; walk in nature; make peace; commit a random act of kindness; speak the truth).

The main challenge is to *remember* to practice. The body and mind are under stress most of the day and are therefore ripe for soothing and self-kindness, but we instinctively apply the majority of our mental and emotional effort to warding off pain and grasping for pleasure that inevitably increases our stress. A formal practice of meditation in the morning is especially helpful to establish a baseline from which to recognize when we're caught up in emotional difficulties and to intentionally offer ourselves a compassionate response.

HAND-ON-HEART

- When you notice you're under stress, take two to three deep, satisfying breaths.
- Gently place your hand over your heart, feeling the gentle pressure and warmth of your hand. If you wish, place *both* hands on your chest, noticing the difference between one and two hands.
- Linger with the feeling for as long as you like.

That simple act helps us find ourselves in the crowd of our thoughts and feelings and reminds us to be kind to ourselves. It's almost reflexive: Just imagine how you might react to really bad news, such as the death of a loved one. You might find yourself gasping (inhaling deeply), putting a hand on your chest, and exclaiming, "Oh my God!" This exercise is an intentional variation on that natural, self-soothing response.

Good Will, Not Necessarily Good Feelings

Progress on the path of self-compassion can be seen as a steady refinement of intention. Over time, we learn to practice self-compassion *not to feel better*, but *because* we feel bad. Why is that important? Because any technique that we practice to *not* feel what we are feeling in the present moment is a form of resistance—and it's destined to fail.

Resistance shows up everywhere in our lives:

- By fighting sleeplessness, we can create insomnia.
- By fighting anxiety, we can create panic.
- By fighting grief, we may develop depression.
- By fighting back pain, we may create a chronic pain syndrome.
- By fighting our daughter's lousy boyfriend, we may get a lousy son-in-law.

The inevitable by-product of self-compassion practice is feeling better; if instead, we meet anxiety or depression with resentment and despair rather than soothing and comfort, we may get stuck in a vicious cycle of striving, frustration, and hopelessness. At its best, compassion is a simple, spontaneous, intelligent response to pain and suffering. We're cultivating good will—an attitude of kindliness and generosity—rather than a demand for our current experience to be other than it is. Compassion gives us the strength to abide with the vicissitudes of our lives—pleasure and pain, sickness and health, gain and loss—until we have an opportunity to change them.

What is true for the relationship we have with our *experience* is also true for the relationship we have with *ourselves*. When we openheartedly accept ourselves—our emotional limitations, intellectual weaknesses, physical flaws—then we can approach our lives with greater humor and grace, see new possibilities, and succeed in key areas of our lives (see broaden-and-build, Chapter 3). Carl Rogers (1959) said, "The curious paradox of life is that when I accept myself just as I am, then I can change"

(p. 17). Therefore, as compassion-based therapists, we cultivate the wish that all beings, including ourselves, be free from suffering even as we open our hearts to our mistakes and inadequacies. As meditation teacher Rob Nairn (2009) quipped, we retain the freedom to be a "compassionate mess."

Individual Differences

When new psychotherapy techniques are introduced to the profession, there is a natural tendency to try them out on everybody. Then we gradually discover, through clinical experience and careful research, how different individuals respond to particular interventions. This is currently happening for compassion-based psychotherapy. For example, depressed people who learned in early childhood to criticize themselves in order to remain in connection with primary caregivers may feel deeply uneasy when they are kind to themselves—it feels viscerally unsafe (Pauley & McPherson, 2010). Some anxious children have more anxiety toward happy faces than fearful faces, which can compromise the therapy relationship (Rich, 2010). Depressed individuals who engage in a lot of ruminative brooding seem to benefit more from breath meditation than loving-kindness meditation, and those with less brooding benefit more from loving-kindness (Barnhofer, Chittka, Nightingale, Visser, & Crane, 2010). We are beginning to learn from such studies how compassion-oriented therapy should be adjusted to suit individual needs. Researchers are also exploring:

- The relationship of self-compassion to attachment patterns (Raque-Boydun et al., 2011; Shapira & Mongrain, 2010; Wei, Liao, Ku, & Shaffer, in press)
- How self-compassion may differentially affect anxiety and depression (Raes, 2010, 2011)
- How to adapt compassion-based treatment to conditions such as mother–infant distress (Cree, 2010)
- Recovery from psychosis (Gumley, Braehler, Laithwaite, MacBeth, & Gilbert, 2010; Johnson et al., 2009)
- Self-attacking in depression (Kelly, Suroff, & Shapira, 2009)
- Bipolar disorder (Lowens, 2010)
- Posttraumatic stress disorder (Thompson & Waltz, 2008)
- Anxiety disorders (Tirch, 2011; Welford, 2010).

Gender also appears to have an impact on how well self-compassion is accepted by patients. Women seem to take to it more easily than men

("Oh, I need *that*!"). Such positive response may be related to women's higher estrogen levels; estrogen enhances the effects of oxytocin, the bonding hormone that generally makes people feel good in connection (McCarthy, 1995). Testosterone, on the other hand, probably suppresses the effect of oxytocin—which could explain why women are more likely than men to seek connection with others when under stress ("tend and befriend") (Taylor et al., 2000). It is noteworthy, however, that women seem to have less self-compassion than men (Neff, 2003a), perhaps due to social pressure to conform to unrealistic stereotypes.

Men are socially rewarded for soldiering on, often at their own peril, in order to shelter and protect others. Hence, compassion for *others* may be a more socially acceptable way for men to begin evoking compassionate mind states within themselves. But men also need to comfort and soothe themselves, as we've noticed in recent years among survivors of war trauma. The language in which we frame self-compassion training is important. For example, self-compassion can be explained to men as a strength that increases their ability to deal with challenges, manage difficult emotions, be honest with themselves, reduce stress, and stand up to the harm they cause themselves or others by overworking, overanalyzing, and overreacting (Russell Kolts, personal communication). Compassion training has been used in the treatment of male domestic abusers (Stosny, 1995), where it's helpful to frame self-compassion in "instrumental" terms—leading to improved caring for others, and earning respect and admiration (Stosny, personal communication).

Backdraft

Most clinicians have witnessed how difficult memories resurface when a patient feels truly seen, heard, and loved in therapy. A metaphor for this process is "backdraft." Backdraft occurs when a firefighter opens a door with a hot fire behind it. Oxygen rushes in, causing a burst of flame. Similarly, when the door of the heart is opened with compassion, intense pain can sometimes be released. Therefore, some patients, especially those with a trauma history, can suffer from "fear of compassion" (Gilbert, McEwan, Matos, & Rivis, in press).

Backdraft is an intrinsic part of healing. Nonetheless, what if a patient leaves the therapy office and does not have the capacity to contain the feelings that arose? Without the skill of self-compassion, a client may find it necessary to fight off disturbing emotions by self-medicating or using other forms of self-harm. A compassion-based therapist needs to have the ability to stop a patient from opening too much in session, especially during trauma treatment. We only need to "contact" underlying emotional pain, not necessarily dive into it, and then find a way to soothe and comfort ourselves (Rothschild, 2000). Soothing and comfort are prerequisites for exposure and desensitization.

Compassion Training Programs

Clinicians can incorporate compassion training into their work with individual patients, or their patients can participate in a compassion training programs. The mindfulness-based stress reduction (MBSR) and the mindfulness-based cognitive therapy (MBCT) programs have been shown to increase self-compassion (Birnie, Speca, & Carlson, 2010; Kuyken et al., 2010; Shapiro, Astin, Bishop, & Cordorva, 2005; Shapiro, Brown, & Biegel, 2007). Self-compassion appears to be a "crucial attitudinal factor" in the relationship between mindfulness training and positive mental health (Hollis-Walker & Colosimo, 2011; Van Dam et al., 2011). Compassionate awareness is implicit in the MBSR and MBCT programs; the amount of *explicit* compassion training (especially loving-kindness meditation) usually depends on each individual teacher.

There are a number of training programs currently under development that are specifically designed to cultivate compassion: compassion-cultivation training program (CCT; Jinpa et al., 2009), Emory compassion meditation protocol (Negi, 2009), nonviolent communication (NVC; Langemann & Yamaner, 2011), compassionate mind training (CMT; Gilbert, 2009a), and mindful self-compassion training (MSC; Germer & Neff, 2011). These manualized programs will provide an opportunity to conduct prospective studies on the impact of compassion training on clinical and nonclinical populations.

COMPASSION-INFORMED PSYCHOTHERAPY

Our patients do not typically come to therapy to learn compassion, nor are they necessarily inclined to learn meditation. They just want to feel better. Therefore, the most common way of teaching patients to be more self-compassionate is through a warm, respectful healing relationship, the primary "intervention" of compassion-informed psychotherapy. Compassion can be transmitted through language, facial expressions, voice tones, and other subtle microcommunications found in human encounters. Given the potential of human connections to mutually affect our brains (Cozolino, 2010; Hein & Singer, 2008; Siegel, 2007, 2010a; Singer & Decety, 2011), the therapy relationship may be considered a key component of all forms of compassion-oriented psychotherapy.

Every practitioner probably has a different explanation for how self-compassion may be transmitted to patients through the therapy relationship. Here's mine:

1. Our patients bring us their emotional suffering, especially the pain they are resisting.
2. We "receive" it with open eyes (mindful awareness) and open hearts (compassion).
3. We "hold" the patient, and the patient's experience, in loving awareness.
4. We "offer" a revised attitude toward suffering back to our patients, who carry it into their lives.

Consider the following clinical encounter:

Maria was the kind of patient I never schedule at 3:00 P.M. when my energy is low. She was the eldest of seven kids who was entrusted as a young woman with the task of caring for her siblings while her single mother worked in a restaurant. Long into adulthood, Maria continued to work hard and had few relationships outside her family of origin. "Superficial" was all I could say about our dreaded meetings. The more I probed for signs of life, the more Maria retreated. Yet Maria returned punctually each week, apparently appreciating (or hoping for) an hour of undivided attention.

At some point, I decided to accept the quiet torture of sitting with Maria—accepting it first as *my* problem, not hers. That simple shift in attention opened up an entirely new world for both Maria and me.

First, I imagined what Maria's life must feel like if this superficial level of connection with me was somehow worth her time, money, and effort. I allowed myself not only to contemplate her experience; I *took it in*. Soon I discovered a hollow feeling in my gut. Then I touched something in common—loneliness, and how lonely life can sometimes be. When I emerged from my reverie, I had a newfound sense of kinship with Maria, feeling almost grateful that she was still there in the room, and her words had a tingling sound like little bells in my consciousness. From then on, I knew where to go—straight into the loneliness—whenever the smokescreen of boredom drew around me. Perhaps Maria could sense my innocent (less therapeutic) curiosity about her, and she gradually brought more of her emotional life into the therapy room. She started to smile more and delighted in sharing insights she had gleaned about other people and herself throughout the week. Learning to cherish Maria, boredom and all, gradually made our interactions anything but boring.

We need to connect with emotional pain for compassion to arise. Life can be shallow if we glide over sorrow, more difficult if we fight it, and simply terrifying when we feel raw and unprotected. A critical skill of therapists is the ability to abide with emotional pain in a safe, non-judgmental way—especially in the crunch moments of therapy—and then model that attitude for our patients. Toward that end, I make a simple vow each morning before I open the door for my first patient: "May I open to sorrow with compassion."

Fostering Compassion in the Therapist

Numerous conditions may impact a therapist's ability to remain compassionate in therapy. In a survey by Vivino, Thompson, Hill, and Ladany (2010), some factors that seem to *support* compassion include:

- Patient in great pain
- Therapist understands and likes the patient
- Patient involved in the therapy process
- Therapist has own therapy or inner practice
- Therapist has/had compassionate role models
- Therapist's clinical experience and training
- Therapist's spiritual values and beliefs

Some factors that *hinder* compassion are:

- Patient aggression or severe pathology
- Boundary violations
- Therapist's personal issues
- Therapist feeling incompetent

Therapists can creatively optimize conditions that foster compassion when they know what supports and hinders compassion in their own lives.

COMPASSION PRACTICES FOR THE THERAPIST

Self-compassion exercises can have salubrious effects on the functioning and well-being of therapists (Kane, 2010; Neff, Kirkpatrick, & Rude, 2007; Patsiopoulos & Buchanan, 2011; Ringenbach, 2009; Shapiro, Brown, & Biegel, 2007; Ying, 2009).

The following self-compassion practice—"Soften, Soothe, and Allow"—works by anchoring difficult emotions in the body and releasing them there, freeing us from excessive rumination. (This and other self-compassion meditations can be downloaded from *www.MindfulSelfCompassion.org*.)

SOFTEN, SOOTHE, AND ALLOW

- Sit in a comfortable position, reasonably upright and relaxed. Close your eyes, fully or partially. Take a few deep breaths to settle into your body and into the present moment.
- Find your breath in the heart region and begin to track each breath with gentle, mindful awareness.
- After a few minutes, release your attention to your breath and let your attention be drawn to the place in your body where a difficult emotion can be felt most strongly. For example, if it's anger, you might feel tension in your stomach. If it's grief, you might feel hollowness in your chest.
- *Soften* into that location in your body. *Let* the muscles be soft without a requirement that they *become* soft, like simply applying heat to sore muscles. You can say "soft . . . soft . . . soft . . . " quietly to yourself to enhance the process. Remember that you are not trying to make the sensations go away—you are just being with them with loving awareness.
- Now *soothe* yourself for struggling in this way. Put your hand over your heart and feel your body breathe. Perhaps kind words arise in your mind, such as, "Oh my dear, this is such a painful experience. May I grow in ease and well-being."
- If you wish, you can also direct kindness to the part of your body that is under stress by placing your hand in that area. It may help to think of your body as if it were the body of a beloved child. You can say kind words to yourself, or just repeat "soothe . . . soothe . . . soothe."
- Finally, *allow* the discomfort to be there. Abandon the wish for the feeling to disappear. Let the discomfort come and go as it pleases, like a guest in your own home. You can repeat "allow . . . allow . . . allow."
- "Soften, soothe, and allow." "Soften, soothe, and allow." You can use these three words like a mantra, reminding yourself to incline with tenderness toward your suffering.
- If you experience too much discomfort with an emotion, stay with your breath until you feel better.
- Slowly open your eyes when you're ready.

"Soften, Soothe, and Allow" as a practice establishes a more compassionate relationship to emotional pain in the physical, emotional, and psychological realms, respectively. After a while, simply saying the words "*soften, soothe, allow*" can evoke a compassionate state of mind.

Another way to cultivate compassion during crunch moments in therapy is called "Breathing Compassion In and Out." It is based on a practice called *tonglen* (Tibetan: giving and taking), attributed to a Buddhist teacher, Atisha, who lived in India in the 10th century CE (Chödrön, 2001b; Tarchin, 1999). The traditional practice involves inhaling the pain and suffering of others and exhaling kindness, warmth, and goodwill, effectively reversing our instinctive, and ultimately ruinous, tendency to battle emotional discomfort. In the current adaptation, we inhale compassion *with* the pain—the medicine along with the toxin—and exhale compassion.

BREATHING COMPASSION IN AND OUT

- Sit comfortably, close your eyes, and take a few relaxing breaths.
- Scan your body for stress, noting any physical sensations of tension. Also allow yourself to become aware of any stressful *emotions* that you may be holding in your field of awareness. If a challenging person comes to mind, let yourself be aware of the stress associated with that person. If you are experiencing the suffering of another person through empathy, let yourself be aware of that discomfort as well.
- Now, aware of the stress you are carrying in your body, inhale fully and deeply, drawing compassion inside your body and filling every cell in your body with compassion. Let yourself be soothed by inhaling deeply, and by giving yourself the compassion you deserve when you experience discomfort.
- As you exhale, send out compassion to the person who is associated with your discomfort, or exhale compassion to the world in general.
- Continue breathing compassion in and out, letting your body gradually find a natural, relaxed breathing rhythm. Occasionally scan your inner landscape for any distress and respond by inhaling compassion for yourself and exhaling compassion for those who need it.
- Gently open your eyes.

You can practice the same exercise during psychotherapy. When you feel distress or discomfort, take a deep inbreath, fill your body with compassion, and then exhale compassion for your patient. Gradually find an easy breathing rhythm, inhaling compassion for yourself and exhaling compassion for your patient. This elegant exercise seems to work by the following mechanisms:

1. Reversing the tendency to resist discomfort
2. Anchoring awareness in the body
3. Facilitating a feeling of connection
4. Evoking a compassionate state of mind

Overall, the undercurrent of compassionate breathing can help us warm up the therapeutic conversation and stay emotionally present with our patients.

Managing Compassion Fatigue

Of course, despite our best efforts, psychotherapy can be emotionally exhausting. We call this *compassion fatigue* (Baker, 2003; Christopher et al., 2011; Figley, 2002; Kahill, 1988). Compassion fatigue doesn't just jump out of nowhere—we can have 100 moments of fatigue in a single therapy hour when our attention glances off unpleasant experiences such as emotional disconnection or boredom. The term *compassion fatigue* may be a misnomer because compassion is usually energizing. Compassion fatigue may be better termed *attachment fatigue*—clinging to certain outcomes, such as enjoyable therapy hours, happy clients, successful treatment, or a lucrative practice—and we tie ourselves into knots when the reality is otherwise. Or perhaps *empathy fatigue*—vicarious suffering without the simultaneous experience of love and equanimity (Klimeki & Singer, in press).

Two mind-training practices that may help to alleviate compassion fatigue involve repetition of key phrases that evoke self-compassion and equanimity.

PHRASES FOR COMPASSION FATIGUE

- *Self-compassion.* When we feel exhausted or irritated by our patients, it's a sign we need to take care of ourselves—we need *self*-compassion. We can begin to funnel goodwill toward ourselves with the following phrases:

  May I be safe.
  May I be peaceful.
  May I be kind to myself.
  May I accept myself just as I am.

  These phrases gradually shape our thoughts, feelings, and actions, such as affirming what's good in us, giving ourselves permission to take naps, getting some exercise, or seeing fewer clients.

- *Equanimity.* The following equanimity phrases are adapted for clinical practice from traditional phrases used in early Buddhist mind training:

  Everyone is on his or her own life journey.
  I am not the cause of my patient's suffering, nor is it entirely within my power to make it go away, no matter how much I wish I could.
  Although this moment is difficult to bear, it remains a privilege to help.

Equanimity and self-compassion phrases should be customized by each practitioner so that they are experienced as authentic, vivid, and alive. Although these particular phrases may appear heartless or irresponsible when we're feeling comfortable and happy, they can have a deep, liberating impact when we're overwhelmed by the suffering of our patients.

Compassion is a fresh new area of psychological study that appears to have important implications for psychotherapy and as well as general well-being. Most of us know how to build muscle tone, but how many of us know how to build *emotional* tone? We can intentionally and systematically cultivate compassion throughout our waking lives, especially while doing therapy, both for the sake of our patients and for ourselves.

CHAPTER 8

The Neurobiology of Compassion

Richard J. Davidson

> At some point the question comes up, "Can we really change our attitude?" My answer on the basis of my little experience is, without hesitation, "Yes!"
>
> —TENZIN GYATSO, the 14th Dalai Lama (2010c)

Imagine it's the early 1970s and you just began your graduate training in neuroscience. You start, like most students, by learning the fundamentals of the field. Among those is the idea that the brain is unlike any other organ in the body; in the adult brain, cells are constantly dying, never to be reborn.

This was an unquestioned assumption of neuroscience until the discovery of mammalian neurogenesis in the early 1990s. Neurogenesis, or the growth of new brain cells, is happening daily, creating 5,000–10,000 cells in the average healthy adult (Aimone, Deng, & Gage, 2010). New cells are continually being integrated into the brain's circuits and play an important role in their functioning. This means that the brain has remarkable potential for structural change, and it is constantly being shaped by what we do, say, and think.

Neuroplasticity is the word we use to describe this potential. It refers to the fact that the brain is an organ built to change in response to experience, perhaps more than any other organ in the body. For example, learning to play a musical instrument such as the piano induces structural changes in several brain regions, including the primary motor cortex and primary auditory cortex (Hyde et al., 2009), and learning to juggle over a period of time as short as 7 days induces measureable structural changes in areas of the visual cortex (Dreimeyer, Boyke, Gaser, Büchel, & May,

---

This chapter is adapted with the author's permission from Davidson (2009).

2008). The mechanisms of these changes in the brain likely include both the growth of new neural connections and the creation of new neurons.

Our scientific understanding of the brain is so different now from what it was in the 1970s that it's like studying an entirely new organ. With this fresh understanding come exciting new possibilities for human development. Among them is the likelihood that *mental* training, such as meditation, shapes the brain just like other types of skill acquisition (Berger, Kofman, Livneh, & Henik, 2007; Kwok et al., 2011; Poldrack, 2002; Tang, Geng, Stein, Yang, & Posner, 2010). And if the brain can be changed through mental training, we may able to shape adaptive human qualities, such as compassion, as well.

Despite growing knowledge of the brain's flexibility, there remains a lingering belief in neuroscience that attributes such as compassion or happiness are relatively fixed. As many have suggested, these attributes have fairly stable set points that persist throughout our lifetimes. On the whole, personal qualities such as compassion are still considered to be less malleable than the brain itself.

In this chapter, I begin by reviewing research that ties compassion to personal well-being—a topic close to the heart of many psychotherapists. Then I describe research from my own lab that demonstrates how compassion training affects brain functioning. Finally, I present evidence that compassion is a skill that can be cultivated even with relatively short periods of practice.

WHAT'S COMPASSION?

The word *compassion* evokes different images and feelings for different people. No doubt our cultural backgrounds and many other factors contribute to the way in which we understand the term. His Holiness the Dalai Lama defines compassion as "the wish that all sentient beings be free from suffering" (2001b, p. 96). More in-depth discussions of the definition of compassion can be found throughout this book (see Chapter 1 for a review).

Compassion *meditation* is the focus of many compassion studies because it provides researchers with the ability to catch people in the act of compassion, which is otherwise hard to do. People who practice this type of meditation can actually "feel" compassion, and they can be studied while doing so. Matthieu Ricard, a very experienced Buddhist monk and author, describes the practice he and other monks use this way: "What we were trying to do . . . is to generate a state in which loving compassion permeates the whole mind with no other consideration, reasoning, or discursive thoughts" (personal communication, October 2001). It is of great benefit to use brain imaging techniques with seasoned practitioners such as Ricard because there is relatively little mental "noise" while they are engaged in compassion meditation.

Compassion and Well-Being

Buddhist Psychology

Within Buddhist psychology, compassion is one of four mental states that contribute to health and happiness: loving-kindness, compassion, sympathetic joy, and equanimity. It is believed that these mental states can all be cultivated with practice. They are collectively known as the *brahmaviharas*, translated literally as "heavenly abodes" (Salzberg, 1997). Some meditation teachers refer to them as "best places to reside" or "sublime attitudes." Whereas compassion is the wish that all sentient beings be *free from suffering*, loving-kindness is the wish that all sentient beings be *happy*, sympathetic joy is taking pleasure in others' happiness, and equanimity is the mind remaining balanced in conditions of both pleasure and pain, fortune and misfortune (see Chapter 4 for more details). Regarding the sense of well-being that comes with compassion, the Dalai Lama (2009a) simply states, "If you want others to be happy, practice compassion; and if you want yourself to be happy, practice compassion" (p. x). Indeed, many people would agree that compassion feels good.

Scientific Psychology

Until recently, compassion has not been a major focus of psychology or science in general. In fact, most psychology books that deal with human emotion do not even mention compassion. Yet compassion may be an important link to well-being through its impact on both happiness and physical health.

Happiness is a state of mind that is experienced by most people as pleasant and therefore desirable, but recent studies have also shown that happiness can actually make us healthier. Steptoe, Wardle, and Marmot (2005) conducted a large study looking at subjective happiness and the physiological stress response. They found that positive affect in middle-age men and women was associated with reduced neuroendocrine, inflammatory, and cardiovascular activity, all of which can be risk factors for physical illness. In a more recent analysis of 30 studies of happiness and longevity, Veenhoven (2008) found that although happiness does not predict longevity in unhealthy people, it is predictive of longevity in healthy people. That suggests that happiness may not make us well when we are sick, but it is protective against illness. Because these studies summarize the results of numerous other happiness studies, it is safe to say that the scientific literature contains sufficient evidence to confirm that happiness has a positive impact on physical health.

Nonetheless, happiness seems to be underappreciated in our modern culture. Indicators of social progress and well-being focus primarily on economic factors, but a comparison of happiness and income levels in America shows that we make more money than ever before yet our average level of happiness has remained relatively stable (Layard, 2010). This finding has been dubbed the "progress paradox" (Easterbrook, 2003). Economic success may be revered as essential for happiness, but research does not support our dedication to the dollar. In fact, once basic needs such as food and shelter are met, more money really does not make people happier (Diener & Biswas-Diener, 2002; Myers, 2000). Scientific research tells us that we do not know much at all about what truly makes us happy. Perhaps it is time to consider some new possibilities.

What might those possibilities be? In a study conducted by Dunn, Aknin, and Norten (2008), the effects of self-centered versus others-centered behaviors on happiness were explored. Their findings lend support to the idea that compassion and happiness may be linked. Subjects were given $50 each and told that they could spend it any way that they wanted, as long as they spent it on themselves. A second group was given the same $50 and told that they must spend the money on others. At the end of the day, both groups returned to the lab and their subjective levels of happiness were measured. Contrary to expectation, the happier group was the one that spent their money on others. Though the study focused more on generosity than compassion, thinking about and acting in ways that benefit others has a lot in common with compassion and compassionate behavior.

Science is only now beginning to explore the beneficial effects of compassion. One question is whether compassion, like happiness, can positively influence physical health. A potential pathway for such a mind–brain–body relationship is the regulation of brain activity involved in the production of the human stress hormone cortisol. Cortisol is released by the adrenal glands, which sit just over the kidneys, and it plays a significant role in physical health. Cortisol release is stimulated by neural impulses from a complex brain circuit that includes the amygdala and the ventromedial prefrontal cortex.

Cortisol normally shows a diurnal variation with high levels in the morning and low levels in the evening. This variation is important because it is associated with a number of health factors. People whose cortisol levels do *not* fluctuate much—who have a flat cortisol profile—are likely to weigh more than those with steep cortisol profiles. They also perform more poorly on measures of explicit memory and report lower perceived social support and higher levels of stress (Abercrombie et al.,

2004). Among women with metastatic breast cancer, those with flat cortisol profiles actually die sooner (Sephton, Sapolsky, Kraemer, & Spiegel, 2000).

Given the harmful effects of too much cortisol, neuroscientists at the Waisman Laboratory for Brain Imaging and Behavior at the University of Wisconsin–Madison were interested in what impact brain and mental activity would have on this key hormone. We looked specifically at the effects of cognitive reappraisals, which require subjects to imagine a positive outcome in response to images of people suffering. Some of the images presented were very emotionally provocative and disturbing, yet cognitive reappraisals reduced activity in the amygdala (Urry et al., 2006). The amygdala is important because it is capable of stimulating the release of cortisol, so reduced amygdalar activity can lead to reduced cortisol levels.

We investigated whether the signals that we recorded in individual brains actually predicted their cortisol profiles, and indeed they did. Some of the subjects had brain patterns characteristic of successful emotion regulation—they were able to downregulate, or decrease activity, in the amygdala after responding to the disturbing images. These subjects had steeper cortisol profiles characteristic of lower perceived stress and better physical health and longevity. Although cognitive reappraisal and compassion are not the same mental function, both involve imagining a positive outcome for a person who has been suffering. It is therefore likely that some of the same effects that occur with this type of cognitive reappraisal might be seen with compassion meditation as well.

A causal connection between compassion and both happiness and health is still far from confirmed. However, existing research suggests that compassion may be one of several mental attributes related to biological markers associated with positive health consequences. This is one reason that compassion should receive additional scientific investigation.

COMPASSION AND THE BRAIN

Our current work on compassion meditation is in many ways a product of earlier research at the Waisman laboratory. After studying affect regulation as well as the effects of meditation, it occurred to us that there was absolutely no reason why we could not bring to bear the rigorous tools of psychology and neuroscience that were being used to study states such as fear, anxiety, and disgust on the study of positive attributes such as compassion. By doing so, we have begun to lay the foundation for understanding what is happening within a brain that is experiencing compassion, and how compassion might be cultivated.

Compassion and the Electroencephalogram

What happens in the brain during the practice of compassion? We first tried to answer this question using the electroencephalogram (EEG). Our study included eight very experienced meditators and 10 novices. The experienced practitioners had logged an astounding amount of meditation practice ranging from 10,000 to 50,000 hours, whereas the comparison group had only a week of meditation training before the study began. We were able to determine when compassion was occurring during the study by using self-report (people told us about their experience). Once a baseline EEG was established, we recorded brain activity during alternating blocks of meditation and rest. During the first block, both the comparison group and the long-term practitioners focused on generating a state of unconditional loving-kindness and compassion, and during the second block they stopped practicing.

The EEG records electrical activity along the scalp produced by neurons in the brain and can reveal what types of brain-wave activity are occurring. The changes we recorded in the advanced meditators were dramatic and could be identified with the naked eye. To this day there have been no reports of this kind of brain activity in any other groups of people. The changes were primarily in gamma-wave activity and neural synchrony. *Gamma activity* is a pattern of brain waves that may be a major factor in the construction of conscious awareness. *Neural synchrony* refers to the coordination of gamma activity in different groups of neurons within the brain, and it may be a factor in the quality of conscious awareness (Engel, Fries, Konig, Brecht, & Singer, 1999; Tononi & Edelman, 1998). EEGs of the experienced practitioners showed high-amplitude gamma activity and large-scale brain synchrony increases during meditation practice. Though gamma activity increased for both groups during the meditation phases, the increase was, on average, 30 times greater among the long-term practitioners (Lutz, Greischar, Rawlings, Ricard, & Davidson, 2004).

We also discovered a relationship between brain activity and the meditators' level of experience. By conducting in-depth interviews with each of the practitioners, we were able to obtain estimates of the total number of hours each subject had practiced. It was a deeply humbling exercise. In order to be included in the study, participants had to have a minimum of 10,000 hours of practice. Ten thousand hours is not just an arbitrary number. It turns out that 10,000 hours is often taken as the number of hours it takes for a person to become accomplished in a high-skill activity such as playing a musical instrument, chess, golf, or tennis (Ericsson, 1998; Ericsson, Prietula, & Cokely, 2007). The average number of hours of practice for our group of expert meditators was 34,000 hours, with a range of 12,000 to 62,000 hours.

We found that the longer the subjects had practiced, the greater was the magnitude of change in their brain activity. Age was not related to the changes that occurred, so the difference in average age of our two groups probably does not explain the results. After this study was completed, we increased the number of both experts and novices in our sample, including some Tibetan novices, and obtained the same basic results.

Compassion and Functional Magnetic Resonance Imaging

Our next step was to understand which brain circuits play a role in the generation of compassion. We used functional magnetic resonance imaging (fMRI), which measures changes in blood flow related to neural activity, to look at brain activity in 15 expert meditation practitioners and 15 novices. As in the EEG study, the experts had accumulated between 10,000 and 50,000 hours of meditation practice and the control group had no prior meditation training, except during the week preceding the study. During compassion meditation and resting phases, we presented subjects with sounds depicting human suffering, such as cries or screams, as an emotional challenge. Not surprisingly, the subjects responded in areas of the brain related to emotion, and no single area alone was linked to the generation of compassion (Lutz, Brefczynski-Lewis, Johnstone, & Davidson, 2008).

The most dramatic changes were seen in the insula, amygdala, and the right temporal–parietal junction. The insula is involved in social emotions and is also a key area for mind–body interactions, like the experience of pain. The amygdala is a critical component of the circuitry of emotion and empathy. Enhancement of the amygdalar signal may play an important role in the experience of suffering, which is a strong motivation for the generation of compassion. The right temporal–parietal junction is a crucial area of the brain in terms of perspective taking (e.g., this area is activated when an adult imagines how a child sees something).

The manner in which our subjects reacted in these areas of the brain was fascinating. Subjects actually responded more strongly when they were practicing compassion than when they were resting, and, just as in the EEG study, advanced meditators showed much stronger brain activity than did the novices. As a whole, these results suggest that cultivating the intent to be loving and compassionate has the potential to enhance the empathic response that we have to others, especially with regard to emotion sharing and perspective taking.

Brief Practice

One observation that people often make when we present our studies on long-term practitioners is that most people will never spend anything close to 10,000 hours practicing. This is certainly true, and it raises the question of whether more limited practice by beginning meditators could still make a difference in some of these same circuits in the brain. To test the effects of brief practice, we chose an extremely short period of meditation practice, which was delivered over the Internet. Participants ($N = 41$) logged onto a protected website and were randomly assigned to a group that received either a guided compassion meditation for 30 minutes a day or to a group that received cognitive reappraisal training for the same duration. Training continued for 14 consecutive days. Participants were told that they would get one of two interventions, either compassion meditation or cognitive training, both of which were designed to promote well-being. Subjects in the meditation group were asked to contemplate and visualize suffering and then wish for freedom from suffering for different categories of people. After completion of the study, both groups were offered the opportunity to donate part of the money they earned from the study to a charitable cause.

The results were intriguing. The level of activity in one of the brain circuits believed to be involved in generating positive emotion quite strongly predicted the amount of money that people donated, but only for the participants in the compassion group. Those subjects who showed the biggest boost in activity in the insula also donated the most money. We may have had even stronger results if the training were extended over a longer period of time.

Research on compassion is still in its infancy, but already some interesting possibilities are emerging. Compassion practice is clearly related to identifiable brain activity and activates areas of the brain implicated in emotional processing. The practice of compassion seems to impact how people respond to suffering in themselves and others. By influencing brain processes associated with affect regulation, compassion training may improve overall health and well-being. The fact that brain function is different among advanced meditators does not yet prove that compassion and other mental attributes can be shaped, but it certainly supports the possibility.

In sum, can meditation training produce the alert, empathic, responsive state of mind known as compassion? Preliminary scientific evidence suggests that we can indeed train the brain to be more compassionate. Mental training may be just like physical training—part genetic predisposition, part environmental circumstances, enhanced by lots of intentional practice. By taking an active role in cultivating compassion, psychotherapists and their clients should be able to enhance well-being not only for themselves, but for society at large.

PART III

The Meaning of Wisdom

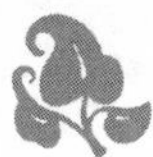

The history of humanity is a tale of human folly. Globally and individually, despite our best intentions, we find ourselves replaying old habits of thinking, feeling, and behaving that we know will only get us into trouble. Wisdom offers an alternative. We have the capacity to stop the madness, turn our attention inward, dismantle our erroneous beliefs and self-deceptions, and build our lives in accord with how things actually are. This is primarily an inside job, but we therapists are uniquely positioned to help others along the way because our clients are desperately searching for new solutions to pressing and persistent problems.

Chapter 9 unpacks, from the Buddhist psychological perspective, how distorted views of ourselves and our world are created in the mind, and how we can disentangle ourselves at the earliest stages of perception. Chapter 10 explores key components of wisdom as they apply to the art of psychotherapy, and how embracing reality–defined as impermanence, the mind's tendency to feel dissatisfied, and the fact that no separate self is to be found–can positively impact treatment. Then we see in Chapter 11 how elusive "personal wisdom" actually is, and why such wisdom may be considered a beneficial goal of psychotherapy. Chapter 12 considers the illusion of a separate self as a widespread form of suffering in our society and how authentic connection in psychotherapy can help to alleviate it. The subsequent chapter offers another way to move to a less egocentric vision of "self"–by learning to listen to, appreciate, and embrace the many parts of ourselves that are crying out for attention. Finally, we discover in Chapter 14 that the subcomponents of wisdom have underlying neurobiological processes, and that both meditation and psychotherapy can induce brain changes similar to those associated with wisdom.

CHAPTER 9

Wisdom in Buddhist Psychology

Andrew Olendzki

> When ignorance is abandoned and true knowledge has arisen,
>
> one no longer clings to sensual pleasures,
> one no longer clings to beliefs,
> one no longer clings to a doctrine of self.
>
> Without clinging, one no longer torments oneself.
>
> No longer tormenting oneself, one inwardly awakens.[1]

Wisdom is the pivotal idea of Buddhist thought, and as such it has a more technical meaning here than is customary in English usage. It is used to describe the understanding of core insights into the nature of experience–insights that provide an antidote to the basic human affliction of delusion. Without wisdom we cannot help but make fundamental errors in understanding ourselves and the world. We cling to a wide variety of erroneous views, are driven by all sorts of unhealthy compulsions, and cause a great deal of suffering for ourselves and those around us through unskillful behavior. With the attainment of wisdom, at first in brief glimpses, then with gradually increasing regularity, and ultimately as a profoundly transformative reordering of experience, we are able to see more clearly the nature of things and dismantle the mechanisms that create our suffering.

Let's look first at the problem to which wisdom is considered a solution, and then examine the specific components of wisdom as they are understood in the early Buddhist tradition. This exploration requires

[1] Retranslated here by the author from The Shorter Lion's Roar Discourse, *Majjhima Nikaya* 11 (Nanamoli & Bodhi, 1995, p. 163).

a review of how Buddhists understand experience to be constructed moment by moment, how habits of belief and behavior are built up and can be intentionally modified, and the role that mindfulness can play in undermining the force of delusion and in paving the way for the emergence of wisdom. We also consider the key components of wisdom as understood by early Buddhist traditions, such as grasping the essential impermanence of all things, the root of suffering, and the contingent nature of the self. Although many of these ideas are challenging to those accustomed to Western views of experience, they have developed in the context of, and are ultimately dedicated to, the alleviation of human suffering at its deepest levels.

THE CONSTRUCTION OF EXPERIENCE

The modern label of *Buddhist psychology* more or less refers to the models of mind and behavior developed in Northern India in the fifth through third centuries before the Common Era, as they are expressed in the body of literature preserved in the Pali language known as the *tipitaka*.[2] This Buddhist psychology is rooted first and foremost in a subjective perspective on experience. Beginning with the fact that each of us is aware and experiences consciousness directly, it proceeds through empirical observation to develop a map of the many physical and mental factors and processes that work together to shape how consciousness manifests in lived experience under ever-changing conditions.

The human body and mind are considered natural components of a natural world. The body is composed of the same basic elements as all other matter, and has evolved gradually over time to have sense organs that are sensitive to particular environmental stimuli (Nanamoli & Bodhi, 1995). These stimuli are "known" as they become objects of conscious awareness, with each moment of knowing dependent upon a particular sense organ and sense object. Thus arises the knowing of a visual form by means of the eye; the knowing of a sound by means of the ear; the knowing of a smell or taste using the nose and tongue; the knowing of touch with other receptors throughout the body. Our human experience consists of these moments of knowing, one following another in a flowing stream of consciousness.

In the Buddhist tradition, the mind is also considered to be like a sense organ. The objects known by the mind include thoughts, memories,

---

[2]The word *tipitaka* means "three baskets" and refers to a collection of about 50 volumes as published in Pali by the Pali Text Society, London, much of which has been translated into English (see *www.palitext.com*).

and images—anything that can be imagined or cognized. The mental organ (we might call it the brain, though it was traditionally regarded as the heart) plays a broader role than the senses, coordinating their inputs in various ways. The objects it knows are internally generated rather than imported from the environment, but the basic model of knowing an object by means of an organ is similar across all six modes of experience. At any given moment, therefore, we are either seeing, hearing, smelling, tasting, touching, or "thinking" (knowing with the mind). Each of these episodes of consciousness involves a very specific, and fleeting, object of experience and follows one after another in rapid succession.

Adding color and texture to these objects, both figuratively and literally, are other mental functions such as perception and feeling. Perception tells us *what* we are knowing, based on prior experience and learned interpretive schemas such as language and concepts. Feeling, used in the limited sense of an affective tone, tells us whether what we are perceiving is pleasant, painful, or neutral. Perception and feeling, along with consciousness and its various corresponding sense organs, operate automatically to shape a world of meaning each moment, as information is received and processed by the mind. We don't really have much influence on how we see or hear things, how we perceive them, or how they feel to us. All these are dealt each moment off the top of the deck, so to speak; our main job is to learn how to play the hand skillfully.

Forming Formations

The mental function that plays the hand, to continue the metaphor, is called *formations*, and has to do with shaping our *reaction* to what is arising in experience. We are not just data-processing mechanisms—we engage intentionally and emotionally with the things of which we are aware. The term for this function (*sankhāra* in Pali) is hard to translate, but it derives from the verb "to make" or "to do" and is directly related to the word *karma*. We need a word in English that can serve equally well as a verb and a noun because it covers both the active making or shaping (forming) of a response to an object in the present moment, as well as the pattern (formation) left behind by that activity—a pattern that will serve as a template for how we respond the next time. As a potter might shape a pot however he or she wishes, and then the fired piece becomes an artifact in a larger body of work, so also each of us is choosing each moment how to respond to all we encounter, and what we have chosen to do in the past shapes how we meet the next moment's experience. It is in this realm of formations that ignorance is met and transformed into wisdom.

An image is offered in the Pali texts of early Buddhism to help us understand what formations are, and I think it is an image remarkably adaptable to our current understanding of the brain and its architecture. Picture a chariot driving across a dusty plain. The chariot may presumably be steered wherever its driver wishes to go, within the constraints of the terrain. It might have to dodge around some rocks or stay away from the swampy areas, but it is under the driver's volitional control. This image captures the first sense of formations: the intention or executive function in the mind that makes moment-to-moment decisions.

Then, as the chariot actually traverses one path or another, it makes an imprint of the wheel upon the earth. This imprint represents the actual carrying out of an action or activity. In Buddhist thought every moment entails some sort of action, by body, speech, or mind, and all such activity is called *karma*, a word that basically just means "action."

The second meaning of "formations" has to do with the fact that volitional activity leaves traces—the tracks of the chariot are embedded in the dust on the plain for all to see. One can gaze out over that plain and have a very good idea of where the chariot has been because it leaves a clear record of its activity carved in the ground. Moreover, if it takes the same route many times over, a path (or even a rut) gets constructed, so the entire history of that chariot's activities is recorded in the patterns it has laid down on the plain.

We might extend the range of this image somewhat by drawing upon another also found in the early literature, where a distinction is made between drawing a line in water, in sand, or inscribing it on a stone (Woodward, 1979). Some habits are so deeply entrenched in solid material that they may be difficult or even impossible to change, whereas other behaviors are more malleable, and still others have little effect and leave no lasting impression.

Reshaping Ourselves

With this idea in mind, let's look at how the brain develops. An infant's brain is populated by a large number of neurons, and as electrochemical currents run through these neurons, certain pathways are formed. As the saying goes, neurons that fire together, wire together. Those pathways that are used regularly connect in relatively stable patterns, whereas those that are used less often are more fragile. Meanwhile, neurons that do not fire actually die off, so that as the brain matures it takes on a particular shape and pattern. These will always be unique because the brain is carved, so to speak, by our distinctive experiences. So the architecture of our brains, just like the network of chariot tracks, consists of both the remnants of past activity and the avenues along which activity is most disposed to proceed in the future.

It is just a metaphor, but it can help us recognize the importance of formations (rather than consciousness, perception, and feeling) for understanding wisdom. Consciousness is the chariot itself, but the formations—the intention that guides it and the pathways established by its passage—are going to condition how consciousness manifests. The mind is not free when it is constrained by its habits, and it is these habits that lead us, time and again, into the territory of suffering.

It is tempting to consider suffering to be something external, and at its worst this perspective comes out as the often-heard misstatement of Buddhism's first noble truth: "Life is suffering." As I understand his teaching, the Buddha was saying instead that our habitual *responses* to life constitute suffering. It is the *attachment* to gratification, the *resistance* to pain, the desperate attempts to hold on to what is slipping away or stave off what is closing in, that not only cause our own suffering but lead us to behave in ways that cause suffering to so many others. These are all pathways of learned behavior, whether carved on a dusty plane or burned into the neurons of our brain, and because they have been constructed by the natural functioning of mind and body, they can also be *re*constructed in a similar way. Because the mind is regarded as a process rather than a thing, the transformation of unhealthy patterns of behavior involves avoiding their repetition and reinforcement, on the one hand, and learning to carve out new tracks, on the other. Although he didn't understand it biologically as we do today, the Buddha clearly believed in neuroplasticity.

Mindfulness

The primary technology for liberating the mind from suffering in Buddhism is meditation, which develops and applies awareness in particular ways. But it is important to recognize that meditation is a means toward an end rather than an end in itself. It is a tool to be used for transforming the formations from maladaptive habits to skillful modes of functioning. Conscious awareness, in the form of mindfulness, is used to reshape the automatic, unconscious structures of the mind. Deeply embedded behavioral patterns need to be altered to promote greater health, but by definition these unconscious patterns cannot be observed directly—they operate outside of our awareness. Mindfulness practice develops the ability to see these dynamics of the mind as they unfold. The practitioner gradually learns to catch a glimpse of what arises from the depth of the unconscious psyche as it passes through awareness on its way to initiating action. Aspects of experience to which we were entirely blind come into view, and the ability to choose one course of action over another becomes strengthened. We learn how to drive the chariot more skillfully, avoiding the deep ruts that lead into danger and trouble, and to forge new pathways that will convey the mind into healthier, more meaningful environs. Ultimately, mindfulness may even liberate awareness from the constraints of formations altogether, allowing us to drive where we will and leave no tracks.

THE CHALLENGE

First let us consider the situation of the average individual, to whom the early Buddhist texts refer as the "unawakened ordinary person" (e.g., Nanamoli & Bodhi, 1995, pp. 83*ff*). Our awareness is generally focused on external objects. The senses see, hear, taste, smell, and touch the world around us, and our awareness focuses upon these sense objects. Think about what you do throughout any given day: cutting a slice of bread, maneuvering a car into a vacant parking space, forming letters and words with a pen or keyboard in hand, walking from here to there, and a hundred thousand similar tasks. We are material bodies making our way through a material world, and it takes a good deal of awareness to do so safely and effectively; it takes holding a detailed perceptual model of three-dimensional space in mind, plotting events on a conceptual timeline of past, present, and future, and generally using our mind to construct and carefully engage with a complex perceptual edifice that we invest with a sense of reality.

With all this outward focus, we usually have little awareness of the internal functioning of the mind. Fortunately we have evolved in such a way that not much is required. The formations take care of this for us. Throughout our lives we have learned various skills, habits, strategies, reactions, and behaviors to respond appropriately to a wide range of environmental situations. The phone rings, we answer it. We notice a police car, we slow down. We see a piece of chocolate, we eat it. These formations are stored in the mind in the form of latent tendencies, and are evoked or triggered when needed by unfolding events. Each of us has a unique set of these dispositions lying in a dormant state, for each of us has had a unique history of what we have encountered and what responses we have learned. These formations, both in a dormant and an active state, are our emotional or behavioral dispositions; and each person's set of underlying patterns is generally called *character*, or *personality*, or even *self*.

When a stimulus presents itself to the sense door or mind door, these dormant dispositions wake up as they become enacted in behavior; they flow from what Buddhist psychology calls a *latent* stage (literally, "lying down") to a *surging* stage (literally, "running away") (see Ledi, 1999, for a discussion of these three stages). It is called surging because these responses arise automatically and get acted out either by the body, in speech, or in cycles of mental activity. There is, however, a third, intervening stage, called the *arising* or *presenting* stage (literally "standing up"). In this stage we have a conscious awareness of the emotions or urges emerging from latency and moving into surging behavior—we can see our reclining habits *stand up* before they *run off*. But without deliberate mindfulness practice, much of the time this middle step is skipped. Again, we are fortunate that this automaticity has evolved, since so often the responses needed to remain healthy in a rapidly changing world do not allow much time or space for conscious engagement. We should be glad that when a truck is bearing down upon us in the street, we don't have to take the time to think about what to do. In fact, most of the time our conscious awareness is "otherwise engaged" in thinking about the past and future, and precious little of it is generally available for monitoring the textures of immediate lived experience.

The Buddha saw this state of being otherwise engaged as a problem for a number of reasons. For one thing, we find there are significant limitations to the information the human mind and body are capable of receiving from the environment. Information is distorted, misapprehended, and misinterpreted, all of which contribute to a generally erroneous view of who we are and what sort of world we inhabit. This is what the words *ignorance* and *delusion* refer to (Ledi, 1999). The lack of conscious awareness between the latent and the surging stages of emotions or behavioral dispositions holds the mind in bondage to its base instincts and allows little room for growth, development, and evolution. It is the absence of wisdom.

This inability to see clearly evokes and reinforces certain primitive instincts that govern our behavior. The impulse to pursue pleasure and avoid pain, in its most primal form, gives rise to a greed and hatred that care only for *my* welfare, and thus causes considerable suffering in a species that needs to live cooperatively in tight-knit social units. When the tendency to pursue pleasure (via greed, attachment, compulsion) and avoid pain (via denial, aversion, hatred) is augmented by fundamental confusion (ignorance, delusion) about what will actually achieve these goals, the detrimental effects are amplified. This confluence of greed, hatred, and delusion (the traditional wording for the primary colors out of which all shades of problematic human emotion are composed) causes considerable suffering all around (Nanamoli & Bodhi, 1995).

Turning Inward

How can mental training help this situation? If the space between underlying dispositions and their surging into action can be pried open, so to speak, so that the intervening gap can be filled with a greater degree of conscious awareness, then the functioning of the model changes significantly. Everything comes into clearer view in the light of awareness. To begin with, the stimulus itself is seen more clearly, since there is a chance to see it consciously, examine it carefully, and perhaps even understand its significance more accurately than when it serves only to provoke an unexamined response. Second, the emotional response is also viewed more clearly as it moves from its latent stage and emerges into view as an arising object. The emotion or urge is now something that is experienced, since awareness is brought to bear upon it, rather than something hidden that passes unseen from the shadows of the psyche into the fog of activity. In addition, the movement into action is also now revealed in the light of awareness and, in the process, loses some of its surging quality. Behavior becomes something you have a hand in initiating, rather than something that feels as if it is happening *to* you. Intention thus also emerges from the darkness and becomes an object consciously regarded. One might even have space to review more than one option and decide consciously how to respond. And finally, awareness buys freedom. It interrupts cycles of conditioned response, compulsive engagement, and primal reflex, allowing us to influence, if not control, how we respond to the stimulus presenting itself in the moment.

With meditation we cultivate the capacity to abide in the arising stage of formations. Thoughts and emotions, responses and aspirations all continue to emerge from the depths of the unconscious mind, but now we are able to see them as they do so. Choices are always made, as we surge into the world with action; the question is whether or not we participate consciously in the process. When awareness is focused outward or is otherwise engaged with something else, then decisions are made automatically and existing patterns of response are strengthened. The person disposed to anger becomes angrier; the person disposed to fear becomes more fearful, and so on. There is little freedom here. The freedom both to see what is emerging from latent states of mind and to make conscious choices about how to respond to these, rises in direct proportion to how much awareness we are able to bring to bear on the present moment.

Yet this clear seeing of what arises and passes away in experience is still only the shallow end of the pool. The Buddhist meditative arts go well beyond this and lead into waters that are deep, still, and exceptionally clear. Much of this territory is described in concentration practices that lead the mind into nonordinary states of consciousness, and although the additional power and capability this gives the mind can be a great asset, this is not directly where the development of wisdom takes place. While it is possible to train conscious awareness in various ways, such as directing it toward and holding it upon a chosen object, this development of mental agility will not, on its own, make changes in the fundamental patterns of behavior that are the source of so much psychological suffering.

Insight Meditation

Insight meditation involves some concentration of the mind, but rather than holding awareness steadily on a single object, it focuses in a disciplined way on the *process* of unfolding experience. We attend carefully to the arising of various thoughts and emotions from latent regions of the psyche, their surging into activities of body, speech, and mind, and their passing out of view as the next event occurs. As an aid to establishing this practice, it is helpful to focus at first on only the physical sensations that arise in the body. The sensations on the skin, the aches and pains within, the dynamic processes of breathing–notice them all, one at a time, with full attention. If awareness wanders to a thought, for example, or a memory, it is gently escorted back to whatever physical sensation is presenting itself with most strength and clarity.

Eventually one progresses through three other fields of exploration, including the feeling tones of pleasure and pain, the quality of consciousness itself that is doing the observing (i.e., whether it is subtly favoring or opposing what it notices, or not), and the multitude of individual thoughts and other contents that arise and pass away in the mind at any time.[3] Each of these foundations upon which mindfulness can be established, as they are traditionally called, constitutes a broad territory to be investigated as one brings as much conscious awareness as possible to every nuance of experience. As with so many skills, the ability to detect subtle variations from one moment to another grows with practice, and it eventually becomes enormously compelling to see just how much is really going on in every moment of the stream of consciousness (see Chapter 2 for another perspective on this insight meditation practice).

CULTIVATING WISDOM

When the ability to notice what is happening has been developed through concentration and mindfulness, the ensuing quality of experience can be remarkable. The concentrated mind feels sharp, clear, and extraordinarily capable. When mindfulness becomes established over an extended period, as it might during a meditation retreat, even the most mundane

[3]See the Foundations of Mindfulness Discourse, *Majjhima Nikaya* 10, translated in Nanamoli and Bodhi (1995, pp. 145–155) for a detailed description of this practice.

occurrence can seem fascinating. Yet as gratifying as these states can be, it is again important to recognize that this is not the end point for which they are intended. The Buddha was very clear in saying that such "peaceful abiding here and now," as he put it, is not necessarily transformative (in the Discourse on Effacement; Nanamoli & Bodhi, 1995, pp. 123*ff*). When the bell rings or the retreat is over, one may still be given to cruelty, killing living beings, or taking what has not been given; to harsh speech, ill will, and gossip; to anger, doubt, revenge, and envy; or to arrogance, negligence, and laziness. There is a long list of such character traits and deep-seated emotional patterns that are unlikely to be washed clean by meditation alone.

The practice of concentration and mindfulness turns into the practice of insight or wisdom when we use the focused mind to penetrate the illusions that grip us. At every step of mindfulness practice, we are encouraged to regard the objects of awareness in four ways in order for the practice to lead into wisdom:

1. By watching the arising and passing away of phenomena, again and again in every aspect of experience, we gradually gain a visceral appreciation of the impermanence of it all—of the world, of our minds, of our views, and of our very selves.
2. By considering all experience from an internal as well as an external perspective, and from the perspective of the interaction of the two, we slowly develop an appreciation of the interdependency of our sense organs and their corresponding sense objects, and of how the world of experience is a cobbled-together, constructed thing.
3. By reducing awareness to its simplest form—to bare attention without elaboration, conceptualization, or interpretation—we begin to glimpse a world below the macroconstruction project through which we create the narrative of our lives.
4. And finally, most importantly, the growth of wisdom allows us to regard every single component of experience without clinging. Craving is effectively undermined by the nimble awareness of experience, for we no longer favor or oppose phenomena when we regard them with evenly hovering equanimity. As it is expressed traditionally, "One abides independent, not clinging to anything in the world" (in the *Foundations of Mindfulness Discourse*; Nanamoli & Bodhi, 1995, p. 146).

This is the sort of deep transformation for which Buddhist meditation experience aims. Heightened awareness is a sort of pry bar or lever used to lift and get under the common assumptions and responses we bring to each moment, loosening the attachment we have to them and the grip they have on us. Wisdom is a wedge that is then inserted into this space and driven in ever more deeply to finally separate the mind from its ignorance. Only wisdom can counter delusion, and thus only wisdom can bring about the thorough liberation of the mind and the robust cessation of suffering. Traditionally, wisdom is said to accomplish this by insight into impermanence, suffering, and non-self (e.g., see the first discourse attributed to the Buddha; Bodhi, 2000).

Impermanence

Understanding impermanence deeply enough to make us truly wise means not just knowing that all things change, but grasping the more intuitively difficult idea that there is nothing whatsoever that is stable. Challenging the dominant religious norm (both ancient and modern) that God provides stability behind the shifting patterns of experience, early Buddhist thinkers opened boldly to the stark view that everything was in flux at all times. Any appearance of solidity or essence was an artificial creation of the mind, to be viewed as a useful adaptive tool, perhaps, but ultimately a fabricated illusion. It is one thing to contemplate impermanence from the stable platform of a transcendent soul or a benevolently created cosmos; it is quite another to encounter the idea from a swirling eddy or a vanishing dewdrop, as the Buddhist poets have put it.[4] Everything we consist of—body, mind, the perceptions of the senses, the linear procession of thoughts, and all the views constructed over time from the cradle to the grave—are vanishing as quickly as they are contrived. Experience itself is thoroughly effervescent, so every notion of the self and the world built upon it is fundamentally unstable and unreliable. Such issues as how it all began or to what end it is all heading, so central to the Western philosophical and scientific agendas, are considered at best unanswerable, at worst unintelligible, and thus in either case largely irrelevant.

It is natural that structures and habits of mind developed to mask this truth in order to ensure that we can maneuver successfully in our environment. At all three levels of scale—perception, thought, and view—one takes very seriously the sound of the twig snapping in the jungle thicket, the thought that it is likely evidence of a hungry tiger approaching, and

[4]This body's like a ball of foam / And feeling is like a bubble; / Perception is like a mirage, / Formations like a pithless tree, / And consciousness is like a trick; . . . No essence is discovered here (*Samyutta Nikaya* 22:95 [Bodhi, 2000, pp. 952–953; retranslated here by the author]).

the view that it is a good idea to avoid becoming a predator's meal. But wisdom involves going beyond the efficiencies of survival to investigate the nature of experience itself, and this is where the fixed vignettes of the mind are seen to be mere constructions that arise and pass away and constitute no abiding reality. It is not that the tiger or the danger it poses are not real, it is rather that our experience of that tiger is entirely constructed as a series of fleeting images flashing though our brains. We generally do not realize this truth, and the masking of it is called *delusion* by the Buddhists. The delusion here is to project onto our world, and onto the self who is conjuring that world, the temporary stabilities that our minds create for survival. Just because we think things are solid or real as a way of making sense of the flux, does not mean that they actually are.

One can begin to see how this common delusion might be the source of a considerable number of problems. If we continually try to capture and freeze frames of meaning from a world that is thoroughly and fundamentally in flux, then by definition we're never going to get it quite right. No matter how skillful the videographer, a film captures only one view per frame, and no matter how engaging the narrative, it remains always only a story. The constructed meanings we create are going to reflect our capacity for creating concepts rather than of accurately describing the world. But the biggest problem this causes is that when we assume something is stable and then it changes, we are setting up the conditions for psychological suffering.

Suffering

The fact that everything is changing all the time should not necessarily be a problem. Impermanence is the rule from the smallest conceivable subatomic activity to the largest possible sweep of the universe. One of the greatest insights of the Buddha was recognizing that suffering is caused not by the fact of impermanence, but by the attitudes toward impermanence that build up in the human construction of experience. Impermanence gives rise to suffering because of the *attachment* we have to things being a particular way. If we feel comfortable or safe or gratified with any object or experience being the way it is, then the changing of that into something else becomes a source of pain. Even imagining that it might change can be the source of considerable anxiety, fear, and stress because of how badly we *want* it to be a certain way. The Buddhist inquiry into suffering thus leads directly to a deep investigation of the workings of desire.

Desire comes in both positive and negative forms and is strongly linked to the dynamics of pleasure and pain. *Craving* is wanting what is pleasurable to occur or continue, whereas *aversion* is wanting what is painful to not occur or to stop. Both cases involve a significant imbalance between what is happening and what one wants to happen. What the Buddhists call the first noble truth of suffering (or unsatisfactoriness) is simply acknowledging that this tension exists, in spite of natural efforts to deny, avoid, distract from, or otherwise pretend this is not the case. The more important second noble truth involves understanding that the cause of such suffering is the craving for things to be other than they are. This understanding is an important component of wisdom and can lead to the third noble truth, which is that suffering can be brought to an end by eliminating its causes. The fourth and final noble truth is that each person can follow a path of behavioral change, mental training, and cultivation of wisdom that can lead to the cessation of suffering (Nanamoli & Bodhi, 1995).

It seems like an astonishing claim, that any human being could overcome entirely the habit of creating suffering by radically transforming his or her understanding, but this is what has inclined people to think of Buddhism as a religion rather than merely a philosophy or psychology. It is more fashionable these days to imagine that some forms of suffering can be assuaged or even eliminated, but that much of it is so deeply seated that we'll never be able to alleviate it. The images of profound happiness found in Buddhist literature and art (not to mention the brain scans of some contemporary Buddhist monks–see Chapter 8), suggest that our potential for well-being may be more extraordinary than we might think. And as much as such deep transformation of suffering may be aided by behavioral changes or intensive mental training, the classical Buddhist tradition always attributes it ultimately to the development of wisdom.

Non-Self

One of the most significant and unique insights of the Buddha, and one of particular interest to modern psychologists, has to do with the nature of the self. In his day, as in ours, there were those who regarded the self as a transcendent sacred essence inhabiting the body but fundamentally nonmaterial and thus imperishable. There were others who saw it entirely as an epiphenomenon of material substances, doomed to dissipate at the moment of death, and thus not in need of moral development or purification, and not capable of release from suffering. The Buddha's approach to the self was described as in between these two extremes. It entailed a dynamic, process-oriented model that regarded mind as interdependent with body, experience as constructed anew each moment, and the lived sense of being a self as something entirely optional to the process.

The Buddha's notion of self is not an alternative philosophical model of identity, but an empirical description of experience. He offers a simple example of someone walking off with a stick taken randomly from the forest—nobody would object to this because that stick is not seen as belonging to anyone (in *Samyutta Nikaya* 35:101 [Bodhi, 2000, p. 1182]). He noticed, however, that when any object or view is regarded as "mine" there immediately arises a fierce impulse to possess and protect it, triggering primitive instincts of greed and hatred. Yet when we view any aspect of experience as "not mine," these reflexes are not activated. It turns out that attachment, the basic building block of suffering, is reinforced by a strong sense of self and identification. Mental training, such as mindfulness meditation, thus invites one to develop a "not me, not mine, not my self" perspective toward all experience. It is not so much a matter of whether the self "exists" or "does not exist." Rather, the self is something we cause to exist when desire is aroused in the moment, and does not exist when instead of wanting or not wanting something, we regard it with equanimity and nonattachment.

The self, in other words, is constructed under certain conditions and not constructed under others. Wisdom involves understanding the utter contingency of what we call the self and having the ability to refrain from the compulsion to fabricate it. The self is not the existential starting point of all experience, but is the final flourish we place upon it when we say, almost in passing, "That's me" or "That's mine." Buddhist wisdom points out that it is not in fact yours, and that regarding it as such merely causes a great deal of suffering. The concoction of any agentic noun—the doer of the deed, the thinker of the thought, the occupant of the body—is ultimately a mistake and will cause more mischief than benefit. The alternative view offered by wisdom is of an interdependent arising and passing away of impersonal natural phenomena. There are many skills that can be learned for working with this flow of consciousness, but the tendency to grasp on to any aspect of it with attachment is antithetical to them all.

BUDDHA'S LEGACY

One of the great strengths of the Buddhist tradition has been its ability to move beyond its original cultural milieu and speak compellingly to evolving human circumstances in different times and places. There is something universal in the Buddha's teachings, something speaking to such basic ways of being human that underlie all people in all cultures. In the matter of wisdom the Buddha engages with the fundamental dynamics of how each individual constructs meaning, by pointing out the specific ways in which we misconstrue reality and offering specific solutions to help heal the afflictions attendant to the human condition. The specific meaning of wisdom has changed somewhat in each later iteration of Buddhism as it has moved over time across Asia and now becomes global, and the specific practices that can help us get free of delusion have also changed.

In its original context, the Buddha (ca. 480–400 BCE)[5] was expressing a perspective on the human condition that was very ancient, perhaps even with its roots in the Indus Valley civilization. This view was radically subjective in its orientation, regarded the capacity for awareness in the present moment as the ultimate religious mystery, and embarked upon a thorough empirical investigation of consciousness in all of its manifestations. Delusion was seen as a toxin that could be purged from the mind and body through mental discipline and deeply transformative understanding. The wisdom generated from this process of purification was not a mystical transcendent vision, but an embodied understanding of the workings of the natural world. The culmination of the path was an experience of profound well-being, here and now, that was imperturbable in the face of any circumstances, even the existential truths of aging, sickness, and death. This early form of Buddhism gradually spread across Southeast Asia and persists throughout the region today.

After an initial period of consolidation culminating in the era of King Ashoka (ca. 250 BCE), the Buddhist tradition adapted over the next several centuries to rapidly changing cultural and historical circumstances in India, particularly at the crossroads of global trade and multiple invasions in the Northwest region (currently Pakistan and Afghanistan). It also evolved as it engaged for centuries with Hinduism, a tradition whose Vedic roots were imported from the Indo-European west and which thus shared some cosmological assumptions with that region. The Mahayana Buddhism that emerged under these influences became more outward-facing and more transcendent in its orientation. Thus wisdom became symbolized by the Bodhisattva Manjusri, a celestial manifestation of great power who could cut through delusion with his sword of deconstructive understanding (e.g., see the *Lotus Sutra* [Watson, 1993] and the *Diamond Sutra* [Conze, 1958]). The early Buddhist insight into the emptiness of self in human experience was greatly expanded to encompass the emptiness of all reality, which brought with it a more mystical and expansive view of wisdom as accessing something ultimately beyond the limitations of time, space, and any attempt at conceptualization (see also Chapter 4).

[5]It has been customary to consider the Buddha to have lived from 563 to 483 BCE, but the recent trend in Buddhist scholarship is to move these dates forward, following the reevaluations of Betchert and Gombrich. See Gombrich (1992).

As Buddhism made its way along the trade routes to China and gradually penetrated that culture's notorious insularity, it picked up some Christian influence along the way and developed into a Pure Land form that placed more emphasis upon devotion than wisdom in the classical sense of the word. This strand of the tradition became very important in Japan and remains strong both in that country and in the United States (Suzuki, 1998). Buddhism was also heavily influenced by Taoism in China, and the Ch'an forms that developed in China as a synthesis of the two perspectives (ca. 600 CE) were exported and altered in Korea and Japan (ca. 1200 CE), where it is known as Zen. Both forms placed a high value on wisdom, which was understood as a direct, spontaneous, intuitive realization of the radical emptiness of phenomena and the utter contingency of all forms of thought and action (Barret, 1996).

In the centuries before its extermination in India at the hands of Muslim invaders (ca. 1200 CE), a Tantric form of Buddhism spread from the Kashmir and Bengal regions into Tibet (ca. 700 CE), where it merged easily with the indigenous shamanic traditions and remained strong and influential through to modern times. Tantric Buddhism, also known as the Vajrayana, involves a return to an emphasis upon direct personal experience, an increase of feminine symbolism, and a rich array of visualization and empowerment practices designed to draw upon transpersonal powers and to use challenges (rather than avoid them) to bring about a transmutation of delusion into wisdom (Powers, 2007). This wisdom is viewed as the natural condition of the mind, which can be directly realized once the habits of constructing conceptual dualities are cleared away.

Buddhist thought and practices were first encountered by Westerners during the centuries of exploration and colonialism (ca. 1600 CE), but it was not until the field of comparative religions was developed toward the end of the 19th century that much real understanding of the depth and significance of its ideas began to be realized (e.g., Sharpe, 1986). Buddhism has impacted the West through the immigration of Buddhist communities (from China and Japan to the U.S. West Coast; from Southeast Asia after the Vietnam war; from Tibet after its invasion by China; etc.), and also by the interest taken in its meditative and psychological practices by Western intelligentsia in the 20th century. While its exotic nature was a draw to Theosophists in the first half of the century and to New Age enthusiasts in the second half, recent decades have shown a gradual maturation of the Western encounter with Buddhist tradition. Its unique perspectives on the nature of wisdom are impacting the fields that strive to support physical and psychological health, effective education, and optimal athletic and artistic performance (Siegel, 2009). In addition, Buddhist perspectives offer useful support for those who are dying, incarcerated, or in recovery, and they provide intriguing perspectives on the nature and function of the brain.

The encounter between Eastern and Western psychological perspectives is still relatively new. What is not new is the human inclination to turn inward in search of essential knowledge about ourselves and our world. It remains to be seen what the current generation can do with the information bequeathed us by the Buddha and the legions of practitioners who have kept his message current over the millennia.

CHAPTER 10

The Wise Psychotherapist

Ronald D. Siegel

> The Way that can be described is not the absolute Way.
> —LAO TSU (Beck, 2002, p. 1)

Why would anyone in his or her right mind write a chapter about being a wise psychotherapist? The enterprise is inherently presumptuous. Writing about wisdom suggests knowing something about it, yet there appears to be an inverse relationship between thinking of oneself as wise and actually *being* wise.

Indeed, when experienced clinicians were asked to describe a wise therapist, one of the most commonly mentioned attributes was awareness of the limitations of one's own viewpoint.[1] This is, in fact, an ancient idea. Confucius suggested that anyone who thinks that he or she is wise, probably isn't (Kupperman, 1990). This notion is backed by a fascinating body of modern research suggesting, more broadly, that people who think they're competent are usually less competent than those who think they're not (Kruger & Dunning, 1999).

With that in mind, this chapter considers some of what researchers have learned about wisdom and its cultivation, what therapists see as attributes of the wise psychotherapist, what wisdom traditions can teach us

[1]In preparation for writing this chapter, e-mails were sent to approximately 30 experienced colleagues asking (1) what it means to them to be "wise," (2) what are the particular qualities of a "wise psychotherapist," (3) what gets in the way personally of being a wise therapist, and (4) whether they consider the cultivation of wisdom in their clients or patients to be a treatment goal.

about cultivating wisdom, and which wisdom skills may be most relevant to the psychotherapy.

WHAT IS WISDOM?

Human beings have mused continuously about wisdom at least since the time of Confucius, and our views have evolved considerably over the years. As discussed in Chapter 1, modern notions of wisdom typically incorporate both ancient ideas and relatively recent understandings of cognitive processes. One way that researchers have tackled the subject is by studying *implicit theories*—the often unspoken assumptions that people have about wisdom (Bluck & Glück, 2005; Clayton & Birren, 1980; Holliday & Chandler, 1986; Kunzmann & Baltes, 2005; Takahashi & Overton, 2005). Using structured interviews and other assessment measures, they've outlined how different people understand "wisdom." These implicit theories offer an interesting starting point for considering what might constitute a "wise" psychotherapist. You may find it helpful, before reading farther, to reflect on your own notions of wisdom and how they relate to your work.

THE WISE PSYCHOTHERAPIST

- Take a few moments to think of a colleague, supervisor, or personal therapist whom you consider to be wise. List his or her most striking qualities.
- Next list several of the most unwise things you've done as a therapist. Is there a theme here? What gets in the way of your being a wise psychotherapist?
- Finally, list several of the things you've done as a therapist that you consider to be particularly wise. What supports your work as a wise psychotherapist?

It turns out that theories about wisdom held by the population at large parallel closely clinicians' views about what would make a psychotherapist wise. Susan Bluck and Judith Glück (2005; developed the MORE definition of wisdom described in Chapter 1) have suggested that these implicit theories describe qualities that cluster into five predictable categories: (1) intelligence, (2) insight, (3) reflective attitude, (4) concern for others, and (5) problem-solving abilities. These are similar to categories of qualities derived by others using factor analytic techniques (e.g., Glück

& Bluck, 2011; Holliday & Chandler, 1986), and were also reflected in clinician responses to a survey (see Footnote 1).

Intelligence

While most people are quick to point out that wisdom goes beyond book learning and analytical ability, Westerners generally see these sorts of cognitive capacities as prerequisites. Scientists describe two types of cognition that are important for wise action: *fluid intelligence*, which involves the ability to think logically and reason clearly, and *crystallized intelligence*, which uses accumulated knowledge and experience to make sound judgments (Cattell, 1971). When asked about wisdom in psychotherapy in an informal survey, many therapists discussed the ability to consider multiple theoretical viewpoints, learn from experience, consider situations from the patient's perspective, and draw on the accumulated knowledge of the field. To do all these well, one needs to appreciate how all experience and behavior are multidetermined—the result of a remarkable number of factors coming together at a particular moment.

Although Eastern wisdom traditions recognize this complex causality (e.g., see Chapter 4), they tend to downplay the importance of fluid and crystallized intelligence—emphasizing instead the transcendence of conventional thought forms to glimpse more enduring truths. As therapists increasingly adopt mindfulness-oriented treatments, they appear to be valuing this latter attitude more. In our enthusiasm to cultivate these transcendent forms of wisdom, however, we should probably take care not to neglect more conventional aspects of therapist training, such as knowledge of lifespan development, diagnostic assessment, therapeutic methods, and cultural differences.

There is a story of a meditation student in Tibet who developed a toothache. He sought the advice of a very wise spiritual teacher. After waiting much of the day, the student was finally granted an interview and presented his problem. The master replied, "How would I know? You should see a dentist." Conventional knowledge and training clearly have a role in wise action.

Insight

Insight begins to take us further from what we can readily glean from books. As a component of wisdom, it involves having intuition into, and a deep understanding of, another's perspective as well as one's own ideas and motives. In supervision, we can learn new ways to view our patients' experiences, but insight requires careful introspection over time—listening with interest to understand exactly what they mean. Being able to sense that a "tired" patient is actually feeling depressed, or a "confused" patient is actually having difficulty tolerating her anger at her daughter, is critical for successful psychotherapy. This sort of insight also includes keen attention to what is loosely called countertransference—monitoring our own emotional reactions with an open curiosity about what they might mean, where they come from, and what they might illuminate about our relationships. Noticing when I'm reluctant to call one patient back or when I'm afraid to be late for another can make me a better therapist (see Chapter 23 for a detailed look at developing this sort of insight). Many therapists suggested in the survey that the capacity to observe one's own inner workings in this way is a necessary skill for the wise psychotherapist.

Reflective Attitude

This component of wisdom involves both thinking deeply about things and thinking before acting. Whereas we might value lively spontaneity in a therapist, impulsivity and compulsivity can be real problems. Indeed, most therapeutic blunders occur when we act first and think later. As the old psychoanalytic maxim puts it, "The right interpretation at the wrong time is the wrong interpretation." Whether we find ourselves suddenly self-disclosing for our own benefit, suggesting that our patient confront his or her fears, or talking about anger that our patient isn't ready to feel, acting without thinking can get in the way of effective treatment.

Related to this point is the near universal tendency, in our quest to be helpful or feel competent, to develop facile, simplistic, or reductionistic understandings of our patients' difficulties. "It's a reaction to childhood sexual abuse," "It's because of his narcissistic father," "She's a borderline," and countless other conclusions help us to feel more secure as therapists while overlooking our patients' complexity. In contrast, a reflective attitude tends to keep the door open to as yet unconsidered possibilities.

Concern for Others

Over and over therapists in the survey cited genuine compassion—concern for others' suffering—as an important quality of the wise psychotherapist. This is no surprise, for we've seen throughout this volume that wisdom and compassion are like two wings of a bird, both necessary for flight. In psychotherapy, concern for others manifests most often by being able to place the patient's needs above one's own desires. Whether it's acting a certain way to be seen as kind or competent, failing to pay attention because we're distracted by personal worries, recoiling from our patient's pain because it hits too close to home, or wanting to fill our practices with gratifying or lucrative patients, concern for ourselves and our loved ones can easily get in the way of our concern for others. Therapists repeatedly commented that it is often their own fears and insecurities that fuel self-centered concern and keep them from acting in their patients' best interest. One therapist put it particularly succinctly: When asked what gets in the way of being a wise psychotherapist, she replied simply, "Me." How might we act differently if we were not as focused on our own comfort or security?

Problem-Solving Abilities

Some clinicians are secretive about how much they problem-solve in therapy. Particularly for those trained in psychodynamic, existential, or humanistic traditions, helping patients to figure out real-world solutions to their problems may seem superficial and not feel like "real" therapy. And yet the ability to come up with practical solutions to problems is widely seen as an important component of wisdom in Western traditions. Indeed, in my own work, I often find myself helping patients find solutions to medical, legal, home repair, automotive, financial, and other problems—usually based on my own successes and failures in these arenas. While at times I feel that I'm overstepping my bounds, it's possible that a willingness to help our patients in whatever area is causing them suffering, if balanced with other more traditionally "therapeutic" work, may indeed be wise action.

The question we face is whether the offering of concrete, problem-solving assistance is coming mostly out of our own needs to feel smart or helpful, or has the potential to be genuinely useful to our patients. This utility can come in the obvious form of solving the real-world problem, but also in the form of deepening the therapeutic relationship as our patients experience us as wanting to be helpful, sharing in life's inevitable challenges, and being accessible as a fellow human being.

Transcending Conventional Concepts

For students of ancient Eastern wisdom traditions, it can come as a surprise that most Westerners only occasionally include spirituality, connection to God or nature, or familiarity with mystical or transcendent experiences as components of wisdom. In fact, transcendent or transpersonal awareness wasn't included as a category in Bluck and Glück's (2005) analysis of implicit theories. And yet, from the point of view of many religious and philosophical traditions, this is at the very heart of wisdom. We look next at how awareness that transcends conventional concepts—especially realizations derived from the therapist's direct experience—can enrich the therapy enterprise.

EMBRACING REALITY

In describing a wise therapist, survey respondents repeatedly mentioned the ability to see reality clearly. But which reality? What each of us sees as "reality" is highly conditioned by our culture, language, and personal history. A Hummer-driving guy listening to conservative talk shows probably has a very different view of reality than a Prius-driving woman listening to National Public Radio.

We can get some guidance here from ancient wisdom traditions. One of the simplest and clearest descriptions of apparent universals in human experience can be found in Buddhist meditative traditions—the same traditions that refined the mindfulness practices that are currently being widely integrated into psychotherapy (see Chapter 2; R. D. Siegel, 2010; and *www.mindfulness-solution.com* for instruction in these practices). These traditions suggest that if we watch our experience carefully, we'll recognize what are called the "three characteristics of existence" (see Chapter 9). These characteristics provide a handy lens for looking more deeply into the "reality" seen by wise psychotherapists.

Impermanence

It's remarkable how reluctant most of us are to notice that everything changes. We become so accustomed to living amidst our relatively fixed concepts of the world that we fail to see it's a very fluid place.

And this fluidity is often not welcome. In her classic book, *Necessary Losses*, psychoanalytic writer Judith Viorst (1986) pointed out that most emotional pain involves reaction to loss. This starts very early: "I don't want to use the potty—I prefer my diapers." Our resistance to change continues throughout our lives as we're separated from loved ones, our children grow up, and our bodies age. Not many of us are happy to surrender our driver's license in old age or enter a nursing home. Because change can be so painful, we don't like to see its inevitability.

The bumper sticker that says "*Whoever has the most toys when he dies wins*" gets to the heart of the matter. We desperately cling to things that bring us pleasure. If we're attentive, we notice that it's actually this clinging that causes our suffering. It's not the changes themselves, but our resistance to these changes that upsets us. In the moments that we manage to let go and allow changes to occur, it's like dropping a hot coal—a relief.

Expecting and embracing change seems to be an important component of wisdom. Countless times I've shut down emotionally in therapy sessions because my patient was describing a change that frightened me. Often it was an illness or other misfortune—that I immediately imagined happening to me or a family member. In the midst of crises we may "get it" for a little while that everything changes, but as soon as we feel more secure again, it's very easy to forget reality.

And yet we seem to be wisest as therapists when we're not so surprised by old age, illness, and death, and when we remember that the wheel of fortune is always turning—what goes up will come down, and vice versa. When we embrace this longer view, we can be more fully present with our patients as they experience joys and disappointments, successes and failures.

Interestingly, research on who will develop wisdom over the course of a lifetime is consistent with the importance of embracing change. Scientists have identified *openness to experience* as a robust predictor of wisdom (Kramer, 2000). And this experience always involves change.

Embracing impermanence can have its pitfalls, however. It can make us miss the mark on another quality of the wise therapist frequently mentioned by survey respondents: understanding what is needed when, and by whom. If my patient is grieving over the loss of a girlfriend, and I suggest that relationships inevitably come and go and there are plenty of fish in the sea, he's likely to experience this response as an empathic failure. Similarly, if my patient is joyous about a new promotion, pointing out that her joy will probably fade as the reality of the job sinks in probably wouldn't be the wisest move. So the wise therapist is faced with the challenge of simultaneously knowing that everything changes—and that we humans are unlikely to remember this most of the time.

Unsatisfactoriness

The second characteristic of existence was aptly summed up by the great philosopher Rosanne Rosanadana, who regularly whined, "*If it's not one thing, it's another.*" If we watch our minds carefully, we notice that they're almost always dissatisfied. This ubiquitous dissatisfaction has many roots. First, all moments of our lives are experienced as pleasant, unpleasant, or neutral. We tend to cling to the pleasant ones, push away the unpleasant ones, and space out during the neutral ones. Most of us don't find unpleasant or neutral experiences to be very satisfying. But even pleasant experiences have a down side. Because we're intelligent creatures, we sense that they're all short-lived—bringing on another sort of dissatisfaction.

When not observant, we assume that our dissatisfaction is due to things not going our way. But when we're attentive, we realize that dissatisfaction is the inevitable result of pursuing pleasure and trying to avoid displeasure. As with *impermanence*, we're able to notice that it's not unpleasant experiences per se that create our suffering, but rather our resistance to them (see Chapter 9). Whether becoming agoraphobic in our efforts to avoid panic, tossing and turning with insomnia because we don't want to feel tired at work the next day, or becoming addicted to intoxicants in our efforts to ward off physical or emotional pain, our efforts to avoid unpleasant experiences can trap us in enormous suffering. Seeing how this works, and becoming willing instead to bear pain as it arises, seem to be important qualities of the wise therapist.

Freud (1933) aptly pointed out that the pursuit of pleasure is part of our instinctual nature. It took later students of psychology, particularly those studying happiness, to identify the futility of this habit. The term *hedonic treadmill* (Brickman & Campbell, 1971) refers to the fact that we tend to habituate to experiences, so that good fortune of all sorts (including becoming wealthy, achieving fame, or marrying a trophy spouse) soon loses its ability to make us happy. We need more and more just to stay in the same place emotionally. And of course this only adds to our dissatisfaction.

As though this weren't enough, it turns out that we evolved to think all of the time, and to think particularly painful thoughts. Our propensity to constantly think stems from its evolutionary value. On the African savannah our teeth, claws, hides, and fur, as well as our senses of smell, hearing, and sight, were pretty pathetic compared to the other wildlife. What we had going for us were our prehensile thumbs (to pick things up and make tools) and our capacity for thought (to learn from experience and plan accordingly).

So it's no surprise that we think almost all the time. Scientists have identified a hardwired "default network" comprised of correlated areas of the brain that become highly active in generating thoughts about the past and the future when we don't need to focus on a particular task (Gusnard & Raichle, 2001; Pagnoni, Cekic, & Guo, 2008). Unfortunately, this network contributes to frequently feeling dissatisfied. Our thoughts make it very hard to just "be" and savor the moment. Instead, they keep us scheming to find ways to feel better.

And to make matters worse, we evolved to think most about bad experiences (Hanson & Mendius, 2009; Lambert, 2007). Since forgetting about dangers such as a sibling being eaten by a lion or a child falling off a cliff might spell the end of a DNA line, it was our ancestors who were best at remembering painful events that survived. They then passed this ability on to us. These ancestors would have done fine had they forgotten about a wonderful sexual encounter or luscious piece of fruit, so the ability to recall pleasurable events was not selected for in the same way. We're thus left with brains that think all the time, readily forgetting the good but reliably recalling and anticipating the bad–not a pretty picture emotionally (R. D. Siegel, 2010).

Many clinicians in the survey suggested that a wise therapist has perspective on his or her thoughts—sees them as culturally and situationally conditioned, recognizes that they change continually, and therefore doesn't take them too seriously. Seeing the insubstantiality of thoughts in ourselves, we are also able to see how our patients' thoughts are mercurial and unreliable. This perspective on thought can be an important fruit of mindfulness practice. When meditating, for example, we observe how thoughts arise and pass away, moment to moment, varying with our moods. We see in action, as Ben Franklin (1793/2005) put it, "So convenient a thing it is to be a *reasonable creature*, since it enables one to find or make a reason for everything one has a mind to do" (p. 46).

Of course, embracing this perspective can also be unsettling. Most of us cherish our beliefs as guides to navigate the world. They're also important building blocks of our identities (more on this next). The experience of really seeing them for what they are feels something like jumping out of an airplane without a parachute. It's terrifying, until we realize that there's no ground. We don't actually go *splat*—instead, we simply experience the next changing moment.

No-Self

This third characteristic of existence is often the hardest for us to see initially. A central tenet of Buddhist psychology is that our conventional sense of ourselves as separate individuals is based on a fundamental misunderstanding, and this misunderstanding is the root cause of all unnecessary suffering in human life. This realization, called awareness of *anatta*, or "no-self" (fleshed out in Chapters 4, 9, and 13), is simple yet elusive. It is essentially an ecological view—noticing that with every bite of food, every breath, and every movement, the organism I think of as "me" reveals itself to be part of the web of life, which in turn is part of the web of matter and energy that makes up the universe (see also Chapter 8). The line of demarcation where elements of an apple I eat or molecules of oxygen I breathe become "me" isn't fixed and clear. Rather, my digestive tract and lungs and are permeable, and what I think of as "me" is constantly exchanging parts with the rest of the world—it is a seamless part of the wider universe.

We can come to see that our sense of "I" is actually just a convenient psychological construct, and that upon investigation we can't locate this "I" anywhere in our direct experience. Rather, what we see (perhaps through meditation practice) is that there is simply a moment-to-moment unfolding of changing experiences. Sensations arise; they're instantly organized into perceptions; these perceptions are experienced as pleasant, unpleasant, or neutral; and the mind endeavors to hold onto the pleasant ones, push away the unpleasant, and ignore the neutral. All of this occurs automatically, and although the mind generates lots of narratives about our experience, there is no independent, enduring "me" to be found in the process (see Chapter 13 for examples of how this realization can be seen in everyday life). Ultimately we find that the world is not populated by organisms or "things" at all, but only by processes in constant flux.

Although this notion can sound rather esoteric, experiencing ourselves in this way has many important implications for psychotherapy. First, it allows us to open to and bear more of our experience. If, for example, someone hurts my feelings and I notice anger arising, there are two approaches I might take. The more conventional is to go with a narrative of "me" and "you": "I can't believe you did this to me after all that I've done for you." An alternative, once I begin to experience *anatta* or "no-self," is to simply notice "anger arising." I notice muscles tensing in the neck and back, the heart beating more quickly, and perhaps images of confronting the person who upset me appearing in the mind. Instead of the experience being about "my" anger (or fear, pain, joy, etc.), it's about "the" emotion arising. Surprisingly, by not getting so caught in thoughts about "me" and "you," it is possible to bear the emotion at much higher levels, and also possible to allow waves of emotion to pass more freely. We see that our narratives about emotional experiences only increase their intensity and duration (Farb et al., 2007).

The ability to bear uncomfortable experience is enormously useful for therapists. Most of us have noticed at some point that our patients will express only those feelings that they feel we can tolerate hearing. If some emotional territory is too raw or difficult for us to bear, our patients will sense this and back away from exploring it. On the other hand, if we are able to tolerate a fuller range of experiences, our patients will be better able to do the same.

Early in my training I had a helpful lesson along these lines. I was working with Jerry, a very depressed young man who was convinced that he had no possibility of happiness, no chance of finding friends or love. Week after week he told me of his hopeless situation, and I made feeble attempts to help. I suggested different ways to handle interactions, reasons why his situation might improve some day. I often left sessions quite depressed myself, thinking of all the careers that might suit me better.

Every once in a while, however, after a particularly depressing session, Jerry would return the next week looking a little brighter. He even occasionally suggested that our previous session was a bit helpful. I would think, "To *you* maybe—it just made me depressed."

Gradually I learned a lesson: If I could accompany Jerry into his darkest places and feel in myself some of the stuckness and helplessness he felt, he'd feel a little less alone, a little more understood, a little more hopeful.

Developing a personal understanding of *anatta* can help us step out of our personal narrative and become less concerned with whether we have pleasant or unpleasant feelings. This shift allows us to embrace stronger and stronger emotions and thereby better accompany our patients wherever they need to go. It enables us to open more fully to all feelings as passing, impersonal phenomena.

Another benefit to seeing *anatta* clearly involves gaining freedom from the limitations of self-esteem concerns. As mentioned above, when asked what gets in the way of acting wisely in their work, therapists often pointed to their own narcissistic preoccupations. And we're constantly reevaluating our status. As my friend Paul Fulton (coauthor of Chapter 13), once quipped in addressing this problem, "I'm only as good as my last session."

Our need to be seen by ourselves or others as kind, intelligent, caring, or even compassionate and wise can be real obstacles to wise action. The universal human desire to be seen favorably by others (Gilbert, 2009a) can make us cover our tracks when we forget what our patient told us last week, don't know as much as we think we should about a particular diagnosis, confuse the names of medications, or become sleepy or distracted in a session. If we were able to experience the moment-to-moment unfolding of a therapy session with fewer concerns for how well we're doing or how we look, we would be free to respond more skillfully and authentically to such lapses. Ironically, not caring so much about appearing competent allows us to actually *be* more competent. A pertinent quote from Rudyard Kipling hangs over the entrance through which competitors enter the Wimbledon tennis courts: "Meet with triumph and disaster, and treat those two imposters just the same" (1910/1999, p. 605). Whether in tennis or therapy, attachment to success often contributes to failure.

Closely related to this observation are the limitations brought about by believing in our identities—limitations also eased by experiencing *anatta* more clearly. One of Carl Jung's important contributions was recognizing that we tend to identify with some attributes as "me" and see others as definitely "not me." Our conscious personalities (*personas*) are made up of attributes we think of as "me," whereas those we think of as "not me" cluster unconsciously into what Jung (1938) called the *shadow*.

For example, if I think of myself as an intelligent, compassionate, generous person (on good days), I'm going to have difficulty whenever I notice my stupid, unfeeling, selfish shadow. Dividing our attributes into "me" and "not me" in this way brings about all sorts of distortions and limitations. It makes it hard to see ourselves clearly, for we get defensive whenever our shadow is illuminated. It also makes us react negatively to others, including our patients, who might embody our disavowed qualities.

Glimpsing *anatta* can help. When through mindfulness practice or other exploration we see that there is no separate enduring self, but rather just a series of changing moments, we become less compelled to seek experiences that reinforce a particular view of ourselves. As great masters have suggested, mindfulness practice is not a path to perfection but a path to wholeness (Brach, 2003). To the extent to which we can see our "self" being constructed moment by moment, we can better embrace all of our experiences and develop a more integrated mind. This in turn makes us less judgmental and more flexible in our responses to our patients.

Another important attribute of wisdom cited both by mental health professionals and by people generally is the ability to see the "big picture" and to act in the interest of the greater good beyond our immediate needs and those of others close to us. This is a broadening of the *concern for others* mentioned earlier. Indeed, there is an extensive literature suggesting that wise professionals across disciplines see their work as extending beyond the individuals with whom they work to the wider world and subsequent generations (Solomon, Marshall, & Gardner, 2005). While we can make this perspective a goal through conscious intentions, directly experiencing *anatta* automatically turns our view to the larger organism of which we are part. Focusing only on our own needs, or the needs of a few close to us, begins to feel as silly as the right hand refusing to help the left when it is injured.

There are, of course, many other ways in which experiencing our interconnection with all things can make us wiser as psychotherapists. Several of these are described in Chapters 4 and 13.

Mindfulness meditation can awaken us to impermanence, unsatisfactoriness, and no-self; contemplative reflection, as presented in the following exercise, can also help:

IF I ONLY KNEW

- Take a few minutes to consider the following questions. It may be helpful to write down your responses.
- How might your therapy practice be different if you were to be fully and continuously aware that everything changes, everything that is born dies, you yourself will also die before too long, and all experience is in constant flux? Are there particular patients or clients you might treat or relate to differently? If so, how?

- How might your therapy practice be different if you were to be fully and continuously aware that the mind perpetually creates dissatisfaction through desire, by wishing things to be other than they are? That it's not events themselves, but our attitude toward events that causes suffering? Are there particular patients or clients you might treat or relate to differently? If so, how?
- How might your therapy practice be different if you were to be fully and continuously aware that your sense of self is a conceptual distortion, that we're all fluid fields of interrelated matter and energy? Are there particular patients or clients you might treat or relate to differently? If so, how?

KNOWING WHAT WORKS

Both Western and Eastern traditions suggest that an important element of wisdom is having an understanding of how people, and the wider world, function. This knowledge often goes beyond the fluid and crystallized forms of intelligence discussed earlier–it includes an intuitive grasp of general principles that apply across situations.

In the psychotherapy field, this involves having a general road map of how suffering is generated and how it can be alleviated across diagnoses and conditions. There are many examples of this understanding.

I heard from one of the developers of the DSM-5 that tension periodically arose between two groups involved in the process: "splitters" and "lumpers." The splitters felt that the problem with the DSM-IV was that it didn't have sufficiently refined categories. Further subdivisions of diagnoses were needed to avoid lumping apples with oranges. The lumpers felt that this approach was wrong-headed, missing the forest for the trees. Our separate diagnoses obscure the commonalities among different forms of psychological distress. The splitters challenged them: What commonalities? The lumpers said: *Experiential avoidance*. The lumpers maintained that all psychopathology involves resisting unpleasant experiences (e.g., see Hayes, Wilson, Gifford, Follette, & Strosahl, 1996). Whether it is the alcoholic drowning sadness with liquor, the phobic person warding off anxiety by staying out of the supermarket, the depressed individual escaping anger or sadness through emotional deadening, or even the psychotic person becoming delusional rather than feeling heartbreak over a loss, most emotional distress involves avoiding something unpleasant. Seeing these sorts of universal patterns can help us act wisely as therapists—trying, for example, to see what painful experience might be warded off with a given symptom, and then gently helping our patient to approach and tolerate his or her discomfort.

There are other general principles that lead toward well-being—principles that may help us to act wisely as therapists. Research in positive psychology has identified both unreliable and reliable pathways to happiness. The unreliable ones almost all involve acquiring pleasant experiences, whether those that enhance our social rank (e.g., power, money, or status) or those that bring other transient pleasures (e.g., tasty foods, sexual encounters, or other desirable sensations). All of these are subject to the *hedonic treadmill* mentioned earlier—after a while we need more and more of the same goodies to feel a certain level of well-being (Brickman & Campbell, 1971).

The more reliable approaches to happiness are not subject to the hedonic treadmill—they're as satisfying the 100th time as they were the first—and engaging in them can dramatically enhance our well-being (Lyubomirsky, 2008). They include *flow* experiences in which we're fully involved in whatever we're doing, with minimal self-consciousness or concern about our performance (Csikszentmihalyi, 1990); moments of *engagement* with other people, animals, or nature; experiences of *savoring* in which we fully feel whatever is happening in the moment and appreciate it; and *gratitude*, in which we acknowledge and express appreciation for our good fortune (see Siegel, Allison, & Allison, 2009, for a review). Also reliable as a source of well-being is *generosity*. Studies have shown that the act of giving to others can go a long way to increasing our own happiness (e.g., Dunn, Aknin, & Norton, 2008).

These are just a few of the general principles that seem to govern psychological distress and well-being. Psychotherapy is itself a wisdom tradition, and there are enduring insights to be found in all our models of treatment, including psychodynamic, humanistic, existential, interpersonal, behavioral, and systemic approaches. A wise psychotherapist probably understands the core healing elements in his or her particular model of treatment from personal as well as professional experience and is able to apply these to a wide variety of patients.

It can be helpful to consciously reflect upon what we understand to be the most important principles of psychotherapy, as in the following exercise.

PEARLS OF WISDOM

- The following questions can help you to reflect on the wisdom you've accumulated about psychotherapy. It may be helpful to write down your responses.

- What three insights about therapy have had the greatest impact on your clinical work or personal life (e.g., the importance of connection, learning to living with uncertainty, the power of transference)? Is there anything you feel you *know for sure* about what matters in therapy?
- What are the key ingredients for living a meaningful life (e.g., love, creativity, accomplishment, generosity)? What do people need to know *to live life well*?
- Imagine you are explaining psychotherapy to someone from Mars. What causes human suffering (e.g., conditioned responses, guilt and shame, unresolved trauma)? How does therapy work to alleviate it?

DISCERNMENT

Although grasping big-picture principles is important, as mentioned before, so is having a sense of what is needed when and by whom. There is a story about the senior student of a Zen master who had the privilege of sitting beside his teacher as he responded to questions. At the end of the day the student was quite distressed. He said to the master, "I'm trying to trust in your teachings, but I'm confused. You seem to give completely contradictory advice to different people." The master said, "I know what you mean. But it's like I'm watching people on a road. I see someone toppling into a ditch on the right and I yell, 'Go left! Go left!' I see another person toppling into a ditch on the left and I yell, 'Go right! Go right!' My advice only looks inconsistent if you don't see the road."

The ability to see different patients' paths, and guide them accordingly, seems to be another important aspect of wisdom. To do this well, a therapist needs to have a road map of psychological and spiritual development and, at the same time, be able to hold his or her theories lightly in order to approach each new situation afresh. Zen teacher Shunryu Suzuki (1973) famously said, "In the beginner's mind there are many possibilities, but in the expert's there are few" (p. 1). The wise therapist tries to discern what level of understanding a particular patient needs at each moment. This ability probably comes first and foremost from our own psychological or spiritual journey—knowing from direct experience what it is like to topple into one ditch or another. It then gets refined through the trial and error of clinical encounters, in which our patients show us what they find helpful and unhelpful.

Just as wisdom itself has many components, becoming a wise psychotherapist appears to be a complex, multifaceted task. It requires finding delicate balances among many apparent opposites: using our heads and our hearts, employing knowledge and intuition, grasping common sense and nonconceptual reality, seeing broad principles and appreciating individual differences. It also requires a deep understanding of the workings of our own and others' minds, all the while appreciating the limitations of that understanding. And of course even the most sophisticated wisdom won't be very useful if it's not also grounded in compassion and a host of others virtues.

So becoming a wise psychotherapist isn't going to be easy for most of us. But having thoroughly explored the alternative, I think it's worth a try.

CHAPTER 11

The Science of Wisdom
Implications for Psychotherapy

Robert J. Sternberg

Although the acquisition of wisdom is not often seen as a main, or even a subsidiary, goal of psychotherapy, it well might be. If we look at how it can be defined (Sternberg, 2005b), then it makes sense to think of wisdom as a beneficial goal of the psychotherapeutic process.

THE NATURE OF WISDOM

Wisdom has many definitions, none of which is entirely agreed on by laypersons or scholars. It has been viewed as the ability to make proper judgments, as possessing a wealth of philosophical or scientific learning, the possession of insight, and the ability to discern inner qualities, relationships, and good sense. How do these general definitions relate to more developed theoretical models of wisdom?

Historically, the concept of wisdom has been the object of philosophical inquiries since the Platonic dialogues in *The Republic* (Robinson, 1990). More recently, with the emergence of psychology as a field of study separate from philosophy, the concept of wisdom has also been explored as a psychological construct, and a number of psychologists have attempted empirical investigation of the concept of wisdom and its manifestations (Ardelt, 2000a, 2000b; Baltes & Staudinger, 2000; Sternberg, 1990a; Sternberg & Jordan, 2005). Wisdom has been studied from a range of psychological perspectives (a summary of the major approaches to understanding wisdom, and references for further reading, can be found in Sternberg, 2001). Some researchers (see Clayton 1975, 1982; Holliday & Chandler, 1986; Sternberg, 1990b) have focused on implicit theories of wisdom; that is, on trying to understand how the layperson perceives and defines wisdom. Other researchers have adopted a developmental perspective to investigate how wisdom develops or fails to develop. Most noticeably, empirical work in this area has been conducted by Paul Baltes and his colleagues at the Max Planck Institute (Baltes & Staudinger, 1993, 2000; Smith & Baltes, 1990). Another developmental approach to defining wisdom is to view it as postformal–operational thinking, extending beyond the traditional Piagetian stages of intelligence (Piaget, 1972). (See also Chapter 1 for details on some of these perspectives.)

Several researchers and theoreticians have focused on the importance of integration and balance as components of wisdom. Labouvie-Vief (1990), for example, has emphasized the balance between different kinds of thinking, suggesting that wisdom constitutes a balance of *logos*, comprised of objective and logical processes, and *mythos*, or subjective and organismic processes. Kramer (1990) has focused on the balance between various self-systems such as the cognitive, conative, and affective domains, arguing that wisdom involves integration of cognition and affect, resulting in a well-balanced personality, where the conscious and unconscious interact in harmony. Still others insist on the balance between different points of view (Kitchener & Brenner, 1990), or on "a balance between the opposing valences of intense emotion and detachment, action and inaction, knowledge and doubts" (Birren & Fisher, 1990, p. 326). This chapter focuses on a theory of wisdom that I proposed and that builds on previous theories by emphasizing the importance of integration and balance in wisdom.

According to a *balance theory of wisdom*, wisdom is the application of intelligence, creativity, and knowledge as mediated by positive ethical values, toward the achievement of a common good. This multifaceted process requires a balance among intrapersonal, interpersonal, and extrapersonal interests, over the short and long terms, in order to achieve a balance among efforts to adapt to existing environments, to shape existing environments, and to select new environments (Sternberg, 1998, 2003, 2005c).

What kinds of considerations might be included under each of the three kinds of interests? *Intrapersonal interests* might include the desire to enhance one's popularity or prestige, to make more money, to learn more, to increase one's spiritual well-being, to increase one's power, to have a happy marriage, and so forth. *Interpersonal interests* might be quite similar, except as they apply to other people rather than oneself. For example, looking out for one's family and one's friends would be an example of taking into account interpersonal interests. *Extrapersonal interests* might include contributing to the welfare of one's school or place of work, helping one's community, contributing to the well-being of one's country, serving God, and so forth. Different people balance these interests in different ways. At one extreme, a malevolent dictator might emphasize his or her own personal power and wealth; at the other extreme, a saint might emphasize only serving others and God.

What constitutes an appropriate balancing of interests, an appropriate response to the environment, and even the common good all hinge on positive ethical values. Ethical values are an integral part of wise thinking (see also Chapter 23). The question arises: "Whose values?" Although different major religions and other widely accepted systems of values may differ in details, they seem to have in common certain universal values, such as respect for human life, honesty, sincerity, fairness, and enabling people to fulfill their potential. Of course, not every government or society has subscribed to such values. Hitler's Germany and Stalin's Russia blatantly did not, and most societies today subscribe to them only to some degree but not fully.

PERSONAL WISDOM

Psychotherapy seems designed to impart something more than wisdom in the abstract: It seems to need to impart what might be called "personal wisdom"—wisdom as it applies to one's own life. How can one find happiness, or at least contentment, through applying the wisdom one has acquired to one's own life? The acquisition of wisdom in the abstract does not necessarily imply the acquisition of personal wisdom (Sternberg, in press).

Consider some individuals who have generally been considered among the wisest of the 20th century: Martin Luther King, Jr., Franklin Delano Roosevelt, and Mother Teresa. King was notoriously unfaithful to his spouse. Roosevelt, like King, was unfaithful to his spouse. He also rejected the opportunity to save large numbers of Jews and members of other persecuted groups from certain death by refusing to accept them into the United States. Mother Teresa's diaries revealed her to be tormented for many of her later years by her lack of faith. Some historical figures have fared no better. Take, for example, Socrates; considered one of the wisest men of all time, he was probably considerably less than a perfect husband or father. Perhaps his scorn of money and material goods would not have been ideally helpful to the family in maintaining an adequate standard of living. If Xanthippe was as ill-tempered as often is suggested, perhaps it was in part because of her husband. And Socrates' drinking of the hemlock by choice may have helped cement his reputation as standing on principles, but it may also have been less than helpful to the family he was supposed to support.

If these individuals, known to be wise, fared less well than we might have hoped with regard to personal wisdom, then many of the seemingly highly successful people of our age have fared even less well. John Edwards, a brilliant trial lawyer, self-destructed as a politician, husband, and friend as a result of a disastrous extramarital affair and the repeated lies he told about it, including that a love child was that of a campaign worker rather than his own. In retrospect, it is hard to think of him as a viable candidate in the American presidential primaries of 2008. Mark Sanford, governor of South Carolina, was touted as a possible Republican presidential candidate. His career, like that of Edwards, imploded not only because of his lack of faithfulness to his wife, but also because of the notably sordid way in which his private life came to light. Eliot Spitzer, former governor of New York State, fared little better: He was a prosecutor of prostitution rings who got caught up in one himself.

One can be wise in the abstract, and perhaps wise with others, but unwise with regard to one's own life. Gardner (1983, 1999, 2006) has distinguished between interpersonal and intrapersonal intelligences, and perhaps wisdom at an interpersonal or more general level needs also to be distinguished from personal wisdom, or wisdom at the intrapersonal level.

Personal wisdom seems to require all that wisdom in the abstract requires, but also something more. What might be this something more? The something more is perhaps an attitude toward life—that one wishes to apply to one's own life the principles that one applies in the abstract. This attitude is not an easy one to acquire.

First, hormones, baser instincts, or whatever one wants to call them, may work against the attitude. Does anyone really believe that Tiger Woods, arguably the greatest golfer of all time, didn't know any better when he became physically involved with multiple women beyond his wife? Certainly President Bill Clinton knew better, and Governor Mark Sanford, who visited his mistress in Argentina while claiming to be hiking the Appalachian Trail. At the extreme, one can live the kind of ascetic life that Mohandas Gandhi eventually claimed to live. But most people try to live normal lives, and in the course of doing so, fight the unacceptable impulses within themselves, with better or worse results.

Second, who among us is never hypocritical, applying to others standards that we fail to observe ourselves? Someone could be wise in giving excellent advice and yet hypocritical in not following the advice him- or herself. For example, a therapist might recommend that a patient stop smoking and then sneak out to have a cigarette himself.

Third, we may have conflicting goals, and lacking external objectivity, fail to apply the same wise standards we would apply to others in seeking a resolution of these goals. No one can view him- or herself in a totally objective manner, and so our perceptions may be skewed and result in our acting in ways that appear very differently to ourselves than to others. For example, the husband who goes out on a business trip might view himself as supporting the family, whereas his wife views him as abandoning the family because the business matters more to him.

Finally, by dint of the "actor–observer effect," we tend to view others' behavior as reflecting their traits and our own behavior as reflecting how we respond to situations (Jones & Nisbett, 1971). Perhaps it is no great challenge to behave wisely when situational variables favor us. But when we lose our jobs or our marriages or our children, we may find ourselves tempted to act in ways that more benevolent situations would not elicit.

In sum, we may fail ourselves, even as we serve others wisely. Personal wisdom goes beyond wisdom in general. Hard though it is to be wise with others, it is probably harder to be wise with ourselves. To be personally wise, one needs to deal, minimally, with hormones, hypocrisy, lack of objectivity, and situational challenges. For psychotherapy to have a successful outcome it must not only impart wisdom, but also, personal wisdom, so that one successfully can apply one's learning to one's own life.

Should Personal Wisdom Be a Goal of Psychotherapy?

There is evidence that wisdom does lead to higher degrees of subjective well-being in older adults, holding constant other variables (Ardelt, 2000a, 2000b). Similarly, Takahashi and Overton (2005) have suggested that wisdom brings an internal sense of reward by helping people better to appreciate the subjective meaning in their lives. Hui and Yee (1994) found that wisdom and life satisfaction are positively correlated in older adults. Although older adults experienced losses, these losses helped them better appreciate what they had and gave them new insights into their lives and what they meant. This in turn increased their satisfaction with their lives. All these goals are consistent with desired outcomes of psychotherapy.

A different view, however, is that of the late Paul Baltes (Baltes & Smith, 1990; Baltes, Smith, & Staudinger, 1992; Baltes & Staudinger, 1993, 2000). Baltes proposed that wise people may experience what he refers to as *constructive melancholy*. People who are wise, in this view, see the sadness as well as the joy in the complex events of life.

The view of Baltes and his colleagues is also different from that of traditional thinkers, such as Erikson (1959), who believe that wisdom involves some degree of emotional distance and detachment. The traditional psychoanalytic view of the therapist, for example, emphasizes the importance of keeping one's emotional distance from the patients one advises, lest one get caught up in their problems and thereby become unable to help the patients overcome these problems. In the Berlin view, wisdom inheres not in detachment but in sympathizing and empathizing with fellow human beings in the crises that beset them (Kunzmann & Baltes, 2005). As also suggested in Chapter 1, here wisdom is inseparable from compassion. Hence, wisdom may bring with it at least as much sadness as joy. People who do good work and apply their wisdom to it may see that others, in contrast, use their intelligence for less positive ends, which may also lead to sadness (Solomon, Marshall, & Gardner, 2005).

The constructive melancholy to which Baltes referred need not be a negative outcome of psychotherapy. A therapist wants a client not only to be happy but also to be realistic with regard to his or her possibilities in life. And sometimes realism engenders a sense of sadness. In the ideal, the psychotherapy will include sufficient optimism and compassion that the client is able to cope with the sadness that realism sometimes engenders.

The data seem consistent with a picture of the ability of the individual to continue to develop wisdom until the latter days in which health problems impair thinking (Sternberg, 2005b). However, a factor that may work against wisdom leading to happiness is the presence of negative stereotypes about aging (e.g., Levy, Slade, Kunkel, & Kasl, 2002). To the extent that people have negative stereotypes, they may find sadness in thinking about their own age-related status, and hence feel the sadness invoked by these stereotypes joining whatever sadness the wisdom of aging may bring. Actual decreases in physical health may also lead to such sadness (Jordan, 2005). However, aging may bring with it not only declines in function but also some kinds of gains—more free time in retirement, the presence of grandchildren who can be a source of joy without some of the encumbrances of one's own children, freedom from certain kinds of work-related responsibilities, and so forth. One can find happiness in aging as well as sadness. For some, psychotherapy will be a means to elucidate the sources of joy with the passing years.

Finally, wisdom may make one more deeply aware of the misery and hardship that exist in the world. Can a wise person ignore the suffering of others while enjoying life, him- or herself? Other contributors to this book argue against this (e.g., see Chapters 4 and 5). But if the person is too cognizant of such suffering, is there a danger that the individual will find him- or herself unable to enjoy life at all? At the same time, it is this understanding that also enables one to give back in later years and perhaps to find ways to donate one's time or money in ways that were not possible before, with the intent of creating a better world.

Therapy is not just about achieving happiness, but also about achieving adequate and realistic adjustment to life's challenges. This means that there will be times when a person will be sad or fearful, but in realistic ways that represent the circumstances facing him or her at a given time. Personal wisdom is a goal not because it always produces happiness, but because it produces a deeper understanding of life's joys and sorrows and a better way of coping with them.

Psychotherapy provides a catalyst to help individuals develop such wisdom. I use the term *catalyst* because, ultimately, individuals must find wisdom as well as happiness within themselves. It cannot simply be "given" to them as a result of psychotherapy or anything else. Whether wisdom actually develops depends not so much on age as upon cognitive variables, personality variables, and life experiences. Most important, the person has to utilize life experience in a way that is consistent with the development of wisdom.

There is a joke about how many psychologists it takes to change a light bulb. The answer is, it doesn't matter, so long as the light bulb wants to change. Similarly, people must want to develop their wisdom-related skills in order for those skills actually to develop, and then they must adopt the attitudes toward life—openness to experience, reflectivity upon experience, and willingness to profit from experience—that will enable this development to occur (Sternberg, 2005b). Psychotherapy may motivate people to want to develop wisdom to clarify the challenges and even suffering in life that may result from foolishness. If one looks at imploded careers, such as those of politicians or even priests who have gone astray, these implosions often result from the lack of personal wisdom.

COGNITIVE FALLACIES

Certain cognitive fallacies can operate against the development of wisdom. These fallacies are as prevalent in bright people as in those with less intellectual wherewithal. Indeed, bright people may be especially susceptible to the fallacies. I have referred to these fallacies as aspects of foolishness—or lack of wisdom (Sternberg, 2002). They can be combated through effective psychotherapy.

1. *Unrealistic optimism.* The person thinks he or she is so bright, or so powerful, that anything he or she does will turn out all right, regardless of how foolish or unethical it may be. When George W. Bush ordered the invasion of Iraq, he expected the war to be completed quickly and even advertised "mission completed" well before hostilities died down. The Vietnam War, of course, was another war in which eager U.S. politicians expected a positive end that never came into sight.

2. *Egocentrism*. The person comes to believe that his or her leadership or power is for purposes of self-aggrandizement. Tyco CEO Dennis Kozlowski, sent to prison for tax evasion, ran this conglomerate as though it was his own personal piggybank. Ethics took the back seat to Kozlowski's desire to enrich himself and his family.

3. *False omniscience*. Some people come to believe themselves as all-knowing. The surprising thing about the behavior of a Bill Clinton or a George W. Bush, in quite different domains, is not that they made mistakes, but rather that they kept making the same mistakes over and over again. Clinton correctly viewed himself as very intelligent, and perhaps thought that his intelligence and excellent education gave him levels of knowledge that he did not have. George W. Bush appears to have believed that he could trust his gut. He was wrong, over and over again, but was so lacking in intrapersonal intelligence (Gardner, 1983) and self-reflection that he learned little, if anything, from his mistakes. Barack Obama, during his presidential campaign, made mistakes, but each time seemed to learn from them and not repeat them, which is one of many reasons he was elected as president. As president, he has not learned nearly as well.

4. *False omnipotence*. Napoleon's failed invasion of Russia stands as one of the great historical monuments to false feelings of power. Napoleon believed himself to be extremely powerful. His invasion of Russia was politically pointless and strategically flawed, but he wanted the prize nevertheless. The invasion was the beginning of the end for Napoleon. Like so many other powerful leaders, he over-reached, and his feelings of omnipotence led to his doom.

5. *False invulnerability*. Perhaps Eliot Spitzer, as governor of New York, felt himself not only extremely powerful but also invulnerable when he secretly patronized prostitutes and used state money to book his travel. He must have felt pretty close to invulnerable because as a former prosecutor of prostitution crimes, he must have known that police agencies had multiple ways of tracking patrons of prostitutes. He nevertheless engaged in a pattern of repeated reckless behavior that eventually cost him the governorship.

6. *Ethical disengagement*. Consider three infamous American televangelists of different eras. How did Jimmy Swaggert go wrong? Or Jim Bakker? Or Ted Haggard? All three preached morality and ended up being shamed for their gross immorality. Or how did any of the countless men of the cloth go wrong who, when given the chance, acted in their own lives precisely how they told their listeners not to act in their lives? They exhibited ethical disengagement, whereby they came to believe that ethics are important for others, but not for them. They came to believe that they were, somehow, above acting ethically—until society decided they weren't.

Foolishness is not a trait. One can overcome it by asking oneself several questions: Is what I am doing promoting a common good? Does it balance other people's interests and larger interests, not just my own? Does it take into account the long term as well as the short term? Does it reflect positive ethical values? One can ask oneself these questions, or come to ask them through the guidance of a psychotherapist.

In conclusion, personal wisdom can enhance one's life, but not necessarily in the sense of bringing only happiness. It brings with it understanding, compassion, and *perhaps* happiness. It prepares one to deal with life in a realistic but optimistic way, knowing that, through perseverance and a positive attitude, much but not all can be accomplished toward a positive end. Psychotherapy can be a means toward personal wisdom. It probably matters little what particular form the psychotherapy takes (although drug therapy, in and of itself, seems a poor candidate to impart personal wisdom). Rather, what matters is the skill with which the therapy is done and the patient's willingness to change. Like the light bulb, the individual can change, but only if he or she wants to do so.

CHAPTER 12

The Wisdom of Connection

Janet Surrey
Judith V. Jordan

To live is to be related.
—VIMALA THAKAR (2003, p. 62)

For the past 30 years, clinicians at the Jean Baker Miller Training Institute at the Stone Center, Wellesley College, have been exploring Western conceptions of self as they create conditions for psychological suffering (Jordan, 1997, 2010; Jordan, Kaplan, Miller, Stiver, & Surrey, 1991; Jordan, Walker, & Hartling, 2004; Miller, 1986; Robb, 2006; Shem & Surrey, 1998). The anguish of the separate self and alienation from deep connection is at the core of many of the psychological disorders prevalent in our society, including anxiety and depression, addictions, posttraumatic stress disorder, dissociative disorders, and abusive behavior. Like water for fish, these conditions of disconnection and isolation are so ubiquitous that we barely glimpse the truth of our situation, nor can we freely imagine and create real alternatives. The belief in the centrality and sanctity of individual "rights" manifests in psychology's emphasis on establishing personal empowerment and self-actualization (the "American dream" and the corresponding self-help movement). This individualism has been basic to American cultural psychology and politics and has clearly shaped our psychological theories of healthy development. At the same time, loneliness, alienation, and the breakdown of marriage, family, and community bonds are prevalent in contemporary American society (Putnam, 2000).

Although a more relational psychology has emerged that more fully recognizes the human need for attachment and optimal relational development (Gilligan, 1982; Goleman, 2006; Robb, 2006; Siegel, 1999), the dominant cultural paradigms and therapy practices continue to support the primacy of the individual as the locus for change and growth. Relationships are seen as buttresses or supports for change in the individual, not the groundwork for psychological capacities that foster mutual relationships or community.

During the Harvard Medical School conference in May 2009, His Holiness the Dalai Lama was asked about the chronic and painful sense of failure, deficiency, and fragility of self- worth so prevalent in Western psychology. He noted that the overemphasis on the individual self creates conditions for overwhelming and immensely unrealistic expectations of self and other–expectations that are doomed to fail. The implication of this overemphasis is that we expect ourselves and each other to be strong, empowered, and actualized in every possible way. We do not feel our basic existence to be part of strong and abiding relationships and communities, to which we contribute in our own unique ways and draw on naturally for strength and wisdom. Our idealized and overblown notion of a separate, individual existence ultimately creates conditions for crises of personal worth and confidence. It also separates us from our deepest resource for cultivating and realizing real wisdom and compassion.

Constant unease over self-worth and self-esteem promotes *power-over strategies* that define personal value as "better than," richer, or greater in some way. Only superiority or "winning" can satisfy the quest for individual value. This mindset leads to a highly stratified society in which certain groups of people are seen as more intrinsically worthwhile or valuable and thus more deserving of recognition, resources, power, prestige, income, and even relationships.

In this chapter, we will present an alternative framework for Western psychotherapists which places relatedness at the core of healing. This model points to the wisdom of connection and offers a way of thinking and working that cultivates authentic connectedness and helps clients see through and move beyond idealized and unhealthy expectations of self and others. It is a path to developing wisdom through relationship.

BUDDHIST DEPTH PSYCHOLOGY

Buddhist depth psychology is still remarkably relevant after 2,500 years. Unlike modern theories, it has already stood the test of time and culture. Buddhist psychology points to the belief in a separate, individual, "essential" self as a primary source of psychological suffering– at odds with our fundamental, interconnected, "true" nature. Seeing through and beyond the idea of separation is at the heart of the Buddha's eightfold path of wisdom and liberation from suffering (see particularly Chapters 4 and 9).

Relationships grounded in competition for resources, wherein others are seen as competitors or suppliers, lead to experiences of chronic wounding and violation. The consequences of such disconnection for children and members of marginalized or culturally stigmatized groups can be seen in clients who develop internalized relational images and "strategies of protection" (Miller & Stiver, 1997) that recreate early damaging relationships. Such strategies fall into three major categories: moving away from relationships (denial of yearnings, numbness, disassociation), moving against relationships (anger, violence, or critical stances), and moving toward control (anxious dependence, accommodation, caretaking) (Horney, 1967). Miller and Stiver (1997) have described the fundamental relational paradox: Although yearnings for connection are basic and natural to all human beings, in the face of wounding, violation, unresolved conflict, or disappointment, people develop protective strategies that actually intensify when intimacy is possible, when yearnings get activated, or when a current relationship triggers old images. They then begin to keep more and more of themselves out of authentic relationship in order to stay in the only relationship available to them. Yearning increases as isolation increases.

Buddhist psychology describes mythical creatures called "hungry ghosts" (Epstein, 1993, p. 28). Because they have narrowed, constricted throats, their thirst can never be quenched. Even when drink is plentiful, they remain thirsty. This is a perfect metaphor for the restless state of disconnection and "burning yearning" (Shem & Surrey, 1998, p. 63) that leads to depressive and anxious states as well as to addictive behaviors, where there is an attempt to take refuge in substances, food, material goods, or technological stimulation in lieu of gratifying relationships. When the going gets rough, a search for new relationships, new communities, or new psychotherapies ensues. The simple release of taking refuge in relationship is lost.

Psychological suffering in this culture can be understood as rooted in an overemphasis on self-development and protection, an unhealthy attachment to self, and difficulties living in mutually empathic, safely vulnerable, authentic relationships. The greater the attachment to a separate self, the greater the psychological suffering (see Chapters 4 and 9 for traditional Buddhist descriptions of this state).

Thich Nhat Hanh is a Vietnamese Buddhist monk who has lived immersed in Western French culture for 40 years and appreciates the primary longing for community and connection that plagues his Western students. He deeply understands the suffering of separation and that wisdom points to psychological release and healing through reconnection.

He promotes relational healing, offering deep insights into our interconnectedness, and stressing the importance of building good enough communities. He teaches meditative practices that nourish love, honesty, harmony, and compassion in order to support individuals' participation in relationships and communities. These practices help us to develop humility, accept and speak from vulnerability, ask for help, be present for the suffering of others, offer service, and experience deep concern and compassion for all beings. One of his key insights is "Happiness is not an individual matter" (Hanh, 2000, p. 227). He would probably add "Nor is wisdom." Thich Nhat Hanh has said that insights that arise and are cultivated in the collective body (the *sangha*, or fellowship) are the most powerful, sustainable, and transformative for all. Separation leads to suffering because insight and transformation are much less possible and wisdom less penetrating and illuminating when we are isolated from one another. Thich Nhat Hanh (2003) suggests that we learn to see with "*sangha* eyes" (p. 86).

RELATIONAL–CULTURAL THEORY

Relational–cultural theory (RCT) suggests that all human beings grow through and toward relationship throughout the lifespan. Our natural state is one of interconnectedness, and our brains are hardwired to connect (Banks, 2010; Cozolino, 2007; Siegel, 1999). Western culture, however, teaches us to be strong in separation and powerful in autonomy. The pain of this mismatch between our biology and our cultural imperatives is particularly evident in the voices of those in nondominant positions in the society, but it ultimately, sadly, affects all people. Wisdom anchored in connection tells us that when threatened and experiencing fear, we can turn to others for comfort. A culture of disconnection and false autonomy leads us to believe that we will be secure only by standing on our own and gaining power over other separate beings.

The Neurobiology of Connection

Our bodies and brains are wired for connection (Banks, 2010; Cozolino, 2007; Eisenberger & Lieberman, 2004; see also Chapters 14 and 18). We are learning that we need relationship to thrive and indeed to survive. When faced with isolation or exclusion, our brains and bodies suffer. Cortisol levels rise, neurons die. Eisenberger and Lieberman (2004) have shown that the pain of exclusion travels along the very same neuronal pathways of the anterior cingulate cortex (ACC) as the pain from physical injury. The pain of isolation is real pain. Whether at a personal or societal level, being excluded or devalued hurts us biologically, neurologically, and psychologically (Eisenberger & Lieberman, 2004; Panksepp, 2011).

There are mirror neurons that fire when we watch someone else taking action. These neurons give us a sense of "being with," of experiencing what the other person experiences. Our nervous systems are primed to function best when we experience a sense of "we," of connection. Being in relationship brings comfort and positive changes in the brain, lessening stress (Banks, 2010). Neurologically primed to connect with others throughout our lifespans, however, we find ourselves in a culture that eschews dependency, connectedness, and emotional responsiveness. Messages abound that we must be strong in separation, stand aside from our feelings, and function in a competitive way.

RCT suggests that we find safety in mutual growth-fostering relationships, not in accruing power over others. RCT points to fear and anger as important relational messages and suggests that the tendency to move toward others for comfort is the soundest response (if a safe and protective other is available). RCT also suggests that people not only want to find relief from their own suffering, but naturally wish to lessen the suffering of others (Jordan et al., 1991). If we are present and open, we will empathically experience connection and be moved to enhance others' well-being.

Relational wisdom recognizes the ultimate interconnectedness of all people and beings. It is founded on the bedrock of hardwired empathy and compassion. It includes discernment, the ongoing ability to be attentive to others. Relational wisdom allows us to see beyond what Albert Einstein called the "optical delusion of . . . consciousness" (Sullivan, 1972) that keeps us from seeing our underlying interconnectedness. It acknowledges the mutuality of growth. At a recent conference on empathy, a woman who is deeply involved in helping the homeless expressed her gratitude for being affected by the suffering of others. The Dalai Lama once said, "If you want others to be happy, practice compassion. If you want to be happy, practice compassion" (as quoted in Schaef, 2000, p. 110). People benefit not just from receiving love but from giving love as well.

It turns out that meditation practices from the world's great wisdom traditions can help us access our sense of interconnectedness and compassion. Research with meditators shows that the part of the brain that keeps track of what is "self" and what is "other" is less active in experienced meditators, and it gets quite still in people during compassion meditation (Begley, 2007; Davidson, 2009; Lutz, Greischar, Rawlings, Ricard, & Davidson, 2004). Researchers in Germany have suggested that clients of therapists who meditate do better in therapy than clients of nonmeditating therapists (Grepmair et al., 2007). There is increasing evidence that being empathically present with our clients creates a sense of safety and brings about healing—fruits of relational wisdom.

Five Good Things and Relational Wisdom

Jean Baker Miller (Miller & Stiver, 1997) spoke of the "five good things" that characterize growth-fostering relationships. These five good things are manifestations of relational wisdom: (1) an increase in a sense of zest; (2) knowledge of self, other, and relationship (clarity); (3) increased sense of worth; (4) productivity/creativity; and (5) a desire for more connection. We can monitor the well-being of our clients by assessing the presence or absence of these five good things in the therapeutic and other relationships (Jordan, 1995):

Does the therapy relationship feel alive and vibrant or deadened and inauthentic?

Do we notice vigor and creative energy, or is there a withdrawal and closing down?

Can the client take small risks toward revealing more authenticity or does he or she become opaque?

Is there expanding engagement in relationships outside of therapy—an increased sense of community—or a movement toward isolation?

We can also draw attention to patterns of connection and disconnection in the therapy relationship, helping our clients appreciate the movement of relationship and what may stimulate them to move into protective withdrawal. Here's an example: One day while I (J. V. J.) was sitting with a client, I was preoccupied with a paper I was writing. I found myself drifting a bit and soon I found it hard to follow her narrative. She began to talk more and more about the usefulness of writing in her journal. I was feeling disconnected. I commented, somewhat covering my own preexisting preoccupation, that "things seem to be getting vague in here today." She looked at me and responded, "With you or with me?" In that moment she helped me come back into the present, to question the quality of my own attention. I thanked her for her question and noted that I had indeed been drifting a bit. I added that she had probably picked up my disconnection and had then also felt a bit cut off and alone. As we named this together, she looked relieved and we both began to reconnect. Had I taken a more traditional route, perhaps by wondering why she needed me to disconnect (the traditional "projective identification" approach), or had I avoided her direct question about the quality of connection, we might not have reconnected as easily. Therapeutic wisdom involves mutual awareness and mutual accountability.

Together, we develop insight into connection, the power of our yearning for connection, and the forces that drive us apart. We respect what Miller (Miller & Stiver, 1997) called the "central relational paradox." As therapists we need to honor both the deep desire for connection and the strategies of disconnection. These strategies developed to protect the client when others were threatening or rejecting, if not outright abusive. We help clients locate and name the relational patterns that led them to need their survival strategies. These include personal, familial histories as well as the societal forces that lead to chronic disconnections and isolation. Racism, sexism, heterosexism, and classism are among some of the more destructive forces.

It is very helpful to have disconnecting societal influences acknowledged by the therapist. While working with a young African American client recently, I (J. V. J.) prematurely shared my feeling that I "got" what it was like for her working in an all-white law firm whose staff were both privileged and totally unaware of their privilege. In that setting all problems were personalized, culture was invisible, and she was frequently treated as "the problem" when she spoke up about social injustice. In our session, when I offered what I meant to be a supportive comment about this, she responded with a good deal of affect, "I seriously doubt that you 'get' it . . . you with all your white and class privilege." I felt ashamed, defensive, but thankfully could also grasp that she was absolutely right. I apologized for my ungrounded assumption, noting that I could not fully imagine what it was like to be the lone person of color in such a setting. The disconnection, culturally determined and played out in the personal realm, needed to be appreciated in its complexity. It was an uncomfortable, uncertain moment. Relational wisdom challenges us to bridge the chasms that exist around race and other cultural identities laced with unspoken dynamics of dominance and subordination.

The work of RCT also involves naming prevalent cultural images (Collins, 1990) that keep us out of the present, out of relationship. These could be images of being a rock–hard, invulnerable, boundaried, or separate and strong–images extolling the virtues of the separate self. Relational wisdom grows when preconceptions and static, controlling images yield to engaged responsiveness.

RELATIONAL–CULTURAL PSYCHOTHERAPY

In relational–cultural psychotherapy, staying empathically present with the suffering of our clients is at the core of treatment. It lessens isolation, the sense of "I'm the only one." However, unflinching empathy is not always easy. For example, our images of the "good therapist" might take us away from this particular moment, with this particular client, in this particular relationship. While we can often stay present when a client is sharing pain about another's empathic failures, when we ourselves are the source of pain or disappointment, we may become defensive, abandoning our client just when relational presence would be most healing. It is also difficult to be present with another person if we cannot alleviate his or her pain. We are challenged, as poet John Keats suggests, to "stay in uncertainty, mystery and doubt without irritable reaching after fact and reason" (1818/1987, p. 43).

When therapists feel uncertain or inadequate in therapy sessions, we sometimes find ourselves turning to theory or distancing ourselves with diagnostic labels. This grasping after fact and reason can take us away from our client and increase the sense of aloneness for both. Instead, we can try to use the impulse to start theorizing as a reminder to come back to the present moment and the relationship with the client. This ability to let go of defensive conceptualizing is another central component of relational wisdom. It is similar to the shift from narrative to here-and-now experiential processing that is typical of mindfulness meditation (Farb et al., 2010).

Early in my work with Molly, a very anxious and guarded client, I (J. V. J.) commented that she seemed very sad about something. At that moment Molly did not feel any sadness, but I failed to appreciate that it was important for her not to be sad. When she reacted vehemently that she was not at all sad and asked if I thought it was part of my job to read people's minds, I found myself getting defensive, thinking how "resistant" she was and how I had probably tapped into some "primitive" anxiety. In this conjecture and theorizing, I completely abandoned Molly. I had to bring myself back to the present, notice my own closing down, admit that I did not read minds, and apologize for my mistake. I added that I appreciated her ability to correct me and thus keep us connected and on track.

It is important that the therapist work with therapeutic transparency, thus providing a window into the ways in which we are affected by our clients. The more the therapist maintains a position of neutrality or opaqueness, the more the illusion of separateness is reinforced. The whole psychotherapy culture of invisible "power over" and Delphic pronouncements (interpretations) regarding the client's functioning contributes to the erroneous notion of one-person individualistic wisdom.

Suffering ensues from living in "condemned isolation" (Miller & Stiver, 1997). In contrast, when a client can see and feel that he or she has had an effect on the therapist, the client begins to feel that he or she matters. This experience heals the suffering of separation, the fear of being unlovable, alone, without empathy from another person. At an individual level, relational psychology supports the primary urge to connect. We help people let go of images of unrealistic independence and self-importance. We assist clients in becoming more present with others. And when we are truly present, we are open to others' suffering and we are moved to alleviate it. We move away from the constructed duality of subject and object. This is *relational mindfulness*, an important foundation for developing relational wisdom.

Psychotherapy informed by RCT and mindfulness is conducted with respect, deep listening, and active attention to one's own experience, the other person, and the relationship (Jordan, 1995; Surrey, 2005). When introducing psychotherapy, RCT practitioners explicitly address the qualities of authenticity and transparency that contribute to the flow of relationship. They share what they believe is healing in therapy. For example, at the end of a first interview, we might ask if the client is interested in hearing about how we work. If we get an affirmative answer, we will explain that we believe a major source of suffering for people arises from our belief that we are separate and alone. And we suggest that in the course of therapy, we will be looking at the ways we are disconnected from one another and how we might begin to question some of the images and beliefs that keep us in isolation. We encourage small steps, small risks in relinquishing the illusion of isolation and moving toward a felt sense of connectedness. Through this process, clients begin to trust their capacity to assess the safety and growth potential of relationships (Jordan, 2010).

Diana was a very creative and successful architect. She came to therapy complaining of difficulty speaking up at work and with her friends. When she and I (J. V. J.) spoke about therapy, we agreed that it might be very useful if we could work together to help her find ways to disagree with me when the occasion arose. She expressed anxiety about this and indeed began her therapy in a compliant position, expressing admiration for me. We looked at her fear and relational expectation that if she expressed anger, I would feel overwhelmed and leave her. She said that her mother, who explicitly said "You can never really count on anyone else," had also taught Diana never to be angry. So Diana had learned not to need others and not to express her anger. Slowly, she and I began to question the certainty of these beliefs, and she became curious about what it would feel like to disagree with people. On the day when I misremembered her best friend's name, and she told me I had gotten it wrong, we knew we were on the way to authentic presence and increasing safety in relationship.

In the therapy relationship both client and therapist come to know at an experiential level that growth occurs within and toward relationship. The ideal outcome of treatment is not the attainment of self-sufficiency. Rather it is the evolving capacity to engage in mutual empathy, where each person is attuned to the other's experience, learning from each person's impact on the other. This approach involves mutual vulnerability and openness to change. It does not mean "equality" or "sameness"—in the therapy relationship, the therapist has a professional responsibility to safeguard the well-being of the client as well as to facilitate the client's healing and growth. In this mutually empathic movement, both the therapist and client are changed, both grow, and collective wisdom is enhanced. In this process, everyone has firsthand experience of wisdom growing from connection. We learn to empathize across differences, stretch to meet one another, feel the tension of trying to find our way toward safe connection. We grow in profound and new ways, learning to question and challenge the beliefs and practices that deprive us of our experience of connection and relational awareness.

RELATIONAL MEDITATION PRACTICE

Traditionally, mindfulness has been cultivated through meditation practices. The extension of mindfulness practice into engaged relationship has been pioneered by Gregory Kramer (2007) in his teaching of Insight Dialogue co-meditation practice. In an otherwise classic silent meditation retreat, Kramer teaches an interpersonal, co-meditation practice where there is face-to-face encounter on the meditation cushion. Listening and speaking are introduced as meditative practices to facilitate mindfulness through and within the relational field. Contemplations are designed to incline the mind toward wisdom, and the practice develops shared insight into nonseparation and seeing through self-images and constructions. Strategies of disconnection are seen and released and experiences of "being with" and "seeing with" are cultivated.

While these practices are perhaps most powerful when there is shared intention (as in co-meditation), we are proposing that they are also of great value in promoting depth and continuity of relational awareness for therapists in clinical practice. The following six co-meditation guidelines offer a framework for deepening the therapeutic encounter. Practicing them can open the therapist to the fluidity and range of connections and disconnections that are the foundation of RCT practice (Kramer, 2007).

CO-MEDITATION GUIDELINES

- PAUSE: This is basic mindfulness practice: noticing the flow of experience, noticing without judgment where attention has wandered and remembering to return to the chosen object. *Remembering, stopping to observe, observing, returning—over and over again.*
- RELAX: This is an invitation to the body and mind to notice and relax, release any stress, tension, or contraction around pain. Noticing tension, worry, obsessions, inviting the mind to release, relax, and accept. *Noticing, releasing, relaxing, accepting.*
- OPEN: This is an invitation toward expansion and spaciousness of mind. Opening awareness to include external objects, sounds, sights—inclining all the senses toward internal and external awareness at the same time, particularly opening to awareness of the other and of the relational space, the space between and the space that holds both persons. It involves exploring the flow and qualities of internal, external, and relational experiences. *Opening into spaciousness, both internally and externally; changing relational awareness, moment to moment.*
- TRUST EMERGENCE: This invites us to release images, agendas, and knowledge rooted in the past—even the past moment—and trust what is emerging. We notice what is arising in this moment as it is co-arising in the relational space. Trust in letting go, not knowing, opening to the as yet unseen, cultivating a willingness to be influenced and touched, to be in the flow. *Letting go, being with what is co-arising as it is coming to be realized in the moment.*
- LISTEN DEEPLY: Listening as meditation, noticing what is happening in the whole body, full receptivity and letting go, attunement, deep receiving, resonance through every sense organ. Noticing what is said, how it is said, what is not said, listening to silence, qualities of speech and voice as well as content. Listening without judgment or self-referencing. *Listening mindfully, mindfulness of listening.*
- SPEAK THE TRUTH: Authentic voice that is aligned with the truth of the moment has physical, embodied qualities that can be mindfully known and felt; noticing the range and fluidity of authentic "real" speaking, present to the moment, seeing and releasing what is heard as false or disconnected. Remembering and encouraging speaking what is true, useful, beneficial, and timely to the movement of the relational moment, courageously stepping into and inviting the unknown. This is the truth of nonconceptual, nondual knowing, moving beyond story or knowledge constructed in the past. *Listening and inclining toward authentic speaking.*

Practicing these guidelines in groups or on meditation retreats has been reported by many practitioners to be of great value. Empathic presence, deep listening, and establishing pathways to connection are fundamental to most treatment approaches (Norcross, 2002) and are of particular value for therapists who place the development of relationship at the center of healing. This practice supports opening to the deep and ever-changing experiences of connection and disconnection. It also offers the opportunity for cultivating the mental factors of awakening found in meditation traditions (compassion, equanimity, mindfulness, energy, tranquility, joy, investigation) in relationship. Perhaps even more than intrapersonal meditation, it offers relational therapists and clients the deep wisdom co-arising from profound moments of insight into the suffering of separation and the potential for wisdom in connection.

Relational Practices: Clinical Training through Role Playing

BREATHING WITH

This exercise involves attuning one's breathing to that of another person. It can be especially useful with anxious, agitated, or physically compromised clients.

- The therapist first follows the breathing of the client and silently notes "breathing in . . . breathing out . . . " for a number of breaths.
- As the breath slows down, the therapist may say silently "Letting go" with each outbreath.
- When it feels natural to be still, the therapist and client sit quietly and savor the silence.
- Switch roles.
- Discuss the experience.

MEDITATION ON THE FLOW OF CONNECTION AND DISCONNECTION

- Therapist and client sit face to face at a comfortable distance.
- Both partners close their eyes and focus on their own breathing.
- Next, they open their eyes and make soft and respectful eye contact for a few minutes.

- While gazing at one another in this way, both partners pay attention to the flow of connection and disconnection; to uneasiness, self-consciousness, and other emotional reactions that arise, allowing all these feelings to arise and disappear.
- The exercise concludes with a discussion of what each noticed about the ebb and flow of connection.

In this chapter we focused on the ways that isolation and separation create suffering at personal, social, and cultural levels. Responding to the pain of disconnection is the practice of compassion, and viewing our suffering through the lens of interconnection is the practice of wisdom. By sharing in this mutual endeavor in relational–cultural therapy, we can grow and thrive, developing compassion and wisdom together.

CHAPTER 13

Self and No-Self in Psychotherapy

Jack Engler
Paul R. Fulton

I know that I exist; the question is, what is this "I" that I know?
—RENÉ DESCARTES (1641/1988, p. 82)

Modern psychotherapists use ancient concepts from Buddhist psychology selectively, naturally favoring those most compatible with our models of health and pathology and omitting others. The most vexing point of departure between these two healing traditions is the nature of self. According to Buddhist psychology, the self that we treasure and protect is significantly less substantial than it appears, and mistaking it as "real" is a major source of psychological suffering. Instead, our sense of self arises when conditions support it and disappears when conditions do not. The self has no enduring essence that stands apart from, or behind, experience—no consistent "me" to whom all experience happens. Therefore, from the Buddhist perspective, our fundamental reality is better described as "no-self," or in Pali, *anatta*.

Although no-self is a relatively new concept in modern psychology and psychotherapy, understanding this idea, especially from firsthand experience, has great potential for alleviating suffering. For Buddhist meditation practitioners, discovering the evanescent nature of the self is the essence of wisdom, and it is accompanied by a profound sense of contentment and well-being. It seems natural, therefore, to consider how the concept of no-self may inform the theory and practice of psychotherapy.

In this chapter, we hope to show how an expanded understanding of the role of self in psychological suffering has direct, practical application to clinical practice. Although it is outside the scope of this chapter to provide a full account of the Buddhist understanding of self (see Olendzki, 2005, and Chapter 9), we attempt to render this elusive concept in experience-near terms and in relation to familiar therapeutic concepts. In the second half of the chapter, we illustrate the therapeutic potential of no-self by considering a relatively new treatment approach: internal family systems.

THE SELF IN PSYCHOTHERAPY AND BUDDHISM

Psychotherapy as a method of healing derives its power and meaning from shared, culturally constituted ideas of what it means to be fully human, healthy, and psychologically developed. Our therapy models contain detailed accounts of causality, such as how psychological suffering results from developmental arrest, failure to adapt, or trauma. How we understand suffering and its alleviation is inextricably bound to what we think is normal and healthy, and what it means to have a healthy sense of self. Whereas a sense of self appears to be psychologically universal, it is not always construed the same way.

In the West, the self is commonly understood as a natural developmental accomplishment dependent on adequate emotional nourishment in early life and ongoing interaction in the social world. In the ideal, healthy, mature individual, the self is viewed as relatively autonomous, independent, separate, and stable. We take these qualities of the self to be natural products of maturation rather than culture-bound products of folk psychology, where they originate. Western psychotherapy rests on our commonly held, cultural view of the self—that *we exist*, and that with optimal development we arrive at a self that is relatively impervious to interference from others, free to act, the locus of moral judgment and control, and of ultimate value.

Buddhist psychology also recognizes a separate self as a persistent category of experience. Indeed, the Buddha's contemporaries showed ample evidence of having psychological selves in our sense of the term. However, rather than taking an enduring and separate self as a hallmark of maturity, Buddhist psychology identifies the persistent *illusion* of a separate, enduring self as a primary source of psychological distress. As a system of healing, then, Buddhist practices do not seek to relieve suffering by improving self-esteem or rewriting personal narratives in a more self-enhancing manner. Rather, they seek to illuminate the self's ultimate ephemerality, and how our restless grasping for pleasure and avoidance of pain reinforce this illusion and give rise to unhappiness. So, in sum, despite all the ways that mindfulness-oriented psychotherapy is consistent with the therapeutic enterprise, there may still be a fundamental, unrecognized conflict in the minds of practitioners regarding the status and role of the self.

In Buddhist traditions, the realization of *anatta*, or no-self, is usually considered an outcome of insight ("mindfulness" or *vipassana*) meditation at a relatively advanced stage of practice (see Chapter 2). In fact, *anatta* is an actual experience we have all the time. At its root, *anatta* is any moment of experience that is not organized around the representation of self as a separate, independently existing entity—any time I am not organizing myself as "me" or "mine," or as any representation or identity at all. When we think of *anatta* this way, we can immediately recall many such moments in which consideration of self is absent. When we reflect on them, we notice that they are actually our *best* moments—the times when we felt freest, most in tune with ourselves, most in a flow with our experience, least anxious and conflicted, most spontaneous and creative.

Here are some examples of naturally occurring moments of *anatta*: hearing one's name called and responding without a second thought; the ecstasy of a child staying on his or her bike for the first time; losing oneself in the contemplation of a work of art; a pianist completely absorbed in the music, playing unself-consciously; a therapist listening in complete attunement with a patient. All of these experiences have at their core a feeling of being completely one with what we are doing. Actually, even that is inaccurate because there is no sense of "I" who feels "one," no subjective distinction between subject and object. Awareness is "nondual": There is just the activity and the awareness of it; the knower, the knowing, and the known are experienced as one. All these types of experience show us that being, feeling, and acting need not be organized around a sense of being a separate self—one who is doing or to whom experience is happening. Even "thinking" can happen quite nicely, and does, without a self or an "I" to do it. In those no-self moments, we tend to function more efficiently and wisely, with natural and spontaneous curiosity, compassion, and joy.

Just as the Buddhist conception of self is not as esoteric as it first seems, the pernicious consequences of holding a mistaken view of self are not hard to identify. With even a modest degree of introspection, we can see how much of our inner lives are concerned with ourselves: nearly constant defensive maneuvering, efforts to maximize our self-esteem, or the incessant tendency to compare ourselves silently (or not so silently) with others. Even the "healthy" narcissism characteristic of a well-adjusted, mature individual is a cause of distress. When we relate to others through the perspective of self, we invite a subtle (and, at times, not-so-subtle) valuation of experience as good *for me*, or bad *for me*. Our likes and dislikes become de facto yardsticks by which all experience is judged, resulting in a degree of restlessness. We come to feel vaguely separate. Like a kitchen appliance running in the background, we may only notice this activity once it stops, however briefly. In these moments we can feel enormous relief; life becomes less complicated, and we begin to learn to rest in our experience without constant clinging to our complaints or opinions.

SELF AND NO-SELF IN CLINICAL PRACTICE

We can begin to understand what *self* and *no-self* mean clinically by imagining a continuum. On one end we have narcissistic disorders. In the middle we find "ordinary" nonclinical narcissism—the daily egocentrism common even in otherwise psychologically healthy individuals. At the far end we find the Buddhist ideal of awakening to the reality of no-self.

Narcissistic disorder — Ordinary "healthy" narcissism — No-self

←——————————————————————————→

	Narcissistic disorder	**Ordinary narcissism**	**No-self**
Object relations	Others exist as narcissistic self objects or "part objects," as a part of ourselves. They are experienced primarily as providers or deniers of narcissistic nourishment and validation. There is an overvaluation of the self in association with an idealized object who validates and reflects one's own (compensatory) specialness. There is a severely diminished capacity for empathy.	"Mature" object relations in which there is the capacity for empathy. Others are seen more in their own individuality and less through the veil of one's own needs for recognition. Others' own narcissistic needs can be recognized. Self is held with appropriate esteem.	Others come to be perceived as abiding in a state of suffering due to their own attachment to an illusory sense of self, allowing for greater capacity for empathy for others. Genuine compassion rooted in recognition of others' fundamental likeness to oneself becomes a natural emotional response to others' suffering.

	Narcissistic disorder	Ordinary narcissism	No-self
Perception	The world is perceived as a reflection of personal needs, highly filtered through individual preoccupations; experience is charged, personalized, idiosyncratic. The world is continuous with oneself, as it is perceived through the lens of one's own egocentricity. The world is populated with others who provide or deny validation of *my* value, *my* importance, and *my* needs.	More of life is experienced as impersonal, independent of self, though still often colored by personal desires and aversions. The world is no longer divided up so fully into suppliers or deprivers of validation and mirroring because desires and drives are no longer the exclusive organizer of experience. One experiences oneself as an individual *in* the world, *with* others.	As the self, its aggrandizement and self-interest abate as an organizing principle, the world ceases to be perceived as a source of nourishment or deprivation, simultaneously becoming impersonal and (because it is not filtered through need states), intimate as well as abundant. As the dualism of "me" and "not me" is abandoned, the self and the world are experienced as "not different," without separation or alienation.
Defenses	Much or most of experience is dominated by conflict, with little room for autonomous ego functioning. Primitive defenses include projective identification, denial, splitting, and idealization. There is highly limited self-awareness or insight.	Mature defenses, such as repression, suppression, sublimation, and altruism (as a defense) are engaged. Meaningful self-reflection and insight are possible.	With growing understanding of the illusory nature of self, the need to defend the self drops, one becomes increasingly less defensive, living with greater receptivity and willing vulnerability. This vulnerability is offset by the understanding that there is "no one" who is hurt, who gains or loses, or who needs protection.

On this continuum, we can extrapolate from what is familiar—narcissistic disorders and healthy narcissism—to deep insight into the illusory nature of the self. It is a progression away from utter egocentrism toward its ultimate absence.

A clinical analogy might be the notion of "conflict-free" functioning. This term, developed by psychoanalyst Heinz Hartmann (1958), describes how individuals—or the same individual at different stages of psychological maturity—have areas of functioning that are relatively free of conflict. For most of us, there are a number of areas in which psychic energy is tied up due to unresolved issues. Successful treatment can be described as expanding the circle that is conflict-free and shrinking the domain of the conflicted.

This process is similar to the movement from egocentrism to no-self. Imagine that we reside at the center of concentric circles, the innermost circle regarded as "me" or "mine"—highly personal, protected, and charged (see Figure 13.1). Outside that circle is what we experience as "not about me"—as impersonal. I may find myself highly possessive about matters in which my sense of identity is at stake, and not so possessive about things that I know are not about me. For example, if I were an artist and visited an art gallery, my experience would probably be colored by a tendency to compare my work to what I see. Growth in *anatta* could be described as shrinking the circle of what is "about me," while simultaneously expanding the remaining space that is "not about me." In the example above, I might learn to see another artist's work with fresh eyes, without reference to my own egocentric concerns.

In treatment, patients may come to understand that something that was once taken highly personally (e.g., a boss's scowling look) may not be about me at all (the boss had a fight with her husband that morning). Relief is found when we see events from a broader, less personal perspective. When insight into no-self grows, more and more of one's experience is seen as impersonal, up to and including one's own mortality. One need not feel that life is a personal oppression or insult; it is only what it is, and our experience can be received without excessive judgment based on whether it is desirable or undesirable *for me*. This perspective naturally leads to wiser behavior because we are holding elements of the entire situation in mind, *as they are*, rather than just our personal desires.

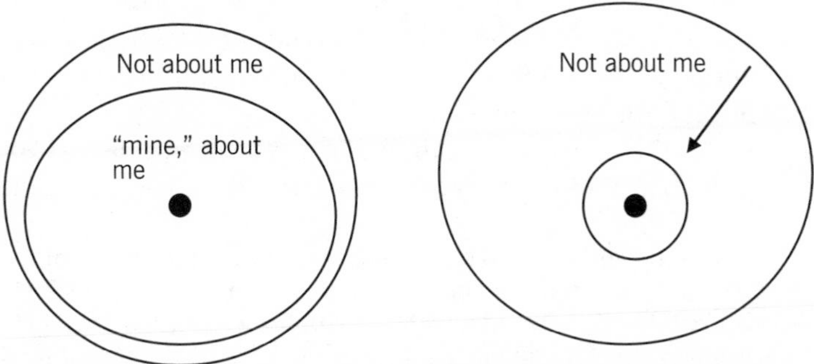

FIGURE 13.1. The movement from egocentrism to no-self.

A CLINICAL APPLICATION

The idea of no-self is beginning to find its way into psychotherapeutic theory and practice. Internal family systems (IFS; Schwartz, 1995, 2001) is a contemporary treatment approach in which accessing no-self is the key to therapeutic change. This approach also illustrates how the liberating experience of no-self can be accessed by specific interventions.

IFS starts from the observation that we have an *internal* family system that is composed of "parts" in complex and dynamic relationships with each other, very much like members of our external family. This means that the self, from the outset, is not a singular entity, a view shared by Buddhist psychology. The first challenge is to recognize these multiple aspects of myself as just parts—not who I essentially am. Normally we are identified with limited parts of ourselves and we take them to be who we are. The second challenge is to *unblend* from them. When I unblend, I am instantly in some degree of no-self or *anatta* and have less need to protect an illusory sense of self. The third challenge is to work with these parts to help them find constructive and preferred roles—ways to live and work in harmony. My parts will only collaborate and trust me to help them if they feel my concern and impartiality. And I can only truly act out of concern and impartiality from a state of no-self.[1]

How does the IFS process work? If I take a moment to "go inside"—as I would be invited to do at the beginning of an IFS session—what would I find? I would find the same stream of thoughts, feelings, physical sensations, anxieties, desires, beliefs, and preoccupations that I would encounter in any type of mindfulness practice (see Chapter 2). Within the IFS model, however, I approach the thought or feeling as a communication to me from some part of myself that is asking for my attention, not just as a momentary event that arises and passes away. In other words, the thought or feeling may be coming from a part of me that has its own history, its own outlook and approach to things, its own idiosyncratic beliefs, its own characteristic moods and feelings, its own relationships with other parts, and most importantly, its own distinct role or function in my life. This is the assumption I am invited to explore.

Assagioli's (1975) notion of "subpersonality" as a full-range inner personality and Jung's (1969) notion of "complexes" both capture something

[1]Following some of the great spiritual traditions, IFS uses the term *Self* with a capital *S* for the unblended state. Schwartz (2001) makes this connection explicitly, though he says he discovered it after developing the core of his system. The overlap between psychological and spiritual terminology can be confusing. The term *Self* as used in IFS denotes the same reality as *anatta* or no-self in Buddhist thought: a state that is not motivated by, or organized around, a sense of a separate, inherently existing agentic self.

of this idea. A "part" in this view is not just a temporary emotional state or habitual thought pattern; it is a discrete and autonomous mental system that has an idiosyncratic range of emotion, style of expression, set of abilities, desires, and view of the world (Schwartz, 1995). This is the normal multiplicity of mind. We know this instinctively when we say, "A part of me wanted to do it, but another part of me didn't."

Now suppose I approach a part of myself that is self-critical, is stubbornly refusing to move forward, or is hurting, with an invitation to tell me or show me what it wants to communicate. The first thing I'll discover is that this part of me, more than anything else, simply *wants to be seen and heard*. But the next thing I'll discover is that, despite the urgent need to be seen and heard, like anyone else this part won't reveal itself or engage with me if it feels me approaching it with preconceptions or judgments—if it feels that I want to fix it, change it, repress it, or get rid of it. On the other hand, if my approach is sincere, the part will often respond to my inquiry and show or tell me what it wants me to understand. This is not simply a "technique" or "exercise"—it is a real-life, real-time encounter in which I engage with parts of myself from the perspective of no-self.

The next thing I'll discover is that this part of me *needs acknowledgment*, and more importantly, *appreciation* for its efforts. These steps are not simply passive, detached observations. I need to fully appreciate the problematic and unwanted parts of myself for them to come forth, as Rumi (1996) encourages us to do with "the dark thought, the shame, the malice" (p. 109) in his poem, "The Guest House." Can I embrace those parts of myself that are in despair, mean, or selfish? That's the challenge and possibility of no-self, where there is nothing to defend or promote.

What I will also discover is that each part has been playing a specific role in my life and has a specific function. Contrary to my everyday experience, no matter how bad the behavior of a part of me looks or feels, if I inquire sincerely, I will find it has *always* had my best interests at heart. Each part has been trying to protect me from further hurt or disappointment, or to help me manage some situation in my internal or external life. In this approach, "benign intent" is a crucial assumption that allows for sustained inquiry into the roles and functions of parts. Understanding the inherent good will of every part makes it possible to work with those elements of myself that other parts might find objectionable or intimidating.

Even with successful treatment, parts do not disappear. They remain part of me. The therapeutic goal of IFS, then, is not to fuse parts into a single personality, or to change, fix, or get rid of them, any more than it would be the intention of a conductor to throw individual instruments out of the orchestra when they aren't playing well. Nor is the goal to "transcend'" unwanted or "unwholesome" parts—a mistaken notion in some spiritual traditions. No instruments, no orchestra. Instead, the goal is integration to help them learn to work together in finding a preferred role that contributes to the welfare of the system as a whole. Though parts may not disappear, they can find new roles for the skill sets they already have, providing I learn to unblend from them, approach them from a state of no-self, and provide leadership that is less conflicted and relatively free of judgment and agenda.

The Wisdom of Nonidentification

From the perspective of no-self, it is possible to relate to all parts of ourselves with genuine curiosity and compassion–to appreciate what each part has endured and how long and hard it has been laboring on our behalf. Care and compassion spontaneously flow toward the wounded parts of ourselves. Nothing actually needs to be fixed or changed; each part knows exactly what it requires to exist productively and peacefully in the internal family system.

Working with ourselves this way has its psychological equivalent in Tibetan Buddhist tantric practices. Instead of trying to extinguish "unwholesome" mind states (*akusala citta*) and replace them with "wholesome" (*kusala citta*) ones, tantric wisdom informs us that all mind states are valuable energies that can be transformed into wholesome qualities: anger into kindness, greed into generosity, delusion into insight. Any troublesome part of ourselves can become a benefactor. Any enemy can become an ally. The parts of myself that are self-defeating, anxious, and traumatized, or violent and destructive, can discover new and more constructive roles for themselves.

Remarkably, even the three traditional Buddhist "poisons" of greed (*lobha*), hatred (*dosa*), and delusion (*moha*) (see Chapter 9) that lie at the root of all unwholesome mental states can be regarded and treated as parts of myself that are actually trying to help me in their own way. Again, the goal is not to get rid of unwanted parts, as it was in early Buddhist practice and often still is in many practitioners' minds today. It is also not to transcend them. It is to integrate them into the internal family by learning how to work with them and appreciating the great power for potential change and good they embody once I stop avoiding them. Greet them, welcome them, treat them as honored guests, Rumi (1996) says. *All* parts are welcome.

Unblending from parts of ourselves is what accesses *anatta* and makes working with these different parts possible. This process is very similar to Adyashanti's (2006) invitation "to wake up from . . . this trance state of identification" (p. 46). Parts are often so insistent–again, with good intentions–that they tend to take over, hijacking us before we know it. And then when we speak or act, we are unwittingly speaking or acting no longer *for* that part, but *from* that part. I say, "I am angry" or "I feel guilty" or "I feel ashamed." Actually, it's a part of me that is feeling angry, another part that is feeling guilty, and probably still another that carries shame. As long as I am merged with a part, I can't engage with it, have a relationship with it, or work with it. So the first step is always to acknowledge the presence or activity of a part, then separate or step back from it, or ask it to step back—not to reject or abandon it, but to engage with it. That's the paradox. I ask it to step back a little bit, and this shift allows us to notice each other.

What do I discover when a part steps back and I no longer identify with it as "me"? As the Indian sage Ramana Maharshi was fond of saying, "Let come what comes. Let go what goes. See what remains" (as cited in Adyashanti, 2006, p. 65). What remains? Something that is completely different in nature from my parts.

As we mindfully observe and unblend from the many different parts of ourselves and gradually unblend from them, we're likely to discover that who we are at our core is not an enduring me or self, but simply awareness itself, without any judgment or agenda. This is not a passive state. Neither is it a transcendent realm of consciousness or a spiritual state without the pain and challenges of life. Living in no-self really means interacting with all parts of myself in creative and healing ways, being an active member of my internal family, encouraging the different parts to be seen and heard, nurturing more constructive roles, and helping them communicate and collaborate with each other. In this state I can be either a witness or an actor, whatever the situation calls for.

As I unblend from my parts, I'm likely to find that my core, my essence, my truest nature, my natural state, is already, will be, and always has been a state of wholeness, not identified with any specific representation of self. This is precisely what Buddhist thought calls wisdom (*panna*)—not just "being wise" as an elder or mentor may be wise, but the very specific realization of being no-thing *in particular*, and therefore capable of compassion toward all things without discrimination (see Chapters 4 and 9).

Inherent Compassion

In a state of no-self, I'm also likely to discover that positive qualities flow more spontaneously within me. I don't actually *become* compassionate and peaceful, for instance; I *discover* that compassion and peace are already there. I discover that wholesome qualities don't come from anyone or anything outside myself either—from a therapist, for instance. They are the same wholesome, healing, and creative qualities that manifest in everyone when we unblend from the parts of ourselves that have unwittingly held us hostage to limited self-images and beliefs. IFS uses a mnemonic of eight C's to identify a core group of wholesome qualities: calmness, clarity or wisdom, curiosity, compassion, confidence, courage, creativity, and connectedness (Schwartz, 2001). But IFS points to additional positive qualities as well: joy, humor, acceptance, forgiveness, and gratitude (Schwartz, 1995). Note that these qualities are similar to those identified in Buddhist psychology as the "perfections" (*paramis*) or "factors of Enlightenment" (*bojjhangas*): mindfulness, investigation, energy, joy, tranquility, concentration, and equanimity. These are the qualities of mind considered necessary for awakening and for truly wise action (Nyanatiloka, 1972). They are like the sun—ever shining. I can add nothing to this state; take nothing away. The problem is only the cloud cover. Part the clouds and I will see the sun. When there is an opening—when I can help a part that has taken me over to step back—the sunlight of *anatta* begins to pour through. At this point, even the sense of being an observing witness drops away. There is just witnessing, just awareness, just connection, with these qualities streaming through.

SEEING FROM NO-SELF

We can know when we are in this state of no-self. I am in this state when I am fully present, but without the accompanying sense I usually have that there is an entity within, a "me" or "I" who is aware. In the state of no-self, odd as it may sound, I am just aware, without any self-consciousness of being or of having a self who is aware. Awareness itself is not just another part of me, as we may be inclined to think of it. It is also not an experience. It cannot be represented as "this" or "that." Rather it is the *condition* of all experience—what makes experience possible. There is a clear awareness of parts of myself and an ability to engage with them, without taking them to be "me" or "mine." Any image or belief I have about myself, on the other hand, can only be a part of me, never who I truly am. When I do not refer my seeing or thinking or doing back to a "me," I am thinking and perceiving from no-self. In IFS terms, when I unblend from any part of myself, partially or completely, there is seeing but no seer, thinking but no thinker, doing but no doer.

IFS PATH EXERCISE[2]

- Find a comfortable position and take a few deep breaths.
- When you feel ready, gradually let your attention turn inside and visualize yourself in a clearing at the start of a path. Invite your thoughts and feelings, your body and physical sensations—all your parts—to gather in the

[2] Slightly modified from the original "Path Exercise" in Schwartz (2001, p. 61*ff*).

clearing. Let them know your intention is to take a walk on the path by yourself, and you want them all to remain here while you are gone.

- If they are anxious about letting you go, let them know you will return, that you won't be gone long, and that this will benefit all of you. Have any parts that may still feel anxious looked after by parts that are less anxious. If the anxious parts are still afraid to let you go, talk with them about their concerns. Once you sense it is OK to proceed, begin walking out on the path.
- As you go, if you find you are watching yourself walking, you are still blended with some part of yourself—perhaps with a watcher or a witness part that still doesn't trust you to be on the path by yourself. When you are truly experiencing from no-self, you will not see yourself because you are the seer, and the seer cannot see itself. Find that part that is afraid to let you be on the path by yourself and ask it to return to the others. If it won't, then take some time to talk with it about why it is afraid.
- As you continue walking, open to all your senses. What is it like to just see, just feel, just hear, just touch, just taste? If you find yourself thinking, ask those thoughts to return to the clearing also, so that more and more there is just pure awareness, pure presence. As each part goes back, notice the space that opens up in your body and mind. Notice the increased flow of energy. What is the core of you like when you are not blended with your parts? (This is a glimpse of no-self, *anatta*.)
- When it feels time to return to your parts, go back to where your parts are gathered. See if you can remain open to the unblended spaciousness and energy as you approach your parts again. When you get back, notice how your parts greet you when you arrive with this energy. Talk with them and see how they did without you. Ask them if there is anything they need from you. Offer to share the spaciousness and energy you have experienced with them. Notice the effect on the parts that are willing to receive it.
- Finally, thank the parts that let you go. And thank the parts who did *not* let you go, for letting you know they were afraid. See if you can bring the spaciousness and energy of no-self with you as you return to your day.

The state of nondual selfless awareness is as important to the IFS model of therapy as it is to Buddhist mindfulness practice. An interesting difference between the two healing paths is that no-self plays a more explicitly interactive role with our inner parts in IFS. No-self not only witnesses, it provides emotional leadership. It not only listens, it conducts. When we are in no-self, we spontaneously bring curiosity, compassion, and wisdom to hear and care for whatever is going on within us. This kind of emotional leadership is trustworthy and effective, coming as it does from a natural, spacious, benevolent state of mind.

Buddhist psychology describes behavior originating from no-self as *asangkarika citta*, or action that is "unmotivated." There is action, but little or no sense that "I" am doing anything. My actions are not experienced as originating in or by "me." They simply occur as a spontaneous response to the situation and need of the moment. Unlike actions initiated and driven by limited parts of myself, no-self is unbiased, impartial, not needing events or outcomes to be this way or that, expressing only interest and concern, compassion and wisdom.

Psychotherapy appears to be on the threshold of a wider understanding of self and no-self. This broader understanding of self may inspire innovative therapeutic models such as IFS and inform psychological interventions of all kinds that might be used to guide patients to an appreciation of no-self that frees the heart. An intuitive realization of no-self is what Buddhist psychology calls wisdom. Such a realization must necessarily inform our understanding of freedom from suffering, which will in turn challenge us to revisit how we practice psychotherapy.

CHAPTER 14

Neurobiological Foundations of Wisdom

Thomas W. Meeks
B. Rael Cahn
Dilip V. Jeste

> Irrigation engineers lead water where they want to. Fletchers make the arrow straight. Carpenters carve and shape the wood. Likewise, the wise ones control and discipline themselves.
>
> —THE DHAMMAPADA (as cited in de Silva, 2000, p. 171)

The quest for a model of the neurobiology of wisdom is daunting. The challenge is apparent when considering the multifaceted concepts of wisdom developed over centuries and across cultures, combined with the astounding biological intricacy of the human brain—with billions of neurons and trillions of synapses. Yet, a number of developments have helped make this once seemingly unattainable idea tantalizingly possible. Technological advances in studying neurobiology have progressed at dizzying rates in recent decades, primarily involving functional neuroimaging (i.e., near real-time observation of changes in brain activity with progressively finer resolutions) and the study of genetics, genomics, and proteomics relevant to the central nervous system.

While these advances are exciting, neuroscience and psychiatric researchers have not utilized these technologies to study the concept of wisdom per se. For many years wisdom was the purview of religion, ethics, and philosophy—and not the so-called empirical sciences. However, since the 1970s, researchers—for example, Clayton, Baltes, and Erikson—in the fields of gerontology, psychology, and sociology (Brugman, 2006; see also Chapters 1 and 11) expressed interest in the concept of wisdom, and publications in peer-reviewed journals on wisdom have increased approximately 15-fold over the past four decades.

Although wisdom has been conceptualized differently by various researchers, our review of the literature revealed that the definitions that have emerged are quite similar to one another and to concepts of wisdom from varied ancient and modern cultures (Jeste & Vahia, 2008). As there were no known neurobiological studies of the concept termed *wisdom*, we took a preliminary step in constructing a neurobiological model of wisdom. First we searched the literature for peer-reviewed publications proposing definitions of wisdom. Next we identified subcomponents of wisdom included in at least three of the definitions (Meeks & Jeste, 2009). These included (1) prosocial behavior/attitudes, (2) social decision-making/pragmatic life knowledge, (3) emotional homeostasis, (4) reflection/self-understanding, (5) value relativism/tolerance, and (6) acknowledgment of/dealing effectively with uncertainty/ambiguity.

Notably, most of these elements of wisdom are similar to those agreed upon by experts on wisdom in a recent study using the Rand Panel or Delphi method (Jeste et al., 2010). Given the similarity of the views expressed by researchers from different perspectives and backgrounds, we believed that researching wisdom from a "bottom-up" approach could at least generate initial theories regarding the neurobiology of wisdom, cognizant that many aspects of any initial model may not stand the test of time. We therefore reviewed the literature on the neurobiology of each of the above-mentioned six domains of wisdom, focusing on their possible neuroanatomical localization, based on functional neuroimaging studies along with investigations of neurotransmitters (Meeks & Jeste, 2009). The putative neurobiological substrates of different domains of wisdom included several common regions: dorsolateral, orbitofrontal, and ventromedial prefrontal cortex; anterior cingulate cortex (ACC); amygdala; and limbic striatum.

A related research area is the nascent field of the neuroscience of meditative states and traits of consciousness. Meditative practices were developed within cultures throughout the world, often conceived as aids in the development of wisdom. There is a growing literature exploring the neurobiological results of meditative practices that overlaps with findings related to the neurobiology of the proposed subcomponents of wisdom. While each of these six domains is related to concepts of meditative practice, there is particularly strong overlap in the neurophysiological research of meditative practices with the wisdom subcomponents of prosocial attitudes, emotional homeostasis, and self-reflection/self-understanding. Interestingly, the above-mentioned brain regions implicated in the neurobiological manifestations of wisdom—the dorsolateral and ventromedial prefrontal cortices in combination with the limbic, striatal, and anterior cingulate regions—are also frequently reported to be involved in meditative practice (Cahn & Polich, 2006).

This chapter explores findings that shed light on the neurobiology of the six subcomponents of wisdom and meditative practices designed to cultivate them, along with research into related neurobiological effects of psychotherapy.

NEUROBIOLOGY OF THE SIX SUBCOMPONENTS OF WISDOM

Prosocial Attitudes/Behavior

Many cultures and researchers have emphasized that wisdom implicitly serves the common social good. We therefore reviewed neurobiological research pertaining to empathy and compassion, altruism, and social cooperation. These are related concepts but also have notable differences. Empathy can be understood as the capacity to understand and share the emotional experience of another. It is adaptive only in the sense that the person empathizing can maintain a sense of separation of self, lest empathy become emotional contagion. Closely related to empathy is compassion (see Chapter 1). Meditative practices in particular have focused on developing this capacity, which involves both empathy and the intention to alleviate the suffering of others. Altruism refers to behavior that may be to one's own disadvantage but that benefits others, and it is thought to be evolutionarily "programmed" more strongly for those genetically close to us. Social cooperation involves complying with actions that serve the common good, not necessarily to one's own disadvantage. In evolutionary biology social cooperation is often thought to result from fear of the consequences of being uncooperative.

A brain circuitry that may have played a role in the development of human empathy is the so-called "mirror neuron system" in the prefrontal cortex (PFC) (Rizzolatti, Fadiga, Gallese, & Fogassi, 1996) (see Figure 14.1a). Ample evidence has accrued for a parietofrontal mirror neuron system that activates both when one is performing an action and when one is watching another person do the same action, and a limbic mirror system that activates both when experiencing a specific emotion and when watching another (presumably) experiencing that emotion (hence the name *mirror*) (Cattaneo & Rizzolatti, 2009). These mirror neuron systems appear to form a basis for empathy and altruistic orientation by helping people appreciate nonverbal communication (Decety & Jackson, 2004).

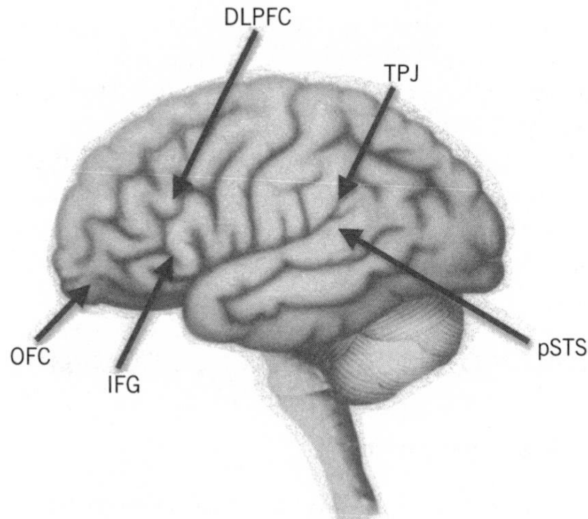

FIGURE 14.1a. Anatomical map of brain regions relevant to wisdom: Lateral (external) view of the brain. DLPFC, dorsolateral prefrontal cortex; IFG, inferior frontal gyrus; OFC, orbitofrontal cortex; pSTS, posterior superior temporal sulcus; TPJ, temporoparietal junction.

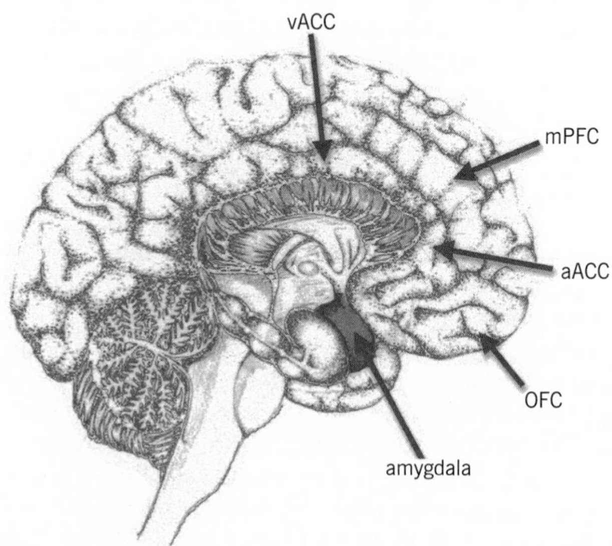

FIGURE 14.1b. Anatomical map of brain regions relevant to wisdom: Midsagittal (internal) view of the brain. aACC, anterior portion of anterior cingulate cortex; mPFC, medial prefrontal cortex; OFC, orbitofrontal cortex; vACC, ventral anterior cingulate cortex.

There is now a growing neuroimaging literature showing that observing others' emotional states activates in observers parts of the neural networks involved in experiencing those same states (de Vignemont & Singer, 2006; Sommerville & Decety, 2006), and it seems that this capacity relies upon the medial prefrontal cortex (mPFC). In support of this finding, a recent functional magnetic resonance imaging (fMRI) investigation showed that the mPFC (see Figure 14.1b) regulated perception of a shared emotional experience (Seitz et al., 2008), and a meta-analysis of 80 studies found that the mPFC plays a major role in human empathy (Seitz, Nickel, & Azari, 2006).

Recent studies have indicated that compassion/loving-kindness meditation practice enhances positive emotions, decreases depression and illness-related symptoms, and increases social connectedness, as measured by both implicit and explicit measures of affiliative tendencies (Fredrickson, Cohn, Coffey, Pek, & Finkel, 2008; Hutcherson, Seppala, & Gross, 2008; see also Chapter 3). Specific neurobiological features of such meditative practice to date include high-amplitude gamma frequency power in long-term compassion meditators, an effect believed to reflect a highly attentive brain state (Lutz, Greischar, Rawlings, Ricard, & Davidson, 2004; see also Chapter 8). In addition, these same practitioners, when exposed to emotional auditory cues, showed increased response in brain areas—the posterior superior temporal sulcus (pSTS) and right temporoparietal junction—implicated in taking the perspective of others (as detailed below in discussions of theory of mind relevant to social decision making), as well as in limbic areas (amygdala and ACC) during compassion meditation (Lutz, Brefczynski-Lewis, Johnstone, & Davidson, 2008). Lastly, these advanced compassion meditation practitioners evidenced significantly increased heart rate during compassion meditation relative to rest periods, and this increased heart rate correlated with increased brain activity in the anterior insula, possibly reflecting the distinct physiological sensations often reported in association with compassion and/or love (Lutz, Greischar, Perlman, & Davidson, 2009).

Social cooperation has been examined in neuroimaging research using a variety of tasks (e.g., trust/reciprocity games, including the "Prisoner's Dilemma") (Knutson, 2004). Functional MRI research has revealed that social cooperation involves brain regions such as the mPFC (similar to empathy) as well as the nucleus accumbens/ventral striatum (see Figure 14.1c), the latter being regions of a phylogenetically more primitive reward neurocircuitry (Decety & Jackson, 2004; Rilling et al., 2002; Singer, Kiebel, Winston, Dolan, & Frith, 2004). Altruism has also shown an interesting, similar pattern in neuroimaging studies, using paradigms such as money donation (vs. taxation), in which the primary brain regions activated were the striatum and nucleus accumbens (Harbaugh, Mayr, & Burghart, 2007; Moll et al., 2006).

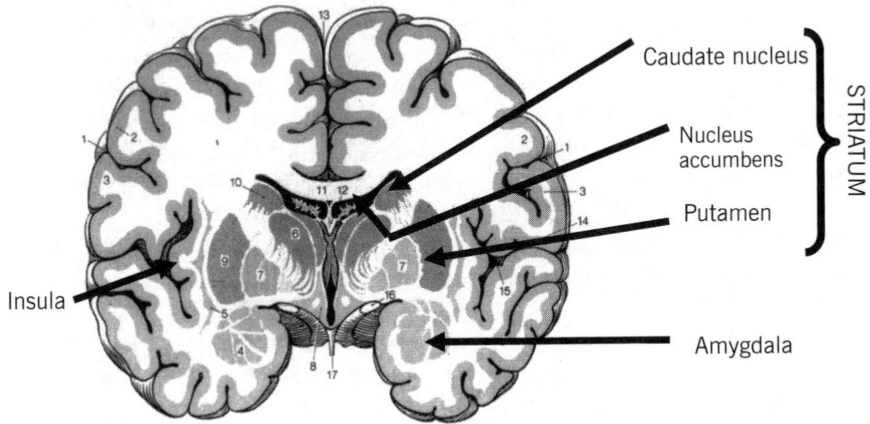

FIGURE 14.1c. Anatomical map of brain regions relevant to wisdom: Coronal cross-section of the brain.

Social Decision Making/Pragmatic Life Knowledge

The concept in neuroimaging literature closest to pragmatic life knowledge and skills is related to social cognition. Perner and Wimmer developed the "theory of mind," which has become a prominent model for explaining how humans understand the mental states of others (Perner & Lang, 1999). Neuroimaging research on theory-of-mind tasks has consistently shown activation in the mPFC and pSTS, with the temporoparietal junction (TPJ) also sometimes implicated (Brunet, Sarfati, Hardy-Bayle, & Decety, 2000; Fletcher et al., 1995; Gallagher, Happé, Brunswick, Fletcher, & Frith, 2000; Goel, Grafman, Sadato, & Hallett, 1995). The mPFC appears more involved in "mentalizing" or conceiving of the inner world of others, whereas the pSTS responds to visual stimuli related to social cues and internal mental states (e.g., body gestures or facial expressions), and the TPJ plays a role in self-versus-other cognitive distinctions. As mentioned above, long-term compassion meditators exposed to emotionally laden auditory stimuli showed greater pSTS and TPJ activity during compassion meditation, supporting a possible enhancement in the biological substrate of this form of perspective-taking and social cognition (Lutz et al., 2008).

Beyond recognizing emotions and motivations in others, one must then use this information to make "wise" social decisions. Montague and Berns (2002) made a key distinction regarding decision making relevant to wisdom. They emphasized that, associated with each decision, is a representation of choices and a short-term (and sometimes longer-range) evaluation of the consequences of those choices. Wisdom may, in part, depend on balancing choices for immediate reward versus potentially more beneficial long-term advantages (see also Chapter 11).

The most common decision-making tasks studied in neuroimaging relevant to wisdom involve "moral decision making." Greene, Sommerville, Nystrom, Darley, and Cohen (2001) reported that personal (vs. impersonal) moral reasoning tasks increased mPFC activation. More impersonal moral decision-making tasks increased activity in lateral frontoparietal regions (often implicated in more rational cognition). Greene, Nystrom, Engell, Darley, and Cohen (2004) examined another aspect in the neurobiology of moral decision making by comparing personal moral decisions versus utilitarian moral decisions—that is, those that require possible violation of personal moral judgments and emotional self-interests for the sake of common social good (e.g., actively sacrificing one person in order to save the lives of several others). These generally more complex utilitarian-based moral decisions preferentially activated the ACC (involved in emotional or cognitive conflict detection) and the dorsolateral PFC, which may be recruited to use more "calculated and rational" thought processes to overcome more automatic emotional responses.

Emotional Homeostasis

A basic brain function necessary for emotional regulation (and also for delayed gratification—part of wise social decision making discussed above) is impulse control. Neuroimaging studies suggest that the dorsal ACC (dACC), lateral PFC, and inferior frontal gyrus are key brain regions modulating impulsivity (Congdon & Canli, 2005). Theoretically, the dACC senses conflict between instinctual emotional responses and more cognitively reasonable social responses, whereas the lateral PFC maintains more socially advantageous responses in working memory and facilitates appropriate action or inhibits inappropriate responses. Simple quantifiable inhibition of behavioral impulses on "go/no-go" tasks is a proxy for general impulse control that is easily tested *in vivo*. The inferior frontal gyrus is consistently activated in "no-go" responses (i.e., those that require behavioral inhibition) (Aron, Fletcher, Bullmore, Sahakian, & Robbins, 2003; Horn, Dolan, Elliott, Deakin, & Woodruff, 2003).

A more challenging task in emotional homeostasis is the cognitive reevaluation of emotions. The effort of reframing negative emotional experiences as less aversive—a cornerstone of many forms of cognitive-behavioral therapy (CBT)—involves recruitment of regions of the more "logic-oriented" PFC to dampen more "emotion-driven" amygdala activity (Cooney, Joormann, Atlas, Eugène, & Gotlib, 2007; Goldin, McRae, Ramel, & Gross, 2008; Kim & Hamann, 2007; Ochsner, Bunge, Gross,

& Gabrieli, 2002; Phan et al., 2005). Neuroimaging researchers have also mapped a form of unintentional emotional regulation in the act of labeling negative emotions with words. This is hardly a revelation for psychotherapists, but to demonstrate this knowledge via imaging is quite another feat. Furthermore, even when not *intended* as a means of self-regulation, this labeling of emotions increased ventrolateral PFC activity and decreased amygdala activity (i.e., the same pattern seen in intentional cognitive reframing of negative emotional stimuli) (Hariri, Bookheimer, & Mazziotta, 2000; Lieberman et al., 2007). Thus, a key neurobiological concept in emotional homeostasis is the ability of the prefrontal cortex to inhibit limbic reactivity.

There is now an extensive research literature relating meditation and a key component of meditative training—mindfulness—to the concept of emotional homeostasis (see Chapter 2). Recent reviews highlight the growing literature relating mindfulness to emotional regulation (Chambers, Gullone, & Allen, 2009; Garland, Gaylord, & Park, 2009; Williams, 2010), and numerous studies have now shown that mindfulness meditation interventions result in improvements both in a broad range of psychological disorders as well as in overall quality of life (Davidson et al., 2003; Kabat-Zinn, 2003; Kabat-Zinn et al., 1992; Teasdale et al., 2000). Furthermore, such interventions, not surprisingly, result in higher ratings of mindfulness, an effect that has mediated improvements in emotional well-being (Carlson, Speca, Patel, & Goodey, 2003, 2004; Carmody & Baer, 2008; Nyklicek & Kuijpers, 2008; Rubia, 2009; Schroevers & Brandsma, 2010).

Related to these results and the previous discussion of the neural circuitry of emotional regulation is a neuroimaging finding that individuals scoring high in mindfulness showed increased mPFC activation and concurrent inhibition of amygdala reactivity to emotionally laden words when engaging in an affect-labeling task (Creswell, Way, Eisenberger, & Lieberman, 2007). Additionally, long-term meditators, assessed for responses to emotionally aversive and distracting sounds during meditation, have been shown to display decreased amygdala activation (Brefczynski-Lewis, Lutz, Schaefer, Levinson, & Davidson, 2007). Of further note, individuals undergoing meditative training as part of the mindfulness-based stress reduction (MBSR) course were assessed relative to control participants for brain activity during both sad video viewing and a cognitive task involving narrative focus (thinking about themselves) versus experiential focus (noticing moment-to-moment sensory experiences) while viewing positive and negative personality adjectives. After MBSR training, active participants showed increased insula activity across both tasks, likely related to increased experiential feelings in the moment, combined with increased lateral PFC activity, likely related to enhanced cognitive control of emotional reactivity (Farb et al., 2007, 2010).

In sum, several studies have shown that meditative training and/or mindfulness are associated with enhanced emotional homeostasis through up-regulating PFC activity and down-regulating amygdala responsiveness to challenging emotional stimuli. A related cognitive and perceptual finding is that meditators have repeatedly shown greater activity in the anterior insula, a region implicated in enhanced experiential awareness of emotions as manifested in the body. Indeed, long-term meditators have been shown to evidence reduced arousal concurrently with improved emotional valence (e.g., ability to discern others' emotional states) specific to visual masked conditions (i.e., under conditions in which the emotional stimulus was vague and likely required subconscious processing) (Nielsen & Kaszniak, 2006).

Reflection/Self-Understanding

Self-knowledge and capacity for self-reflection are common in various researchers' and cultures' concepts of wisdom. Uddin, Iacoboni, Lange, and Keenan (2007) reviewed the concept of a "default mode" of the brain. The *default mode network* refers to a set of brain areas that is more active during nontask periods than when one is engaged in particular cognitive or emotional tasks (Gusnard, Akbudak, Shulman, & Raichle, 2001; Raichle et al., 2001). This network involves a set of midline structures, including dorsal and ventral medial PFC, posterior cingulate, precuneus, and inferior parietal lobule. The *default mode* refers to what has been termed "task-unrelated imagery and thought," such as autobiographical reminiscence, self-referential thought, and inner speech. Greater activity in this default network is associated with more active periods of "mind wandering" (Mason et al., 2007).

On neuroimaging, reflecting on one's own current experience has been repeatedly shown to cause activation of the mPFC (Lieberman, 2007), and tasks that require self-judgment likewise activate the mPFC (Fossati et al., 2003). Having a continuous and coherent sense of self (a painstaking goal for many individuals in psychotherapy and a key concept in many treatment approaches) requires cohesive autobiographical memory, and, consistent with the above studies, autobiographical memories activate the medial and ventromedial PFC, versus the dorsolateral PFC activation in *non*autobiographical episodic memory (Gilboa, 2004). Although certain kinds of self-reflection in moderation probably foster wisdom, it also seems clear that excessive self-directed internal thought can be maladaptive, as happens in perseverative worry or rumination, obsessions, or narcissistic self-absorption—all of which are antithetical to wisdom. Such excess self-absorption may be mediated by overactive default mode network activity, and some evidence suggests that the lateral

PFC may help inhibit excessive mPFC-related self-absorption (Samson, Apperly, & Humphreys, 2007; Samson, Apperly, Kathirgamanathan, & Humphreys, 2005; van den Heuvel et al., 2005).

Meditators and individuals scoring high in mindfulness have been shown repeatedly to evidence less default mode activity than control subjects. For instance, Zen meditation practitioners and matched control participants were presented with nonsense versus real words during functional neuroimaging and asked to categorize the words as real or nonsense while maintaining a breath-focused, present-moment awareness (Pagnoni, Cekic, & Guo, 2008). The Zen meditators showed a faster return to baseline activation in the default mode network, which, on the other hand, tended to remain active longer in response to word presentations among control participants, who presumably were unintentionally thinking about the words presented. In response to distracting sounds, long-term meditators relative to novices exhibited less brain activation in default mode network areas, including the posterior and anterior cingulate cortex and the precuneus. In another study, when participants completed MBSR training, default mode network structures, including the mPFC, superior temporal sulcus, and the precuneus, were less active in response to emotionally challenging stimuli (Farb et al., 2007, 2010).

These findings in aggregate suggest that the brain activities most clearly associated with normal self-referential thinking (the default mode network activity of medial brain areas) are likely reduced through the practice of meditative techniques and the development of mindfulness. This research may help us to understand the difference between the kind of self-reflection thought to be an important component of wisdom and the more commonplace narrative self-talk related to the default mode network and susceptible to maladaptive self-absorption.

Value Relativism/Tolerance

Acceptance that the world consists of diverse people with different beliefs and value systems, without judging them as "right" and "wrong" (*value relativism*), has traditionally been considered an important component of wisdom. Beyond *believing* in this abstract concept, tolerance requires the considerably more difficult task of *acting* on it. This may not be a universal a goal of psychotherapy, though one might argue that such tolerance is a basic component of health. And even if not taught directly, many therapists cultivate it in their clients through modeling—by accepting all that the client "brings to the table."

Neuroimaging studies of tolerance have primarily focused on the most prominent societal prejudices, such as race and ethnicity. Some investigations have demonstrated that the regulation of "automatic" prejudicial responses follows a neurobiological pattern similar to that already described for impulse control: The dACC presumably detects an undesirable attitude surfacing, at which time the lateral PFC inhibits the expression of the undesirable attitude and likely leads to downstream deactivation of the amygdala (Amodio et al., 2004; Cunningham et al., 2004). Other relevant evidence comes from theory of mind, which proposes, in part, that the lateral PFC inhibits excessive focus on oneself (see discussion in the section on self-reflection) in order that one may consider someone else's state of mind or view. Research on persons with lesions in the lateral PFC confirms this notion: These persons were very self-focused, preventing them from accurately interpreting social cues from others (Samson et al., 2005, 2007). Lieberman (2007) reviewed how the ability to recognize others' views and values may be linked to general inhibitory control provided by the lateral PFC, stating "a failure of this process may play a role in 'naïve realism,' when individuals assume that others see the world the same way as they do and have difficulty acknowledging alternative viewpoints" (p. 263).

Acknowledgment/Dealing Effectively with Uncertainty/Ambiguity

The inherent uncertainty of life causes angst for therapists and clients alike. Tolerance of ambiguity is an important theme not only in mindfulness-based psychotherapy, with its roots in Buddhist psychology, but also in psychodynamic, cognitive-behavioral, and other more traditional approaches. This subcomponent of wisdom has received sparse attention in biological studies. There have been some neuroimaging studies of persons confronted with risky versus ambiguous decisions. Krain, Wilson, Arbuckle, Castellanos, and Milham (2006) reviewed this issue by contrasting decision making related to risk (i.e., when outcomes have known probabilities and persons choose between "safe" and "risky" decisions) versus decisions made amidst ambiguity (i.e., when the probability of specific outcomes is either unknown or close to chance and the choices do not differ in reward value). They reported that making decisions in the face of ambiguity most consistently activated the dorsolateral PFC, dACC, and insula. In contrast, risky decisions activated the OFC, mPFC, caudate, and ventral ACC. Another investigation supported these finding in that persons who preferred ambiguous over risky decisions had higher activity in the lateral PFC, whereas ambiguous versus unambiguous decisions activated the dACC and dorsolateral PFC (Huettel, Stowe, Gordon, Warner, & Platt, 2006).

NEUROBIOLOGY OF WISDOM: LINKS TO CURRENT PSYCHOTHERAPIES?

In recent years, there have been several neuroimaging studies of patients undergoing psychotherapy. During a 16-week randomized, controlled trial comparing CBT with the antidepressant venlafaxine for major depression, both treatments had equivalent efficacy and showed several similar changes in neuronal activity in treatment responders as assessed by neuroimaging (Kennedy et al., 2007). These included decreased activity in the lateral PFC, medial PFC, and the OFC. Decreased medial PFC activity is congruent with this region's association with self-referential thinking, which in major depression is likely ruminative self-denigration. As hypothesized before, appropriately modulated mPFC activity may, together with emotional homeostasis, promote healthy self-reflection, but in excess may facilitate emotional distress inconsistent with wisdom.

Another treatment for depression is interpersonal psychotherapy (IPT). An early study (with the caveat of several methodological issues) compared IPT to paroxetine over 12 weeks for major depression (Brody et al., 2001). Those receiving IPT, similar to the CBT results above, showed decreased lateral and ventral PFC activity, which correlated with improvement in several depression symptoms. CBT is also extensively used for anxiety disorders, ranging from panic to social anxiety. De Carvalho and colleagues recently reviewed fear neurocircuitry and its relationship to panic disorder, noting patterns of decreased PFC and increased amygdala activity (de Carvalho et al., 2010). They reported on the limited evidence from two small trials of CBT for panic disorder, noting that in one open-label trial, responders had increased mPFC activity. This pattern is opposite that observed above for depression, but problematic methodology and small sample sizes limit interpretations of whether CBT has differential positive effects in depression versus anxiety. The model posited above regarding emotional homeostasis as a subcomponent of wisdom (i.e., lateral PFC down-regulation of amygdala hyperactivity) was supported by an experiment using cognitive reappraisal skills akin to those used in CBT among persons with social anxiety disorder (SAD) versus healthy subjects (Goldin, Manber-Ball, Werner, Heimberg, & Gross, 2009).

An open trial of MBSR for SAD assessed neuroimaging patterns of participants while performing an emotional regulation task (reacting to statements of negative self-beliefs for 12 seconds) before and after 2 months of weekly MBSR (Goldin & Gross, 2010). In descriptions of MBSR, concepts related to wisdom are quite apparent—emotion regulation, control of self-focused attention, and nonjudgmental awareness. When practicing breath-focused attention (a core technique of MBSR) after the therapy, improvements in SAD symptoms were correlated with increased activity in brain regions associated with attention, delayed peak amygdala activation, and lower baseline right amygdala activity. These changes appeared consistent with both a core mechanism of the therapy (attentional focus) and with the notion that decreasing amygdala activity would correlate with improved emotional homeostasis.

CONCLUSIONS

There are surprising similarities in the basic concepts of wisdom across cultures and over millennia, suggesting that the potential to develop wisdom is part of our shared biology. Indeed, age-related increase in human wisdom may have evolutionary significance in that it may serve to compensate for the biological losses that are characteristic of middle and old age, thereby enabling older adults to better utilize their remaining resources and age successfully (Jeste & Harris, 2010). Elements that are common to several modern definitions of wisdom include prosocial behavior/attitudes, social decision making/pragmatic life knowledge, emotional homeostasis, reflection/self-understanding, value relativism/tolerance, and acknowledgment of/dealing effectively with uncertainty/ambiguity.

Recent neuroscience research suggests that each of these traits may be related to the functioning of specific areas of the brain. The two regions of the brain closely involved in all of these components of wisdom are the prefrontal cortex and the limbic striatum, phylogenetically among the newest and the oldest parts of the brain, respectively. A balance between these areas seems to underlie wisdom. Recent studies have also shown that meditative techniques—and practices that developed in cultures throughout the world to support the development of wisdom—actually produce neurobiological outcomes that correspond with a number of the domains of wisdom, including prosocial behavior/attitudes, emotional homeostasis, and reflection/self-understanding.

Psychotherapy, which often involves one or more components of wisdom and increasingly involves meditation-derived practices, also has a significant effect on brain functioning as judged by functional neuroimaging. Future advances in neuroscience may suggest ways of developing psychotherapeutic interventions that cultivate wisdom while creating lasting and positive changes in brain function and structure.

PART IV

Clinical Applications

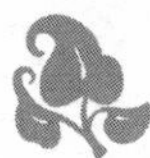

How are wisdom and compassion applied in the treatment of actual patients? Should we expect compassion and wisdom to naturally arise in any good therapy, or might we intentionally build them into treatment? The following chapters explore how wisdom and compassion may be implicitly or explicitly cultivated in treating a variety of psychological conditions.

Chapter 15 describes how radical acceptance (compassion) plus real guidance (wisdom) are necessary to help suicidal patients build a life worth living. The following chapter reframes substance abuse treatment as learning to make wise choices through careful observation of one's own experience without shame and self-blame. Chapter 17 applies similar principles to the treatment of anxiety disorders, emphasizing how the alternative–avoiding our experience–only intensifies anxiety, and how important it is to model mindfulness and compassion through the therapy relationship. Depression is the focus of Chapter 18, which explores how evolution has created a brain that can become depressed, despite our best efforts to the contrary, but we can also alleviate depression by tapping into our mammalian caregiving system. Chapter 19 describes how compassion and wisdom allow us to accompany and guide those who have endured extreme suffering in the form of trauma. Finally, Chapter 20 shows couple therapists how to help their clients grow in love by safely expressing their vulnerabilities and by sharing the depth of human experience–sorrows, fears, and joys–with one another.

CHAPTER 15

Compassion, Wisdom, and Suicidal Clients

Marsha M. Linehan
Anita Lungu

> It is not enough to be compassionate.
> You must act.
> —TENZIN GYATSO, the 14th Dalai Lama (2008, p. 70)

Every other year at the University of Washington I (M. M. L.) teach a graduate course on assessment and intervention with suicidal individuals. The course is open to clinical psychology graduate students and residents in psychology and psychiatry. The class always begins the same way: pizza on a Friday night, wine available to those who wish, and three questions: (1) "What is death?", (2) "Do individuals have a right to commit suicide; do you have that right?", and (3) "Does anyone have the right to stop another person from committing suicide; do you have that right?" Each person takes out a pad of paper and writes consecutively for 5 or 10 minutes on each question followed by sharing and discussion. Everyone then tears up their papers, letting go of the verbal products of their minds—products that are quite a valuable commodity for individuals still in academic training.

Working effectively with suicidal individuals requires this letting go of preconceived ideas about suicide, about people, and about the individuals who talk to us about the most important decision of their lives—to live or die. It also requires psychotherapists to integrate the knowledge gathered from clinical training and the research findings of the many studies of suicide and of complex disorders with the intimate knowing of the suicidal individual whose words are heard and face, body, and posture are seen. The suicidal person is like someone trapped in a small room with high, stark white walls but no lights or windows. The room is hot, humid, and excruciatingly painful. The individual searches for a door out to a life worth living, but cannot find it. Scratching and clawing on the walls do no good. Screaming and banging bring no help. Falling to the floor and trying to shut down and feel nothing give no relief. Praying to God and all the saints one knows brings no salvation. The room is so painful that enduring it for even a moment longer appears impossible; any exit will do. The only door out the individual can find is the door of suicide. The urge to open it is great indeed. The task of the therapist in this situation is to somehow find a way to get inside the room with the person, see the world from that person's point of view, and find that door to life that the therapist knows must be there. This view does not champion the idea of the therapist as the only expert in the room. Both must look for the door together.

This book is about compassion and wisdom in psychotherapy. In this particular chapter we're going to discuss compassion and wisdom in the context of working with suicidal individuals with severe and chronic multidiagnostic conditions. In doing so we're going to give an overview of dialectical behavior therapy (DBT; Linehan, 1993a, 1993b), a treatment rooted in behavior therapy, dialectical philosophy, and Zen practice developed to treat these severe and complex clients. After a brief description of empirical support for DBT and a rationale for how DBT concepts are related to compassion and wisdom, we'll go into more depth about core DBT concepts.

Initially proposed for treating severely suicidal and complex clients, DBT was subsequently expanded and tested for a variety of clinical populations: individuals meeting criteria for borderline personality disorder (BPD), for BPD and severe suicidality (Linehan & Shaw-Welch, 2002), for BPD and substance dependence (Dimeff, Comtois, & Linehan, 1998; Linehan & Dimeff, 1995), and for eating disorders (Safer, Telch, & Chen, 2009). Adaptations of DBT are ongoing for suicidal adolescents (Miller, Rathus, & Linehan, 2006) and children (F. Perepletchikova, personal communication, 2010). DBT was designated an empirically supported treatment by APA Division 12 and by the Substance Abuse and Mental Health Services Administration (SAMHSA), and the efficacy of the treatment has been assessed in 11 randomized, controlled trials across seven independent research sites (Clarkin, Levy, Lenzenweger, & Kernberg, 2007; Koons et al., 2001; Linehan, Armstrong, Suarez, Allmon, & Heard, 1991; Linehan et al., 1999, 2002, 2006; Linehan, McDavid, Brown, Sayrs, & Gallop, 2008; Mcmain et al., 2009; Soler et al., 2005; Turner, 2000; Verheul et al., 2003). Throughout these studies, DBT was found to improve a variety of behavioral outcomes, including decreases in suicidal behaviors, in nonsuicidal self-injury, depression, hopelessness, anger, eating disorders, substance abuse, and impulsivity, as well as increases in general and social adjustment and self-esteem (Lynch, Trost, Salsman, & Linehan, 2007).

We want to highlight, from the beginning, that DBT is not a treatment for suicide prevention—for keeping people alive at any price. Our goal is not to convince suicidal individuals to keep living lives of emotional agony. There would be little compassion or wisdom in such a treatment target. Indeed, one of the assumptions in DBT is that the lives of suicidal individuals are unbearable *as they are currently being lived.* DBT's ultimate goal is to help people build lives they experience as worth living, or in the terms of our metaphor, to effectively help them find that door out of excruciating emotional pain and back to life. The greatest compassion, therefore, is to find a way to help individuals change in ways that bring them closer to their own ultimate goals. The greatest wisdom is to provide an effective and efficient intervention to help clients reach their own ultimate goals. Such a venture requires that therapists believe that clients themselves have the capacity for wisdom.

It's hard to imagine a place where *compassion* is more critically needed than in working with individuals with severe disorders who are also suicidal, people who find life to be a living hell. How could therapists tolerate the hardship and emotional roller coaster involved when working with these clients without compassion? Indeed compassion, conceptualized as sympathetic consciousness of others' distress together with a desire to alleviate it (Merriam-Webster, 2006), is what drives therapists to get in that excruciatingly painful room in the story above. Feeling deep sympathy for another and a desire to help, however, are not sufficient to radically change the lives of severe, chronically suicidal people. As a former client recently said at a national meeting, love may have kept her alive but it did not treat her suffering. This point is made in a more poetic voice by Georges Bernanos (2002): "I know the compassion of others is a relief at first. I don't despise it. But it can't quench pain, it slips through your soul as through a sieve" (p. 261). Offering compassion without simultaneously offering concrete help in changing current behavioral patterns and circumstances is similar to going into that high walled room with the person, feeling the person's pain, feeling a deep desire to get the person out, but doing nothing to search for a door back to life. To use another metaphor, compassion without actual help would have the same effect that a fireman or -woman would have if, climbing the ladder to the window of a burning building, he or she empathized with the person about to burn to death instead of carrying the person to safety.

In sum, the most compassionate thing a therapist can do is effectively assist a client to achieve his or her own treatment goals. This approach requires a certain amount of faith in the client because without it, clinicians often impose their own goals on the clients they treat. Wisdom in this instance requires humility on the part of the therapist and a willingness to forgo the belief that he or she knows better what is good for a client. Like other professionals, therapists are paid to know how to help someone reach their goals. They are not paid to set the goals. Therapists are not parents, employers, guardians, or legal overseers of the clients they treat. They are their servants.

BEHAVIOR THERAPY, ZEN, AND DIALECTICS

DBT emerged out of a number of failed attempts to apply the standard behavior therapy of the late 1970s and early 1980s to treat individuals who were highly suicidal with multiple Axis I and Axis II disorders. The clinical research was funded by a small grant from the National Institute of Mental Health and the aim was to develop an intervention for highly suicidal individuals and then conduct a randomized clinical trial to determine whether it was, in fact, effective. That the treatment would blow up and fail was not in anyone's mind. But it did. There may be many reasons why the treatment failed, but the primary reasons reflect key dilemmas that emerged in therapy.

First, almost all of the clients were extremely sensitive to any approach that appeared invalidating or suggested that they, the clients, should change. Thus, a behavioral intervention that focused on helping clients change their own behaviors and emotional responses was experienced as extremely invalidating. A metaphorical way to describe their experience is to say that they didn't have emotional skin. Emotionally, they were like persons who have suffered third-degree burns throughout their body. Furthermore, not only was even the lightest touch excruciatingly painful, they also often lived in environments where everyone kept poking. In the context of this extreme emotional sensitivity, suggestions aimed at change were perceived as attacks or as further invalidation. Arousal and a sense of being out of control went up, collaboration went down, and no new learning occurred.

Switching to an approach of acceptance and validation of suffering did no better. The therapist's focus on acceptance and empathy, in the absence of change, felt invalidating of the clients' suffering. Acceptance alone communicated passivity or hopelessness on the part of the therapist. The therapist did not "get" the extreme suffering of the client and the client's desperate struggle to escape it. This approach generated such increased arousal and sense of being out of control that no new learning or collaboration was possible for the client.

Truth can be found in both of these approaches, since neither change nor acceptance alone is sufficient. Offering change without acceptance can feel rejecting, invalidating of one's experience, and painful. Acceptance without change can feel hopeless, invalidating of one's suffering, and again painful. The solution was to apply an approach that balanced acceptance and change strategies (Linehan, 1994). The key here was *balance*. The treatment dilemma was solved by developing a dialectical strategy of constant movement between acceptance and change strategies. Balance in this context is defined by what is needed in therapy, moment by moment, to go forward; it varies from client to client and for the same client from moment to moment. It is not necessarily created by an equal amount of acceptance and change. Lack of balance between acceptance and change leads to both the therapist and the client becoming stuck and consequently makes progress in therapy very difficult. In DBT, this interweaving of acceptance and change strategies, referred to as movement, speed, and flow, permeates the treatment. Compassion from the therapist requires radically accepting the client and the therapy itself as they are in the present moment, while at the same time working diligently to create the change that will allow clients to move toward their goals. Dialectics provides the theoretical framework for holding together the seeming opposites of acceptance and change. Wisdom within DBT requires applying the full array of necessary and effective interventions for change while simultaneously maintaining a dialectical stance: finding and keeping the balance between acceptance and change.

A second dilemma was that these clients had almost no ability to tolerate distress without escaping via dysfunctional behaviors. Suicide may have been viewed as a problem for the therapist but it was viewed as a solution for the clients. Drugs, sex, shoplifting, angry outbursts, self-mutilation, and countless other dysfunctional behaviors each functioned to immediately reduce unbearable suffering. The multiplicity of behavioral and emotional problems clients presented with—major depression, panic attacks, eating disorders, posttraumatic stress disorder, joblessness, homelessness, loneliness, and unbearably painful life events—could, and often did, create a chaotic therapy. It was immediately clear that without client abilities to radically accept one set of problems while they worked on others, therapy could not progress. It was equally clear that many aspects of clients' lives could not be changed and therefore had to somehow be accepted—their own past lives, their present circumstances, unwanted limitations on their future. The solution here was to find a way to teach these clients how to practice acceptance (a major change in itself) as well as how to change both themselves and their environments. A technology of acceptance as well as a technology of change were needed.

Here again there is wisdom in focusing on both sides of the dialectic: acceptance and change. Both the ability to make necessary changes as well as the ability to accept reality as it is are necessary for well-being. Teaching how to accept and tolerate intense pain, and also how to change painful circumstances, had to be brought together in a coherent balance.

The third dilemma was that therapists confronted with such high risk for suicide, combined with lives of immense suffering and tragedy, found themselves vacillating between overemphasizing change on the one side or overemphasizing compassion on the other side. The high risk of imminent client suicide often led to emotional dysregulation on the part of the therapist. Fear could easily morph into frustration and anger, and both would lead to angry attacks and efforts to control the client—almost never good ideas. On the other side, the immense suffering and tragic lives of the clients could also lead to therapist hopelessness, grieving, and falling into the pool of despair with the client. In both cases—anger and efforts to exert control, and hopelessness and grieving—effective therapy is abandoned.

Once again, there is truth in both sides. Clients must be pushed and chided at times. Contingency management, for example, is one of the most effective therapeutic strategies we have. On the other hand, warmth, joining with the client, and active compassion are also necessary. What was needed with out-of-control high-risk clients was a way for therapists to keep to the middle path between all out attempts at control on the one side and letting go and giving up on the other. For therapists working alone, with no support from their peers, consistently maintaining that middle path was difficult. We needed a community of therapists who could bring together acceptance and change and help each member keep a balance in their work. Therapists themselves needed to practice both acceptance and change. To create this balance on the middle path, DBT requires an active treatment team. DBT therefore can be defined as a community of therapists treating a community of clients.

Acceptance in DBT

The Role of Zen

The technologies of change afforded by behavioral interventions are, for the most part, highly effective and efficient. However, once it became clear that acceptance was needed, it also became clear that teaching distress tolerance and acceptance were not the forte of behavioral or cognitive therapies in the early 1980s. Thus, the question arose: Where to learn an approach to acceptance that could then be reformulated and taught to both clients and therapists? Mindfulness, widely incorporated into psychotherapies today, was not part of behavior therapy or even discussed as a possibility except behind closed doors. Behavior and cognitive therapies at the time focused on change—not on acceptance or even tolerance of distress (T. Wilson, personal communication). Alan Marlatt, a colleague at the University of Washington to whom this book is dedicated, published the first randomized trial on meditation in 1986 (Murphy, Pagano, & Marlatt, 1986) but did not find it effective for decreasing alcohol consumption. Jon Kabat-Zinn was teaching *vipassana* meditation plus yoga to people with medical disorders (Kabat-Zinn, 1982; Kabat-Zinn, Lipworth, & Burney, 1985).

At that time, mindfulness was not incorporated into nonbehavioral psychotherapies either. The most accepting Western psychological treatment for mental health problems was the Rogerian approach to therapy that emphasized unconditional positive regard (Rogers, 1959). There were two problems with this approach, however. First, the Rogerian approach emphasized the process of actualization. Such a process implies that individuals are "on the way" to actualization and perfection but are not there yet. Radical (i.e., complete) acceptance, however, required an approach that emphasizes that one is perfect as is, not that one is becoming perfect. Second, while the Rogerian approach placed enormous emphasis on acceptance and unconditional positive regard on the part of the therapist, it did not have a transparent method of teaching this same acceptance and unconditional positive regard to the client.

Alternative approaches were Western spirituality and Eastern approaches to both psychology and spirituality. However, an approach to acceptance that relied on religious concepts ran the risk of alienating atheists and individuals of alternative religious beliefs. A treatment was needed that could be accessible to individuals of all faiths and of no faiths. Across all religions, both West and East, at the mystical/contemplative level one finds love, compassion, and wisdom as core teachings and beliefs. Drawing from the contemplative rather than the ritual level of spiritual approaches seemed promising. Meditation and other contemplative practices exist across all religions; the idea was to find a way to learn these practices and then translate them into behavior therapy.

By happenstance and by following recommendations on who were good teachers of acceptance, the basis of the acceptance teachings in DBT are primarily drawn from Zen teaching and practice. Although not incompatible with any other contemplative practices, the simplicity of Zen practice made it a good match for behavior therapy. Three aspects of Zen in particular match well with behavior therapy.

First, neither Zen nor behavior therapy emphasizes the construct of an individual self (see also Chapters 4, 9, and 13). Indeed, neither even has the construct of an individual self within its theory (behavior therapy) or beliefs (Zen). (Both Zen and behaviorism would be easier to grasp if the entire language consisted only of verbs.)

Second, both view the universe as unified and connected, while at the same time recognizing individuality. Behavioral theory emphasizes the inextricable link between the individual and the context (or environment) and the inability to unlink one from the other. The following is a DBT exercise for developing awareness of our connection to the universe.

CONNECTION TO THE UNIVERSE

- Focus your attention on where your body touches an object (floor or ground, air molecules, a chair or armrest, your bed sheets and covers, your clothes, etc.).
- Try to see all the ways you are connected to and accepted by that object.
- Consider the function of that object with relation to you. That is, consider what the object does for you. Consider its kindness in doing that.
- Experience the sensation of touching the object and focus your entire attention on that kindness until a sense of being connected or loved or cared for arises in your heart.

The fundamental enlightenment experience of the Zen student is the experience of the unity of all things. At the same time, neither dismisses the individual. Behavior therapy pays exquisite attention to assessment of the individual and development of ideographic treatment plans. Its battle with the link between a categorical diagnosis and recommended treatment is, and always has been, on the failure of such systems to focus on the individuality of the client. In Zen, like the thread that makes up the one carpet, the individual is not ignored or dismissed. Koan practice, for example, is based on the individual relationship of the student with the teacher. As Willigis Jaeger Koun Roshi has noted, when saying "the wave is the ocean," one is not saying there is no wave (Jager, 1994; Jager & Quarch, 2000).

Third, practice prescriptions and proscriptions in Zen are highly compatible with behavior therapy. Consider this principle: "The first truth . . . is that life is suffering. Avoidance of suffering leads to worse suffering" (Aitken, 1982, p. 49; see also Chapters 4 and 9). This is the consistent theme of behavior therapists working with clients whose disorders are so often the result of avoidance of painful emotions and thoughts. Exposure to such emotions, thoughts, and events is part and parcel of most evidence-based behavioral interventions. Statements such as "Practice these things [wisdom, compassion, freedom] as if you already have them"

(P. Hawk, Roshi, personal communication) and "Act as if you always had compassion and then you will find you always did" are common in the teaching of Zen. Compare these to the treatment of phobia by getting clients to act the opposite of their urge to avoid and run away, and to *opposite action* in DBT where, when treating emotions that are ineffective, clients are taught to identify their urges and then to do the opposite, all the way. When afraid, act as if you are unafraid. When angry and judgmental, act as if you are compassionate and accepting.

Translating Zen into behavior therapy started from two different points. The first was teaching clients that they indeed had the capacity for wisdom. Similar to the idea that one already is enlightened, the idea was that each of us, including our clients, are already wise (see Chapter 4). The difficulty is experiencing our own wisdom, not attaining it. The skill of "wise mind" was developed by teaching clients how to go within themselves to access their own inner wisdom. Although not obvious to the naked eye, the idea also was that by going inside ourselves, each person has access to the wisdom of the universe. The second approach was to teach clients meditation and other Zen practices using instructions and terms that were compatible with the multiplicity of views of reality and the universe held by participants. This latter effort fell apart when participants refused to meditate, saying that they "did not do breathing" and other similar statements. At that point the task became how to deconstruct meditation into small pieces that could be taught. The focus was on the practices of both radical acceptance and entering into "just this one moment" that make up the essence of Zen practice, translated into behavioral skills. *Mindfulness* was a term already in use in psychology (Langer, 1989) and was also popularized by Thich Nhat Hanh in his book *The Miracle of Mindfulness* (1976). Thus were born the DBT mindfulness skills of observing, describing what is observed (without adding), participating, nonjudgmentally, one-mindfully, and effectively (using skillful means).

Drawing more from Christian contemplative practices, a second set of skills encompassing reality acceptance was also developed to help clients accept the lives that they had, even when those lives were not the ones they wanted. Similar to the concept of "Thy will be done," the skills of *willingness* (May, 1982) and *radical acceptance* go together with the skill of *turning the mind* to remind participants that both acceptance and willingness are active behaviors that have to be repeated—that is, turned to—over and over.

Radical Acceptance

The Middle English root for the word *accept* is *kap-*, meaning to take, seize, or catch. This root meaning more closely embodies the spirit of this discussion and is more accurate for our purposes than the modern meaning for acceptance, "receiving." *Receiving*, an aspect of acceptance, fails to convey how the practice of active acceptance requires careful observation, openness to experience, and tolerance of all that life presents. Acceptance is the developed capacity to fully embrace whatever is, in the present moment. It requires a spacious mind, an open heart, and strength to bear one's experience. A strict definition is required to avoid misunderstanding. Acceptance, although at times it might imply the following, does not necessarily mean resignation, agreement, approval, or passivity.

In DBT we use the term *radical acceptance* to more precisely define the kind of acceptance we strive to reach for ourselves as therapists and to teach our clients. When combined with the word *radical*, acceptance takes on a more complete meaning. It is *radical*, that is, far-reaching and thorough, affecting the fundamental nature of one's relationship to reality as it is. Synonyms for radical include such terms as *thoroughgoing, thorough, complete, total, comprehensive, exhaustive, sweeping, far-reaching, wide-ranging, extensive*, and *profound*. Radical acceptance does not come easily for the timid.

> It costs so much to be a full human being that there are very few who have the enlightenment or the courage to pay the price. . . . One has to abandon altogether the search for security, and reach out to the risk of living with both arms. One has to embrace the world like a lover. One has to accept pain as a condition of existence. One has to court doubt and darkness as the cost of knowing. One needs a will stubborn in conflict, but apt always to total acceptance of every consequence of living and dying. (West, 2003, p. 254)

The discipline of radical acceptance is not for the faint-hearted. Review the life of any major contemplative, any sturdy practitioner of acceptance, and you will discover an individual with deep reserves of mercy, patience, and compassion that they have come by the hard way. Gandhi, Martin Luther King, Jr., His Holiness the Dalai Lama, and Thich Nhat Hanh all adopted peaceful protest in their crusades for social justice. In doing so, they have demonstrated tolerance and understanding of their "enemies." None of these individuals can be described as passive. It is more accurate to view them as actively opening to life as it is, all the while seeking change.

Their example returns us to the root meanings of acceptance. It is receiving, seizing, and catching reality as it is. But, why bother radically accepting reality? Why tell our clients to confront helplessness, terror, losses, and accept other painful facts of their lives? Lack of acceptance of the facts of reality is deeply connected to avoidance, escape, and a prolonging of fear and suffering. Paradoxically, to change one's life is to first accept one's life as it is in the present. In DBT, acceptance strategies help therapist, client, and treatment teams tolerate themselves and one another, as they struggle together for change.

From the perspective of the therapist, acceptance includes radically accepting the client as he or she is in the moment. Change, including improvement, can be frightening to clients. Therapists must know their clients intimately and have the capacity to simply be present with them as they struggle with fear of change or hopelessness or terror of the unknown. And thus the therapist must accept the slow and episodic rate of progress in therapy. Often the most difficult thing for therapists to accept, though, is accepting the real risk of the client committing suicide and their lack of ultimate control over the life of the client. Although this is extraordinarily difficult to radically accept, lack of acceptance can result in the therapist's becoming rigid and controlling, perhaps thereby alienating and even rejecting the client as he or she is.[1]

On the other side, what is there to accept for the client? We can enumerate here some universal truths that are difficult for almost everyone to accept: the inevitability of pain, suffering, disease, old age, and death. For our clients, though, there may be other facts of their lives that they struggle to accept: the impossibility to change what was done to them in the past, such as abuse, trauma, invalidation, losses; the impossibility to change what they did to their children or to other people they care about; lost opportunities for achieving their goals and living fulfilling lives; limitations on what the future may bring. In the process of therapy our clients also need to accept and tolerate one set of problems in order to work effectively on another, as constant switching between problems in sessions is rarely productive.

As mentioned earlier, finding the balance between acceptance and change is the fundamental dialectic in DBT. If we could simply push our clients nonstop into a life of less pain and greater satisfaction, we would do so; however, the therapist who relentlessly emphasizes only change may discover too late that the client has had enough and is dropping out, literally or figuratively. Acceptance strategies, balanced against change, permeate the treatment in DBT. They inform the therapists' verbal and nonverbal styles of communication, their relationships with clients' environments, and the fundamental interventions implemented in individual psychotherapy sessions.

---

[1]This discussion of radical acceptance is adapted from Sanderson and Linehan (1999). Copyright 1999 by the American Psychological Association. Adapted by permission.

Validation as Acceptance

Validation is the central acceptance strategy in DBT and has been thoroughly described elsewhere (Linehan, 1997); here we give only a brief definition and describe the motivation for using validation in psychotherapy:

> The essence of validation is this: The therapist communicates to the client that her [*sic*] responses make sense and are understandable within her [*sic*] *current* life context or situation. The therapist actively accepts the client and communicates this acceptance to the client. The therapist takes the client's responses seriously and does not discount or trivialize them. Validation strategies require the therapist to search for, recognize and reflect to the client the validity inherent in her [*sic*] response to events. With unruly children parents have to catch them while they're good in order to reinforce their behavior; similarly, the therapist has to uncover the validity within the client's response, sometimes amplify it, and then reinforce it. (Linehan, 1993a, pp. 222–223)

Validation has a number of functions in psychotherapy. It balances the emphasis on change, preventing clients from feeling pushed too far too fast. It teaches clients self-acceptance and balanced self-assessment; as a result, they experience increased confidence in their judgment. Validation can strengthen behaviors through the principles of positive reinforcement. And finally, with validation of normative responses, the therapist communicates to clients when and how their behavior is reasonable, appropriate, and sensible. Taken together, these functions strengthen the alliance between therapist and client.

Reality Acceptance Skills

Acceptance skills are taught to both therapists and clients. These principles teach that emotional suffering often is created because we cling to things as we wish they would be, or think they should be, instead of accepting things as they are. Our attachment to our wishful thinking, our longings, our ideas of fairness and of what others should do, think, and feel can trap us in cycles of pointless longing and despair. The practice of nonattachment is frequently misunderstood as some effort to extinguish love, interpersonal attachment, warmth, and personal meaning. Attachment here, however, refers to the mind's habitual clinging to feelings, thoughts, and behaviors that are ineffective or not reality-based. Emotional suffering is created through this form of attachment and is distinct from the pain of accepting that what one wants cannot be. In addition to orienting therapists and clients to these principles, DBT leads them in guided practice of behaviors that enhance acceptance. These include mindfulness practices as well as exercises designed to cultivate a willingness to "be" with whatever reality presents.

Dialectics and DBT

As mentioned above, the theoretical framework holding the apparent opposites of acceptance and change (and others) together is *dialectics* (Linehan, 1995), also referred to as the logic of process (Wells, 1972). Dialectics in DBT is elaborated elsewhere (Linehan & Schmidt, 1995), so we will mention only a few key points here. Although most recently associated with Karl Marx, the philosophy of dialectics extends back thousands of years. Georg Wilhelm Friedrich Hegel is the one generally credited with restoring the dialectical philosophy. He discerned that specific forms or arguments come and go in a complex interplay, each argument creating its own contradiction, and each contradiction in turn being negated by a synthesis that often includes or enlarges upon both preceding arguments, beginning the entire process anew. What remains consistent, and thus becomes worthy of study and philosophical explication, is the process of change. From this perspective, it is not surprising that dialectics found a home within psychotherapy, since psychotherapy can ultimately be seen as a change process often resulting from the interplay of contradictions between therapist and client.

A dialectical worldview on the nature of reality and human characteristics has three primary characteristics: (1) The principle of interrelatedness and wholeness maintains that everything and every person is connected in some way (e.g., what clients do in their environment impacts how the environment responds, and vice versa); (2) the principle of polarity holds that everything is made of opposing forces or sides (e.g., there could be no concept for "right" without a corresponding "left"); and (3) the principle of continuous change and synthesis of polarities (e.g., when a client and therapist become polarized on a subject, the goal in DBT is to look for what is left out in each perspective and to reach a synthesis that incorporates points from both sides, thereby generating change in the system).

For our discussion of compassion and wisdom in psychotherapy, the third principle is the most relevant. It is the tension between polarities (*thesis* and *antithesis* in dialectical terms), such as parents and children, patient and therapist, positive and negative, in every system that creates change. The most fundamental dialectic in any therapy is that change requires acceptance of "what is," and acceptance of "what is" itself changes.

Wisdom in DBT

As with compassion, it is hard to imagine a place where wisdom is more necessary than in psychotherapy with severe, complex, and suicidal people. Therapeutic wisdom requires that therapists have the requisite knowledge and skill to apply treatment interventions that work, the ability to provide these interventions in a manner suited to the individual and his or her goals, and the willingness to admit when the therapist's interventions are not the most effective and efficient available. For a DBT therapist treating high-risk clients with complex, severe disorders, wisdom involves finding the middle path between change and acceptance. The Serenity Prayer is very relevant here:

> God, give us the grace to accept with serenity the things that cannot be changed, courage to change the things which should be changed, and the wisdom to distinguish the one from the other. (attributed to Reinhold Niebuhr [Bartlett, 2002])

Both client and therapist present with their own strengths, weaknesses, foibles, triumphs, senselessness, and inner wisdom. Both have goals that rest on change, and both present as individuals who must be accepted as who they actually are at this moment. The client comes to the therapist for wisdom, and the therapist must discover and bring out the wisdom that is inherent in the client.

Dialectics again provided an appropriate framework for a concept in DBT that is tightly connected to this process of bringing out of the wisdom inherent in the client: the concept of *wise mind*. This concept arose out of working with individuals with recurrently suicidal, dysfunctional, off-the-wall behaviors. These clients were so severely distressed that most people looking at them saw only abnormality, craziness, and disease. Being so stigmatized had a powerful iatrogenic effect in that the clients came to see themselves in this pathologized way. The concept that absolutely everyone is capable of inner wisdom countered this view. The term *wise mind* gave a name to the state of wisdom that, given the right tools, could become accessible to the person. The practices of both contemplative prayer (similar to centering prayer [Pennington, 1980]) and Zen suggest that wisdom is inherent in everyone.

Wise Mind

DBT presents to both clients and therapists the concept of "wise mind" or "wise knowing"—the inner wisdom within each person. Wise mind is in contrast to "emotion mind" and "reasonable mind." *Reasonable mind* is cool, rational, thinking, and logical. When completely in reasonable mind, one is ruled by facts, reason, logic, and pragmatics; values and feelings are not important. Reasonable mind is not balanced by emotions and values. *Emotion mind* is active when one's emotions control thinking and action. When completely in emotion mind, one is ruled by moods, feelings, and urges to do or say things; facts, reason, and logic are not important. In the spirit of dialectics, wise mind is the integration, the synthesis of, emotion mind and reasonable mind, and further includes intuitive, experiential, and/or spiritual modes of knowing.

A further definition of wise mind is the state of being wherein wise behavior (i.e., behavior that is just what is needed at the moment in the present context) is experienced as effortless even when the behavior is difficult. Wise mind is also the integration of "being mind" and "doing mind," concepts described by Jon Kabat-Zinn (1990) and expanded in the mindfulness-based cognitive therapy (Segal, Williams, & Teasdale, 2002). Here wisdom involves being aware and present while doing what is needed, employing what in Zen traditions is called "skillful means" (Gudo Nishijima & Chodo Cross, 2006).

In wise mind, we are open to reality in the here and now, as it is. Wisdom, wise mind, or wise knowing involves integrating all ways of knowing: knowing by *observing*, knowing by *analyzing* logically, knowing by what we *experience* in our bodies (kinesthetic and sensory experience), knowing by what we *do*, and knowing by *intuition*. It has qualities of direct experience, immediate knowing, understanding the meaning, significance, or truth of an event without having to analyze it intellectually, and feelings of deepening coherence.

It is sometimes difficult for clients (and therapists) to grasp what wise mind is, how to find his or her wise mind, how to tell when he or she is in wise mind. The following exercise illustrates one way to experience wise mind.

WISE MIND PRACTICE

- Imagine that you are by a lake on a warm, sunny day. It is a large, clear, very blue lake, and the sun is shining warmly on the lake.
- Imagine now that you are a small stone flake from a piece of stone near the lake and imagine being thrown out onto the middle of the lake, skimming onto the cool, clear, blue waters.

- Next imagine that you are slowly, very slowly, floating down in the lake, noticing all that is in the lake as you gently float down, floating down in the cool, clear blue waters, gazing at what is around you, and now settling on the clear bottom of the lake, at the center of the lake gazing at the clear waters and what is nearby.
- When you are ready, open your eyes, come back to the room, trying to maintain your awareness of that clear center that is within you.

We also use metaphors to describe wise mind:

> Wise mind is like a deep well in the ground. The water at the bottom of the well opens into the ocean of the universe which is wise mind. But on the way down there are often trap doors that impede progress. Sometimes the trap doors are so cleverly built that you actually believe that there is no water at the bottom of the well. The trap door may look like the bottom of the well. Perhaps it is locked and you need a key. Perhaps it is nailed shut and you need a hammer, or it is glued shut and you need a chisel. When it rains emotions, it is easy to mistake the water on top of the trap door for wise mind. (Linehan, 1993b, p. 66)

Or to describe finding and experiencing wise mind:

> Learning to find wise mind is like searching for a new channel on the radio: First it's like hearing a lot of static and you can't really make out the lyrics of the music, but over time if you keep tuning in, the signal gets louder, you know right where the station is, and the lyrics of the music become even a part of you, so that you can access them automatically, just like you can finish the lyrics immediately if someone starts singing a song you know really, really well.[2]

Clients who suffer from excruciating emotional pain require not only compassion (the feeling of deep sorrow for another and the desire to help) but also effective help to build meaningful change in their lives. DBT is a treatment that balances acceptance and change strategies within the theoretical framework of dialectical philosophy. Wisdom helps to maintain a balance between acceptance and change as our clients learn to find and experience their own wise mind.

[2]This metaphor was contributed by a participant to one of M. M. L.'s DBT trainings.

CHAPTER 16

Substance Abuse and Relapse Prevention

G. Alan Marlatt
Sarah Bowen
M. Kathleen B. Lustyk

> When we pause, we don't know what will happen next. But by disrupting our habitual behaviors, we open to the possibility of new and creative ways of responding to our wants and fears.
>
> —TARA BRACH (2003, p. 52)

We make hundreds of choices every day—from small decisions, like choosing what to wear, to big ones, like changing careers. Every choice bears consequences, and our smaller choices may lead to enduring patterns of behavior, some healthy, some detrimental, and most somewhere in between. For those who struggle with addictive behaviors, there is often an ongoing battle between the daily choices that may feel good in the moment and their frequently harmful consequences. Having a drink at the end of a stressful day may soothe the mind, but if one drink leads to several, the results are potentially far-reaching. Understanding the mechanisms that underlie these decisions and their consequences while creating balance between the challenging and rewarding experiences of our clients has been the hallmark of our work.

In our view, we can help people step out of the cycle of addictive behaviors by bringing awareness to the series of smaller daily choices that leads to enduring and often destructive patterns of behavior. First, however, people must be willing to enter treatment, which requires a compassionate, inviting approach to individuals who often feel blamed, shamed, and stigmatized by others' views of their behavior. Potential clients often avoid seeking treatment, for example, out of fear of being confronted, condemned, or even ending up in jail. There is a strong need for "low-threshold" treatment options that invite patients in, meeting them "where they are" rather than "where they should be." Once in a safe, nonjudgmental environment, we can begin to work on interrupting patterns and teaching skills to make wise choices. To change these well-worn behavioral grooves, we need both wisdom—to make considered choices—and compassion for ourselves and for those around us.

As many of the contributors to this book have pointed out, mindfulness provides an entry into making more skillful choices. In that mindful moment of a choice point, there is the potential to decide differently, even if we don't do this every time. Step by step, we can slowly create for ourselves a path that leads to less destructive behavior, accruing along the way a better sense of self-efficacy, positive growth, and confidence. We can begin to live our lives with a clearer intention, such that the tail is no longer wagging the dog.

A primary goal of our work has been to develop effective ways to help people with addictive disorders learn new strategies, behaviors, and attitudes to cope more skillfully with the inevitable ups and downs of life. Through raising awareness of, and compassion toward, our own behavior, we begin to make wiser choices and seek help and support when needed. This chapter illustrates how we have incorporated the critical elements of wisdom and compassion to help people with addictive behaviors learn to avoid the trap of seeing their behavior as "bad" and blaming themselves—judgments that motivate substance use. Our program for mindfulness-based relapse prevention (MBRP) is an empirically grounded therapy built upon principles of wise choice and self-compassion. It is designed to work with clients "where they are" while also helping them make changes that will bring greater freedom in their lives.

We begin with a case that illustrates how mindfulness meditation can enhance treatment outcomes by offering a metacognitive coping strategy for relapse prevention. We then describe a variety of strategies used in MBRP that are consistent with the principles of compassion and wisdom. Interwoven in this section are neurobiological findings that help to illuminate mechanisms by which mindfulness meditation may be helpful in reducing the risk of relapse among individuals who have struggles with addiction.

OUR FIRST MBRP CLIENT

We began the practice of using mindfulness meditation for treating addictive behaviors several decades ago with a single client. It all started when I (G. A. M.) received a phone call from a psychiatrist. I was asked to do an evaluation of Susan, whom he was treating for depression. After he had seen her for several sessions, she revealed that she also had a drinking problem. He told Susan that he could not continue to treat her depression until she had sought out treatment for alcohol dependence, and he referred her to a local inpatient alcoholism program. When she arrived for her appointment with me, she had already talked to intake workers at the residential treatment center. When I asked her how things were going, Susan replied:

"Everyone is telling me different things about the cause of my problems. My psychiatrist told me that I was trying to self-medicate my feelings of depression so that I could feel better in the short run. But then, when I went to the alcoholism clinic, they told me that it was the other way around: that my alcoholism was causing my depression, and that unless I stopped drinking, the depression would remain a serious consequence."

I asked about her thoughts regarding alcoholism treatment. Susan described her unwillingness to check in for a 28-day program, in which she would undergo detox and recovery training beginning the first day of admission. Knowing that she would be required to give up drinking on day one, she questioned whether she was willing or able to give up alcohol entirely.

"Drinking is the only thing I know that helps me overcome feelings of depression. Even though I know that in the long run my drinking problem is contributing to my depression, I can depend on it for short-term relief. It helps me relax and takes my mind off other problems in my life. It's the only thing that works and I can't give it up, even though my psychiatrist told me that he could no longer see me unless I was on the wagon."

It was clear that Susan was a prime candidate for harm reduction therapy (Marlatt, 2002), which is often indicated for those with co-occurring disorders who are unable or unwilling to pursue an abstinence-based treatment program. I explained to her that this approach was designed to reduce the harmful consequences of her drinking by helping her learn new skills both to handle her stress and depression and to moderate her drinking. I explained that she would learn to recognize cognitive and emotional factors that might enhance her craving (primarily based on the need to self-medicate her symptoms of depression) and begin to develop alternative coping strategies rather than "drowning her sorrows" in drink. Susan agreed to work with me on a weekly outpatient basis. Her first task was to keep track of her daily drinking using our self-monitoring forms (listing time of each drink, her mood level before and after each drink, and the setting). Based on this information (and her gender and weight), her daily blood-alcohol level chart could be plotted.

As our therapy progressed, it became clear that Susan's husband played a strong role in triggering her depression. Concerned about her drinking, he attended Alanon meetings (based on the 12-step disease model of alcoholism and designed for family or friends of alcoholics) and became convinced that his wife's behavior had to change. He accused Susan of being an alcoholic who was "in denial" and asserted that she should start attending Alcoholics Anonymous meetings and sign up for a residential rehab program. She described his anger toward her whenever he "caught" her drinking, and she expressed her overwhelming feelings of guilt, shame, and blame, all of which increased her depression, which in turn intensified her craving for alcohol. When asked if he would consider marital therapy as an option, her husband refused, saying, "My wife is an alcoholic–it's a chronic, progressive disease, and has nothing to do with our relationship."

The goals of our therapy included helping Susan acquire new coping skills to help handle more effectively her negative emotional states, including her anger at her husband (anger management training), and ruminations associated with feelings of guilt and depression. Many of these sessions were based on cognitive-behavioral theory and its applications for relapse prevention and harm reduction. In addition, we practiced some basic mindfulness-based meditation skills (breath meditation and the body scan exercise) to help with stress management; to begin to raise her awareness of her physical, cognitive, and emotional experience; and to provide an alternative to relying on alcohol to relieve tension (see Chapter 2).

A crisis occurred when Susan was arrested for a DUI. Although she was not driving at the time of the citation, her car engine was running as she waited to pick up her two children from school. After a serious argument with her husband earlier that day, she had consumed over half a bottle of sherry before driving to the school parking lot. Once there, Susan slumped over the wheel and was spotted by a passing police car and was arrested (her blood-alcohol level was over the legal limit). After meeting with her attorney and upon my recommendation, she agreed to sign up for a month-long residential treatment program, an abstinence-based approach that focused on cognitive-behavioral interventions, social support, and family therapy (although her husband refused to attend the family therapy weekend).

Following completion of treatment and a 2-week period of abstinence, Susan experienced another crisis. While driving through her neighborhood, she spotted her husband kissing another woman in his car. She drove straight to the nearest liquor store and bought a bottle of sherry, which she drank in its entirety, seeking refuge from her anger and rising feelings of anxiety and depression. After finishing off the bottle, she sought support from her best friend, a woman who also was an active practitioner of mindfulness meditation. After explaining what had just happened, her friend recommended that the two of them sign up for a 10-day *vipassana* (mindfulness or insight) meditation retreat. Within a few days, after Susan filed for divorce, they arrived at the retreat center. Once there, the participants were asked to take the "precepts," including the commitment to abstain from any intoxicants during the retreat.

After the retreat, Susan told me that when she took that precept, she knew without a doubt that she was going to follow it throughout and beyond the end of the retreat—that she was ready to give up drinking, once and for all. She said that when I first taught her meditation during our outpatient therapy, she found it to be the most helpful alternative coping skill in that it enhanced her feelings of relaxation and self-acceptance. Also, she said, it gave her a new perspective on recognizing urges and craving and applying mindfulness and nonjudgmental awareness as a metacognitive coping skill. Instead of giving in to the craving, she stayed with her experience, focusing on her breath until the urge passed. During our final meeting, I asked her if she still experienced feelings of depression and whether those feelings triggered thoughts about drinking. Susan replied:

> "Yes, I still sometimes get depressed and have thoughts about drinking. But you know, since practicing meditation, I no longer have to be dictated to by my thoughts. As you know, the word *addiction* and *dictator* have the same underlying meaning: Your mind or brain is telling you to do something, like take drugs or drink alcohol. But now, I'd rather practice meditation than rely on self-medication."

SUBSTANCE USE DISORDERS

As Susan's story so clearly illustrates, substance use disorders are essentially "chronic relapsing conditions" (Connors, Maisto, & Donovan, 1996). Although relapse appears to be an integral part of the recovery process—60% of individuals relapse following treatment (McLellan, Lewis, O'Brien, & Kleber, 2000)—significant shame, loss of confidence, and a sense of failure often occur following a lapse. This is an especially slippery time for individuals struggling with addiction. The negative thoughts and emotions following the first use after a period of abstinence are often very compelling, plunging an individual into feelings of self-hatred that can lead to further use. Coping in a compassionate way with lapses and the shame and doubt that follow is thus a crucial part of any relapse prevention program.

Understanding the neurobiological changes that ensue with substance abuse may help clinicians and loved ones develop greater compassion for the user, and may help the user cultivate self-compassion in the event of a lapse. Substances of abuse increase the release of dopamine within a complex neural circuit associated with pleasure and reward.

This circuit, often called the pleasure circuit, involves three regions: (1) a region within the midbrain (or mesencephalon) named the *ventral tegmental area*; (2) an area further up in the brain, the *nucleus accumbens*; and (3) a part of the cortex that lies behind the forehead, the *prefrontal cortex*. Collectively, these regions which make up the pleasure circuit are termed the *mesocorticolimbic* system. Irrespective of the primary pharmacological effects of abused substances, research teaches us that substances of abuse increase the release of dopamine within the mesocorticolimbic system, and this dopaminergic activity is rewarding or pleasurable. With repeated exposure to a substance, the pleasure circuit is less and less activated by the substance. At the cellular level, this decrease in the reinforcing properties of the drug reflects tolerance, which is subjectively experienced as the failure of the substance to meet expectations. To gain the desired effect, a higher dose is needed, which in turn results in more cellular adaptation and system dysregulation (for a review, see Kauer & Malenka, 2007). Thus, with substance abuse, the pleasure circuit becomes hijacked and abusers experience less pleasure from their drug of choice as well as a reduction in the subjective experience of "natural" pleasures. This diminution of pleasure can give way to pain, which may cloud one's judgments and abilities to make wise choices.

MINDFULNESS-BASED TREATMENT FOR ADDICTIVE BEHAVIORS

The MBRP program (Bowen, Chawla, & Marlatt, 2010) is designed to integrate mindfulness practices with cognitive-behavioral skills from Marlatt and Gordon's (1985) relapse prevention model to help addicts in early recovery maintain their treatment gains. Much of the program is based on the content and structure of mindfulness-based cognitive therapy (Segal, Williams, & Teasdale, 2002), and its intentions are to develop awareness of environmental triggers and internal cognitive, physiological, and affective reactions. Clients learn skillful responses in the face of these challenges through meditation and other mindfulness-based practices.

The meditation practices in MBRP are rooted in the *vipassana* (or insight) tradition. The word *vipassana* means "seeing things as they really are." This clear seeing comes from repeated observation of our experiences, as we learn to differentiate what is actually happening from the delusions our minds are so skilled at creating. This is a time, more than any, to counter the self-doubt ("I am a failure") with wisdom ("I made a mistake, and that is often where we learn the most") and compassion ("This is a difficult and painful journey; the kindest thing I can do right now is offer myself compassion").

Cultivating Wisdom and Compassion

MBRP begins with the assumption that wisdom emerges from observation of one's own experience. Observing the nature of mind and body in meditation allows awareness to develop. Over repeated observations, clients gain wisdom into their own minds and into the nature of being human. The practices and discussion throughout the course center on two basic questions: What is actually happening? What does my mind do with what is happening? By learning to differentiate between what arises (e.g., a physical sensation or an emotion) from how we relate to it (e.g., with judgment, aversion, clinging), we develop flexibility–whatever arises, we have a choice in how we respond (see Chapter 9). This is where we find freedom.

The MBRP program begins with simple observation of sensations, emotions, and thoughts through a series of practices and exercises. Clients are instructed to notice, too, how the mind is reacting to their experiences, and to practice, as best they can, a nonjudgmental stance toward whatever arises. The pervasive judgment and self-doubt so common in clients with addictions often appear in meditation practice, too. After a period of sitting practice, a client may comment that the mind wandered and there was pain in the body, accompanied by a sense of restlessness. Then perhaps a thought arises, such as, "I can't do this–I've messed up my mind so badly, I can't meditate." Here we have the opportunity to differentiate what actually happened (a sensation in the body followed by restlessness and distraction) from what the mind does with this experience ("I can't do this–I've ruined myself and can't do what normal people can do"). By bringing nonjudgmental (i.e., compassionate) awareness to this process, clients learn to observe the habits of the mind and to discern between observing and responding versus habitually reacting (see also Chapters 2 and 9).

The Neurobiology of Addictive Behaviors

If we turn again to the neurobiology, there is much we can learn about the habitual patterns of individuals struggling with addiction. Following the adaptation taking place within the pleasure circuit during early substance abuse, as described earlier, another pathway from the midbrain comes into play that further drives repeated substance use (Belin & Everitt, 2008). This pathway involves a brain region known as the *dorsal striatum*, which includes the caudate and putamen. Again, using dopamine as the chemical messenger, this pathway is implicated in a simple form of instrumental or reward-based learning. This kind of learning is behind the behaviors we call habits. According to Barry Everitt and colleagues

(2008), "drug addiction can be viewed as the endpoint of a series of transitions from initial voluntary drug use through the loss of control over this behavior, such that it becomes habitual and ultimately compulsive" (p. 3125). Interestingly, Rajita Sinha and her colleagues at Yale University have shown that in humans, the dorsal striatum, as part of the putative habit circuit, is activated during stress (Sinha et al., 2005). Thus, people with substance use disorders are likely motivated at the cellular level to habitually seek out and use their substance of choice when stressed. Moreover, this stress could be coming internally from craving, which may result from withdrawal sensations between periods of use. In response to this latter scenario, people with substance use disorders may habitually use substances to avoid negative sensations. So what might start with a conscious choice—Had a bad day? Have a drink. Just got out of a stressful meeting or presentation? Step outside for a smoke—over time becomes automatic, performed without engaging in a process of conscious choice.

In healthy individuals, the prefrontal cortex (PFC) can inhibit the habit circuit, contributing to our ability to make wise choices. In fact, the PFC is involved in many cognitive regulatory processes that are collectively called *executive functions*. Examples of these functions include cognitive flexibility, impulse control, emotion regulation, and planning. Thus, although we may be motivated to engage in a habit such as biting our nails or twirling our hair, we can consciously temper that motivation and desist from engaging in the persistent behavior. To do this, we recruit our PFC. Fibers from the PFC use the neurotransmitter gamma-aminobutyric acid (known as GABA) to inhibit various subcortical regions, including those involved in the putative habit circuit. Unfortunately, research indicates that individuals addicted to alcohol or other drugs experience gray matter loss in the PFC (Franklin et al., 2002). This anatomical deficiency is met with functional deficiency known as hypofrontality (Bolla et al., 2004; Mathalon, Pfefferbaum, Lim, Rosenbloom, & Sullivan, 2003). This means that the very region of the brain that might help a person with an addiction curtail his or her habit is deficient. This loss of functionality likely contributes to the pattern whereby persistent habitual drug use operates on "automatic pilot." Understanding the neurological mechanisms of addiction can also alleviate the shame associated with it.

While this cortical atrophy may seem grim at first blush, due to the neuroplasticity of the brain, regular activation of the PFC through meditation may actually help to restore this region. *Neuroplasticity* means that the cells comprising our brains can change with experience. Two independent studies (Hölzel et al., 2008; Lazar et al., 2005) have shown that prefrontal cortical tissue was significantly thickened in long-time practitioners of mindfulness meditation. Although these studies did not specifically assess individuals with substance use disorders, it is reasonable to expect that neurogenesis that results in functional cells capable of engaging in PFC activities, such as executive functions, would be profoundly beneficial in recovery from addiction and maintenance of abstinence.

Work from Richard Davidson's lab, described in Chapter 8, demonstrates that neural responses to emotional cues are modified by a compassionate state. The degree to which those observations translate into increased self-empathy might be particularly relevant to individuals struggling with addiction. As mentioned previously, individuals in early abstinence often suffer greatly in the wake of a lapse. This abstinence violation effect is characterized by feelings of guilt, shame, and self-degradation. Meditation practices that cultivate self-compassion are thus potentially therapeutic for these individuals (see Chapters 6 and 7). Since compassion practice is capable of increasing activity in brain circuits involved in empathy, it seems reasonable to expect that routine activation of the empathy circuit via compassion practice could induce self-empathy in individuals struggling with addiction.

Urge Surfing as a Practice of Compassion

In the second session of MBRP, clients practice an exercise called "urge surfing," adapted from Marlatt and Gordon (1985). This practice offers an alternative to the notion of "willpower" and is, at its core, an exercise in compassion.

URGE SURFING

- Bring to mind a situation in which you feel triggered or in which you experience urges to react in a way that is not in your best interest, whether engaging in substance use, lashing out, or perhaps withdrawing or isolating.
- As you imagine this scenario, pause right at the point at which you would typically react and observe the physical sensations, emotions, and thoughts that arise in that moment.
- Explore what it is like to pause right at that edge, without reacting. As best you can, soften into the experience rather than bracing against it.
- Notice how the wave of sensations, emotions, or urges swells in intensity. Rather than trying to fight the wave or being wiped out by it, see if you can stay with it, riding it to its peak as though surfing. Use your breath to stay with the experience, to stay steady, until eventually the wave begins to subside.

Clients often believe that the wave of intensity will continue to grow until they do something to stop it. In reality, these waves naturally arise and pass. This exercise gives them the opportunity to experience this ebb and flow for themselves.

There are, of course, times when it is skillful to take action, such as extricating oneself from a high-risk situation or engaging in another activity. However, through the practice of "staying with," rather than fighting or reacting, clients may gain the space within themselves to choose a response rather than reactively seeking an escape. They develop the capacity to hold all of this experience in their awareness without reaction, and the wisdom to see that these are all passing moments, and that no matter what the mind may say or the body may feel, they have a choice in how they respond.

Loving-Kindness Meditation

Practices of compassion, particularly self-compassion, may be especially challenging for those with addiction histories. Loving-kindness or *metta* meditation (see Chapter 3) can, for this reason, be an especially transformative practice for individuals—introducing kindness and well-wishes into the repertoire of potential responses to a situation or challenge. Beginning with exploring loving-kindness for a person or being that is easy to love, such as a child, a spiritual figure, or even a pet, can help open the doors of the heart. Clients then practice sending wishes for safety, strength, ease, and freedom from suffering to themselves, then to those around them. This offers an alternative to the often defensive, fear-based reaction to self and others. As one woman tearfully explained after a 10-day *vipassana* retreat in a women's prison, "I finally love myself." She had forgiven herself for what she saw as shameful behavior, hurtful toward herself and others, by developing her capacity to feel kindness toward herself.

Group Therapy

In sharing experiences with mindfulness practice in a group setting with others who have wrestled with addiction, clients often begin to take their particular stories a little less personally. This experience of shared struggle offers a sense of support that *sangha,* or community, can provide. Clients begin to see similar struggles and habits of mind in their peers, and they start to recognize that, although the daily-life manifestations may be different, the underlying patterns and tendencies of the mind are universal. They may begin to see their experiences as part of being human rather than as personal shortfalls; this is just how the mind works. Now, however, they have some choice. No matter what arises, they can *be* with the experience in a different way, allowing them to respond rather than react.

Generalizing Practice to Daily Living

Bringing this practice out into the day-to-day struggles of early abstinence, clients learn to recognize triggers and the subsequent physiological, cognitive, and emotional reactions. They learn to note these triggers, to pause where historically they have behaved reactively, and to observe their experience in that moment. They develop more skillful means for responding to urges, and they learn new strategies to cope with high-risk situations. Through practice, they discover that although the weather around them may be fierce and the stories the mind is telling may be compelling, there is still choice in every moment. By stopping and observing, there is an opportunity to recognize what is actually happening, "reground" themselves in the present using the breath, and respond from a place of wisdom rather than habitual reactivity.

Therapeutic Dialogue

MBRP therapists work with clients in a nonconfrontational, nonjudgmental, and compassionate manner. Informed by the approach of motivational interviewing (Miller & Rollnick, 1991), they help clients identify treatment goals and approach therapy with a collaborative, curious, and open-minded way. For example, clients are seldom taught *about* mindfulness. They are offered exercises and meditation practices, followed by an "inquiry" process (Segal et al., 2002) through which they discover and share their own experiences. They develop a personalized awareness and wisdom through a series of open questions from the therapist. Inquiry following a sitting meditation might look like this:

THERAPIST: What did people observe during that practice?

CLIENT: My mind wandered. I kept thinking about how I was late to group.

THERAPIST: Ah, yes. What happened when those thoughts came up? Did you follow them for a while? Did you come back to the meditation practice at any point?

CLIENT: I'd stay with the thoughts for a while, then I'd hear your voice again and try to come back to the exercise.

THERAPIST: So you're sitting here listening, trying to focus on your breath, then these thoughts arise and you get a little caught up in that story. Then you hear my voice and return to the practice again. Then what happened?

CLIENT: Then I'd focus for a second, then start thinking again.

THERAPIST: And then what? What did you notice?

CLIENT: Well, then I felt bad.

THERAPIST: Say more about "bad."

CLIENT: Guilty about being late, then frustrated that I couldn't focus. Then sort of defeated. Then I'd start thinking about that—about how maybe I can't do this meditation thing.

THERAPIST: Our minds can be pretty relentless sometimes, can't they? It sounds like you noticed a lot about your mind and what it tends to do, including the emotions that follow thoughts. Is any of this familiar to you? The mind getting sort of stuck in a story about something that's happened, even when you're asking it to stay focused on something else?

CLIENT: Yes! It sort of drives me crazy.

THERAPIST: Ah, so the frustration is familiar too? Do you remember how we talked about how meditation doesn't mean getting rid of thoughts? What we are doing here is getting to know our minds a little better, watching how they tend to react to events or sensations, and how that affects us. What you've described here is a beautiful example of how minds often work. The practice is the willingness to stay with it, to keep bringing the focus back to the breath as best we can, noticing when the mind wanders—because it will—then beginning again. And again and again and again.

Here the therapist explores the client's experience without agenda or judgment, approaching it with curiosity and acceptance. She reflects the client's experience in terms of the nature of mind rather than as a problem needing to be fixed. She offers compassion for this process by suggesting that it is just what minds do, and that practice is really the willingness to observe. The therapist models the qualities intended to be fostered through mindfulness practice: open-minded observation of all experience, acceptance of whatever arises, curiosity, and a nonjudgmental stance.

Outcome Research

Learning to respond to unpleasant experience in a mindful and accepting way, versus attempting to reduce, avoid, or resist the experience, shows promise across many populations (e.g., Dahl, Wilson, & Nilsson, 2004;

Gifford et al., 2004; Levitt, Brown, Orsillo, & Barlow, 2004). In the particular case of substance abuse, Witkiewitz and Bowen (2010) reported that following a mindfulness-based treatment for relapse prevention, those who completed the program, as compared to those in a control group, showed a weaker relation between depressive symptoms and craving. In other words, although they still experienced depressive symptoms, those symptoms did not lead as reliably to craving. In the control group, however, the experience of depressive symptoms remained significantly predictive of subsequent experiences of craving. Another study (Bowen & Marlatt, 2009) showed a similar pattern in college-student smokers: Those who participated in a brief mindfulness intervention, as compared to those in a control group, still experienced urges to smoke, but reported smoking fewer cigarettes over a weeklong follow-up period.

Still, the effects of compassion or loving-kindness practices, in and of themselves, on the neurobiology of addiction are unknown. However, researchers have begun to investigate the neurobiology of compassion meditation. This burgeoning area of research points to the recruitment of neural circuits that, in theory, could benefit an individual with addictive behaviors.

The short-term aim of compassion meditation is to generate a state in which an "unconditional feeling of loving-kindness and compassion pervades the whole mind as a way of being, with no other consideration, or discursive thoughts" (Lutz, Brefczynski-Lewis, Johnstone, & Davidson, 2008, p. e1897). The long-term goal of the practice is to enhance empathy for oneself and others and to inspire altruism, which requires focus on paying deep attention to experience. This attention should be aimed at understanding experiences in a heartfelt and nonjudgmental way. This type of attention can be characterized by attuning or assimilating. According to Buddhist philosophy, when we cultivate our ability to attend to, attune to, and empathize with suffering, we are more likely to engage in altruistic acts aimed at easing suffering.

It requires both wisdom and compassion to respond skillfully to adversity. We cannot eliminate all triggers, cravings, and challenging mood states that lead to addictive behaviors. We do have a choice in how we relate to these experiences, however. By practicing compassionate awareness and wise responding in their meditation practice, clients can successfully expand these skills into their daily lives.

CHAPTER 17

Anxiety Disorders
Acceptance, Compassion, and Wisdom

Lizabeth Roemer
Susan M. Orsillo

> When we simply experience fear just as it is—without our opinions, judgments, and reactions—fear is not nearly so frightening.
>
> —EZRA BAYDA (2005, p. 91)

Fear and anxiety are universal human experiences. Our bodies naturally ready themselves when threat is detected and prepare for potential threat with constant vigilance and tension. These responses are adaptive and have helped our species survive. However, our ability to imagine innumerable possible threats, and our potential for erroneously learning to fear harmless situations, people, and even thoughts or feelings, puts us at risk to develop a chronic and pervasive struggle with anxiety that can seriously diminish life satisfaction. Genetic vulnerabilities, traumatic experiences, and modeling of anxious responding are among the many potential risk factors for anxiety disorders. Despite these varied pathways, research suggests that anxiety problems may be perpetuated and increased by our common human tendencies to judge and avoid our own painful emotions.

Over the past 10 years, we have been developing and refining an acceptance-based behavioral therapy (ABBT) aimed at targeting these common processes and enhancing quality of life and satisfaction among individuals struggling with anxiety (Roemer & Orsillo, 2009; Roemer, Orsillo, & Salters-Pedneault, 2008). Our approach, grounded in cognitive-behavioral theory (e.g., Borkovec, Alcaine, & Behar, 2004) and informed by Rogers's (1961) emphasis on validation and unconditional positive regard, draws from other acceptance-based approaches such as acceptance and commitment therapy (Hayes, Strosahl, & Wilson, 1999), mindfulness-based cognitive therapy (Segal, Williams, & Teasdale, 2002), and dialectical behavior therapy (Linehan, 1993a, 1993b).

This chapter provides a brief overview of our understanding of anxiety and a description of how ABBT targets the key maintaining factors that may underlie anxiety. (Readers with interest in a more detailed discussion of the treatment should see Roemer & Orsillo, 2009, as well as Orsillo & Roemer, 2011, for a self-help approach.) Inherent in our approach is an emphasis on helping clients to (1) develop wisdom, or to come to see their experiences and lives more clearly, with reduced reactivity; (2) cultivate compassion, or a genuinely kind and accepting stance toward themselves and their suffering; and (3) flexibly choose skillful actions based in their enhanced understanding (i.e., act wisely). We discuss more explicitly how compassion and wisdom are addressed and cultivated in our treatment approach at the end of this chapter.

AN ACCEPTANCE-BASED BEHAVIORAL MODEL OF ANXIETY

Extensive research and theory come together to suggest a number of common, human processes that seem to underlie anxiety problems—factors that can be targeted with acceptance-based behavioral strategies.

Problematic Relationship with Internal Experiences

Many theories of anxiety highlight the ways that anxious symptoms themselves (e.g., worry, increased heart rate, tightness in one's chest, obsessive thoughts) occur commonly in the general population. Ongoing difficulties with anxiety seem to be associated with the *reactions* people have to these symptoms (e.g., judging them as catastrophic or negative, or seeing them as self-defining), rather than the symptoms themselves (e.g., Borkovec & Sharpless, 2004). For instance, people with and without generalized anxiety disorder (GAD) worry about the same things, except those with GAD also worry about their worry and view it as dangerous (Wells, 1999). Similarly, people with panic disorder respond to natural bodily sensations as though they are dangerous, paradoxically increasing the intensity and frequency of those sensations (Barlow, 2002). People with posttraumatic stress disorder similarly react negatively to their memories of traumatic events, as if they were happening again, increasing their distress (American Psychiatric Association, 1994). Furthermore, these "reactions to reactions" (Borkovec & Sharpless, 2004) generalize beyond symptoms of anxiety to emotions in general (e.g., Mennin, Heimberg, Turk, & Fresco, 2005).

These findings suggest that the problem isn't internal experiences (sensations, thoughts, emotions, memories) themselves, but the way that people relate to these experiences. Sensations of arousal, worried thoughts, and anxious feelings at times do signal true danger, which makes it easy to learn to fear them and harder to simply acknowledge their presence when they arise in nonthreatening contexts. Furthermore, these internal experiences are uncomfortable, often unwanted, and can require attention and resources, making it difficult to engage in the task at hand, so it is natural that people come to judge them as negative or threatening. This can lead to even more judgments and fear of the responses, increasing the spiral of distress and reactivity. People with anxiety disorders frequently describe this cycle, wherein any hint of anxiety evokes intense reactions that increase their fear and distress.

In addition to responding to internal experiences with distress, criticism, and judgment, people with anxiety disorders often become *fused* with their anxious experiences (Hayes et al., 1999). In other words, people come to define themselves by their symptoms, using language such as "I'm an anxious person," rather than "I'm a person who experiences anxiety at times." In this way, people become entangled in their own thoughts and reactions (Germer, 2005a). Seeing symptoms as all-encompassing further intensifies their negative impact, in part by increasing their seeming threat, making it even harder to continue to live a meaningful life in the face of anxiety and distress. This fusion with experiences of anxiety also often feeds self-criticism as people learn to see their anxious symptoms as defining signs of their inherent weakness. That's when a compassionate response to suffering is especially important, both by the therapist and by the client him- or herself.

This cycle also leads to confusion as it becomes difficult to accurately identify one's feelings because the reactivity to these experiences leads to general, undifferentiated distress, rather than to a clear emotional response. Because clear emotions give us important information about what's happening in our lives (i.e., enhance wisdom), these habitually muddy responses interfere with people's ability to live their lives in ways that are meaningful and satisfying.

Avoidance of Internal Experiences

Naturally, this tendency to view internal experiences as dangerous and threatening leads people to develop a habit of trying to avoid them. People struggling with anxiety often engage in a variety of internal strategies aimed at quieting their mind or dampening down their arousal. They try distraction, self-criticism ("Stop being a baby—get a hold of your nerves"), or positive thinking ("There is nothing to be afraid of"). Unfortunately, trying to change or avoid internal experiences (i.e., experiential avoidance; Hayes, Wilson, Gifford, Follette, & Strosahl, 1996) can paradoxically increase their frequency and intensity, feeding the cycle of distress rather than ending it. People with anxiety disorders often describe trying to put worries out of their mind or quiet their autonomic arousal, only to find themselves more upset. These failed efforts at control actually lead people to judge internal experiences more harshly as they seem to be out of control and unmanageable. They can also motivate experiential control strategies that are somewhat more effective in the short term, but self-harming in the long run, such as excessive engagement in "mindless pleasures" like shopping, Web surfing, television watching, overeating, or substance misuse.

Experiential avoidance interferes with the wisdom that comes from fully participating in the present moment. Engaging in cognitive avoidance strategies such as distraction or becoming caught up in worrisome thoughts about the future diverts attention away from the present, making it difficult to notice and attend to other important interpersonal or contextual cues. In addition to reducing the inherent satisfaction with living in the present moment, this cognitive and attentional avoidance or narrowing interferes with people's ability to learn from their current experience and deepen the emotional dimension of their lives and relationships.

Restrictions in Behavioral Engagement

People struggling with anxiety also aim to avoid experiencing painful thoughts and feelings by restricting their behavior, making matters even worse. Behavioral avoidance is a defining characteristic of anxiety disorders. People with social fears avoid public speaking or social events, people with agoraphobia avoid public places, and so on. Sometimes this avoidance is subtler. For example, someone with GAD may refrain from engaging in personally relevant experiences, such as opening up in a relationship or taking a risk at work, in order to avoid experiencing painful thoughts or emotions. Unfortunately, avoidance is strongly reinforced by the immediate, though short-lived, relief a person feels when he or she makes this choice.

When avoiding situations and experiences that could evoke anxiety becomes the central motivator of behavior, people's lives become narrower and less satisfying. Rather than allowing self-knowledge or wisdom to guide actions that could be valued and life enhancing, people become habitually focused on avoiding pain and staying safe.

TREATING ANXIETY

An acceptance-based behavioral approach to treating anxiety disorders explicitly targets the clinical processes we've been describing. Many other approaches to treating anxiety disorders similarly target these elements. For instance, traditional exposure-based approaches directly target behavioral avoidance and also implicitly target experiential avoidance by teaching clients that they can tolerate distress while they approach things that elicit fearful responses (e.g., Arch & Craske, 2008). In addition, the monitoring and psychoeducation commonly used in these treatments likely help clients to develop a different relationship to their internal experiences (one of observation and curiosity, rather than judgment and reactivity). We draw from these traditional behavioral elements, as well as mindfulness- and acceptance-based approaches, in our treatment of anxiety disorders.

Developing a Decentered, Compassionate Relationship with Internal Experiences

Psychoeducation

A central goal of our approach is to help clients to relate differently to their internal experiences. We use a number of strategies to accomplish this goal. A first, important element is psychoeducation about the nature of anxiety and worry, so that clients can begin to see their experiences as natural and understandable, as opposed to frightening and dangerous. Presenting a basic behavioral model of anxiety can help a client to view his or her own symptoms with more compassion and care, rather than seeing them as a sign of weakness or inability. When anxious responses are understood as a learned habit, it becomes much easier not to judge or react negatively to the experience.

Drawing from dialectical behavior therapy (Linehan, 1993a, 1993b; see Chapter 15), we also teach clients more broadly about the function of emotional responses. Often people come into therapy wanting to get rid of their distressing emotions, and they can't imagine how sadness, anger, or fear might be useful. By exploring the ways that these emotions give us important information about our own responses to situations (e.g., when our needs aren't being met or someone has taken advantage of us) and also other people's responses (through nonverbal communication of emotions), clients begin to see that emotions themselves are not a problem, but that instead it is reactivity to these emotions, or efforts to avoid them, that lead to difficulties. We make a distinction between *clear* emotions, which are a direct response to a current situation, and *muddy* emotions. Emotions may become muddy due to (1) failures in self-care (e.g., lack of sleep, unhealthy eating), (2) leftover responses to past situations (e.g., someone reminds us of a parent or past partner, or something upset us earlier in the day so that we respond with heightened intensity to a less significant event), (3) anticipation of future threats (e.g., worry), (4) judgment and reactivity to our clear emotions, (5) fusion with our emotions, or (6) efforts to avoid our emotions. By drawing this distinction, clients can begin to see that despite the core function of our emotions, careful attention and compassion are sometimes needed when muddy responses arise in order to clarify what, if anything, is being communicated. This awareness allows us to draw wisdom from our emotional responses, rather than being deluded or confused by them.

Self-Monitoring

Although psychoeducation can help to lay the groundwork, experiential learning is the most powerful way for clients to change the relationship they have with their internal experiences. One method we use from traditional behavior therapies is monitoring. We ask clients to monitor the signs of their anxiety (thoughts, sensations, behaviors) in a compassionate way, and to gradually add in monitoring emotions more broadly as well as efforts to control internal experiences. In doing so, they begin to develop an observational relationship with these internal experiences so that they can notice them as they arise and then write them down on a sheet of paper, rather than reacting to and becoming entangled with them. This simple process allows clients to *decenter* from these responses and to see them as experiences that naturally arise and dissipate, rather than as permanent truths or defining aspects of the self (Segal et al., 2002). In the context of this book, decentering from our experiences through monitoring is a wisdom practice (see Chapter 10). We not only develop a more flexible sense of self, but we have the possibility of responding to our discomfort in more skillful (i.e., wiser) ways.

Mindfulness Practices

Mindfulness practice provides another central experiential learning opportunity. We use a wide range of practices to help clients cultivate this new relationship with their internal experiences. Mindfulness, the process of paying attention, on purpose and with compassion in the present moment (Kabat-Zinn, 1994), provides an excellent opportunity to learn to notice when we become entangled with our internal experiences and how to disentangle ourselves, again and again (see Chapter 2). We ask clients to set aside regular time for formal practice (i.e., a planned time to practice the skills of mindfulness) and give them a progression of exercises designed to help them build these skills. We begin with physical sensations (mindfulness of breath, sounds, eating, bodily sensations), as these are often the easiest targets of attention.

We encourage clients to bring "beginner's mind" to routine tasks like eating and listening so that they can start to see the ways that judgments and reactions arise automatically, coloring their experience of even relatively neutral targets (e.g., "That sound is screeching brakes—people drive so poorly!" "That's a person laughing—why don't I ever laugh anymore?"). Once people notice how frequently the mind automatically judges even the most benign experiences, they can begin to feel kindness and compassion toward themselves for this very human habit. We encourage clients to gradually bring this practice of noticing things as they are, without judgment and criticism, to more complex, emotionally charged situations, such as difficult conversations with a partner or boss.

Next, we have clients bring their awareness to emotional responses. We might ask them to vividly imagine a time when they were sad and to bring awareness to any other emotions that arise, how these emotions rise and fall, and any efforts to avoid, during their recollection. We also use Rumi's poem "The Guest House" (Rumi & Helminski, 2000) to provide an image of welcoming and allowing emotions, rather than trying to bar the doors to keep them out, as so many of us have learned to do. Similarly, we introduce an exercise called "Inviting a Difficulty In," adapted from mindfulness-based cognitive therapy, in which clients recall a difficult situation and imagine softening their bodies to allow whatever responses arise for them. Each of these exercises encourages an opening up and turning toward emotions, rather than a bracing against and turning away. By engaging in this practice repeatedly, clients often discover that their emotions are less all-consuming than they had imagined. They also learn that they can tolerate the distress they have been avoiding for so long. This acquired wisdom allows them to live their lives more fully.

Several other exercises can help clients learn to decenter from their thoughts and emotions, observing them, rather than becoming caught up. Clients can imagine placing their thoughts on leaves as they float by on a stream (Hayes et al., 1999), or that their thoughts are clouds and they are the sky behind the clouds, to practice this new relationship to thoughts and feelings. Our clients also find the mountain meditation (Kabat-Zinn, 1994) to be a very helpful practice for connecting to a sense of stability in the face of changing moods and contexts.

In addition to formal practice, we emphasize the value of informal practice, which involves cultivating mindfulness while engaging in daily activities. Here again a progression can be useful. Clients often begin practicing being mindful while washing dishes, taking a shower, walking, or brushing teeth—times when they are likely to be somewhat less reactive and entangled with their experience. Our ultimate goal is for clients to be mindfully engaged in their life. Thus, over time, clients expand their practice to being mindful during a job interview, a stressful meeting, or a difficult conversation with a loved one.

Several challenges frequently arise when teaching mindfulness skills to clients who struggle with anxiety. First, it can be difficult for clients to fit regular formal practice into their lives. We are sure to explain why we think practice will be helpful, often using the example of training for sports where it is useful to do specific drills so that you are easily able to flexibly apply the skills during a game. We also suggest that briefer practices are more useful than no practice at all, and encourage clients to cultivate self-compassion as they develop this new habit. When clients truly cannot make time for any formal practice, we encourage informal practices so they can still engage in a regular practice each day, developing new skills of paying attention, in the present moment, with compassion toward oneself. For instance, busy parents of toddlers can shower mindfully or fold laundry mindfully to develop these skills.

Second, clients struggling with intense anxiety, who are critical and avoidant of their internal experiences, are seeking relief from their symptoms. Many clients initially find formal mindfulness exercises such as mindfulness of breath calming and relaxing, which can lead to unrealistic expectations or attachments to this state. We validate this reaction and also continuously emphasize that mindfulness involves bringing a compassionate, welcoming stance to the full range of internal experiences, including distress, enhancing one's engagement in life.

The Therapeutic Relationship

The therapeutic relationship is a powerful vehicle for changing the relationship clients have with their internal experiences. Self-compassion is actively and intentionally cultivated through a relationship in which the therapist validates the client's experience and accepts whatever responses and reactions the client expresses as part of being human. Therapists also strategically provide examples from their own lives that model the humanness of critical thoughts and judgments and the possibility of being kind to oneself in response to these reactions, rather than responding to judgment with more judgment and to criticism with more criticism. As with mindfulness practice, an emphasis on process is important here—we can cultivate self-compassion again and again and again, no matter how often judgments arise.

Flexibility and Experiential Acceptance

As clients begin to cultivate an accepting and compassionate relationship with their internal experiences and toward themselves, habitual attempts at experiential avoidance naturally diminish. Mindfulness exercises that focus on turning toward emotions or noticing thoughts and physical sensations help promote clients' willingness to approach rather than avoid their responses. This shift in turn allows for more wisdom and flexibility in behavioral responding, as clients can now choose their actions rather than habitually attempting to reduce distress.

Psychoeducation and experiential exercises that demonstrate the ways that efforts to control our thoughts, feelings, sensations, or memories can paradoxically increase the intensity and frequency of these responses, as well muddy our emotional responses, can also help to reduce experiential avoidance. For instance, we might ask clients to consider what it would be like to be Juan, who is having this experience—"I'm noticing some anxiety about asking Lena out. I really want a relationship so I'm taking a risk"—versus Carlos, who is having this experience—"I'm an anxious loser. Why can't I just get over this anxiety and ask her out? I'm so weak." Clients are also asked to mindfully monitor the consequences of experiential avoidance, and with time, they often come to learn that these efforts are neither successful nor life-enhancing.

We also try to promote emotional willingness by emphasizing that emotional responses evoke action *tendencies*, or impulses to act in particular ways, but they do not necessitate specific actions. Often clients respond to their emotions with heightened distress due to fear they will act from these emotions. For instance, Randy was extremely critical of his own anger because he was afraid it would make him yell and punch walls like his father did. He worked very hard not to feel anger, yet when his avoidance attempts backfired, he often found himself responding with exactly the kind of explosive rage he feared. Of course, this sequence only contributed to his sense of anger as an overwhelming and dangerous emotion and his intense self-criticism. Through monitoring and exploration, he began to see how his fear of his own anger, and subsequent attempts to suppress it, were actually intensifying his reactions and increasing the risk that he would act in unwanted ways. His therapist suggested that allowing anger to be present and bringing compassion to himself when angry, while still refraining from angry actions, might be a better strategy for living the life he valued.

Sometimes clients mistakenly believe that acceptance involves needlessly immersing themselves in emotional pain. To the contrary, acceptance requires us to use clarity and wisdom to know when an action is worth the pain it may elicit. A useful metaphor (adapted from Hayes et al., 1999) clarifies this concept. Imagine we are on our way to a beautiful mountain and we come across a swamp. If the swamp is to the side of our path, there's no need to jump into it and roll around—there's nothing particularly noble about purposefully wallowing in dirt and mud (or emotional pain). However, if the swamp is between us and the place we want to go, we'll need to walk through it to lead the life we choose. We can certainly go ahead and throw on some waders (if we have them) or put a plank across the swamp to try to minimize contact with the muck. In other words, we acknowledge that at times breathing can calm anxiety or a conversation with a good friend can lift our mood. And yet, sometimes there won't be any tools to lessen the messiness, or sometimes we'll trip and fall face first into the mud despite our best efforts. In these cases, we can just pick ourselves up, bring compassion to ourselves for enduring the challenging journey, tend to our wounds, and keep going toward our mountain. We can be willing to encounter any internal experiences that arise as we make our way through life in valued ways. Discerning an optimal path is a component of the wisdom cultivated in this approach.

Living a Life That Matters

We explicitly target the behavioral restriction associated with anxiety and anxiety disorders by helping clients clarify what matters to them and helping them commit to taking actions that are consistent with these values (drawing from acceptance and commitment therapy; Wilson & Murrell, 2004). By *values*, we mean personal choices regarding what is important, not externally imposed moral rules. As clients simultaneously develop mindfulness skills, we use writing assignments and exploration within sessions to help clients gain clarity into the ways that anxiety negatively affects their lives (in relationships, work/school/household management, and self-nourishment/community engagement), and articulate the ways in which they would optimally like to live in each of these domains. As clients come to appreciate the wisdom in their own emotional responses and gain a sense of strength from honoring their personal values, specific actions are identified that they can take each week between sessions to engage in their lives more meaningfully (e.g., sharing emotional vulnerability with a partner, being creative at work, engaging in community activities they value). We explore any obstacles that may prevent these actions and encourage clients to use self-awareness, acceptance, and compassion to effectively address them.

Throughout our work aimed at clarifying and promoting valued action, we emphasize the ability to choose actions regardless of internal experiences, an important element of wisdom (Olendzki, 2010; see Chapter 9). For instance, Soojin really wanted to develop close friendships and be honest and open with people in her life. Yet, she experienced such strong thoughts of self-doubt and inadequacy in social situations that she had learned to avoid speaking up or initiating social contact in an effort to avoid this distress. Inevitably, she continued to experience self-critical thoughts, including judgments about how socially isolated she had become ("I'm such a loser. I don't even have any friends"). Through her work with us, she learned to notice these thoughts and the feelings associated with them, as well as the action tendencies that were so strongly evoked when she felt discomfort. As she began to see these responses as natural and transient responses learned through the constant harsh and critical parenting she received from her foster parents, Soojin began to cultivate self-compassion and she committed herself to engaging in value-consistent actions even when her mind responded in its habitual way. She started small, asking people for notes after class to get more used to social contact, and then began to open up emotionally and pursue more meaningful contacts over time.

CULTIVATING COMPASSION AND WISDOM WITHIN THIS APPROACH

As noted throughout the chapter, ABBT aims to elicit the self-compassion clients need to accept their internal experiences and the wisdom they need to guide their behavior. Compassion is more explicitly addressed than wisdom, in that we help clients promote self-compassion as a direct counter to the habitual self-criticism and judgment that are closely tied to the experience of anxiety. Although we focus less explicitly on compassion toward others, we often find that as clients cultivate more kindness and understanding toward themselves, and as they start to see their emotions and self-judgments as part of the human experience, they naturally begin to apply this understanding to others, seeing people in their lives as human beings doing the best they can—just like they are doing. Often this clear perception promotes feelings of connection to others and reduces fears of others' judgments.

INVITING A DIFFICULTY IN AND WORKING WITH IT THROUGH THE BODY

- Before you begin this exercise, think of a difficulty you're experiencing right now. It doesn't have to be a significant difficulty, but choose something that you find unpleasant, something that is unresolved. It may be something you are worried about, an argument or misunderstanding you've had, or about which something you feel angry, resentful, guilty, or frustrated. If nothing is going on right now, think of some time in the recent past when you felt scared, worried, frustrated, resentful, angry, or guilty, and use that.

- Notice the way you are sitting in the chair or on the floor. Notice where your body is touching the chair or floor. Bring your attention to your breath for a moment. Notice the in-breath . . . and the out-breath. . . . Now gently widen your awareness, take in the body as a whole. Notice any sensations that arise, breathing with your whole body.
- When you are ready, bring to mind whatever situation has been stirring up difficult emotions for you. Bring your attention to the specific emotions that arise and any reactions you have to those emotions. And as you are focusing on this troubling situation and your emotional reaction, allow yourself to tune in to any *physical sensations* in the body that you notice are arising . . . becoming aware of those physical sensations . . . and then deliberately but gently directing your focus of attention to the region of the body where the sensations are the strongest in the gesture of an embrace, a welcoming . . . noticing that this is how it is right now . . . and *breathing into that part of the body* on the in-breath and breathing out from that region on the out-breath, exploring the sensations, watching their intensity shift up and down from one moment to the next.
- Now, see if you can bring to this attention an even deeper attitude of compassion and openness to whatever sensations, thoughts, or emotions you are experiencing, however unpleasant, by saying to yourself from time to time, "It's OK. Whatever it is, it's already here. Let me open to it."
- Stay with the awareness of these internal sensations, breathing with them, accepting them, letting them be, and allowing them to be just as they are. Say to yourself again, if you find it helpful, "It's here right now. Whatever it is, it's already here. Let me be open to it." Soften and open to the sensation you become aware of, letting go of any tensing and bracing. If you like, you can also experiment with holding in awareness both the sensations of the body and the feeling of the breath moving in and out as you breathe with the sensations moment by moment.
- And when you notice that the bodily sensations are no longer pulling your attention to the same degree, simply return 100% to the breath and continue with that focus as the primary object of attention.
- And then gently bring your awareness to the way you are sitting in the chair, your breath, and, when you are ready, open your eyes.

A challenging aspect of cultivating compassion (toward ourselves or others) is that judgments automatically arise when we notice how judgmental our thoughts are. Daniel, who was unemployed and very worried about his economic situation, noticed that he had intense negative reactions toward any person he saw driving a nice car or wearing nice clothes. He then had a lot of negative judgments about himself for these thoughts, mirroring the critical message he received from his parents any time he disclosed feelings of jealousy. Through validation, psychoeducation about the nature of thoughts and emotions, and mindfulness practice, Daniel developed self-compassion and was able to see the humanness of his responses, given his own circumstances. Once he was able to let go of the hatred and self-loathing he felt when these thoughts about others arose, he became less entangled with the judgments and more able to have compassion for others as well, including his parents, who had learned to respond critically from their own challenging histories. Beginning with validation and kindness toward ourselves, regardless of the kinds of thoughts we frequently have, is often a vital first step in loosening the hold those thoughts have on our minds, as well as our judgments of others (see Chapters 6 and 7).

Though we have not previously written about the concept of wisdom in ABBT, throughout this chapter we have attempted to demonstrate how ABBT allows our clients to tap into and benefit from their inner wisdom. Linehan (1993b) describes using mindfulness to cultivate *wise mind*, a perspective that balances the rational and the emotional in order to promote adaptive living. Similarly, we see cultivating a compassionate, open relationship with internal experiences, developing experiential willingness, and intentionally choosing mindful, meaningful actions as important aspects of wisdom (see Chapters 1 and 10). Reducing reactivity and entanglement with internal experiences allows people to understand situations and their own responses, and to respond with intentional choices that are consistent with what matters most to them. These wise actions are the ultimate intention of our treatment.

Several of the methods we've described facilitate the development of clients' wisdom. Psychoeducation lays an important foundation for understanding human responses by illuminating experiences of anxiety, our range of emotional responses, and the factors that contribute to ongoing suffering. This groundwork is fertilized with clients' own self-discovery through monitoring of their experiences, formal and informal mindfulness practices, experiential exercises, clarification of values, engagement in valued actions between sessions, and interactions within the therapeutic relationship. As clients develop their ability to turn toward their own experiences with increased compassion, they are more and more able to connect to their own inner wisdom (rather than their reactivity or preconceived notions) and use it to guide their actions. As Andrew Olendzki puts it in his discussion of Buddhist psychology, "Freedom means being able to choose how we respond to things. When wisdom is not well-developed, it can easily be circumvented by the provocation of others" (2010, p. 101). Our approach to treatment helps clients develop their wisdom so that they have the freedom to respond intentionally, rather than react automatically.

CLARIFYING VALUES IN RELATIONSHIPS

- Please set aside 20 minutes during which you can privately and comfortably do this writing assignment. In your writing we want you to really let go and explore your very deepest emotions and thoughts about the topic. You may want to take several minutes to practice mindfulness before you start, so that you can approach this task with openhearted awareness.
- As you write, try to allow yourself to experience your thoughts and feelings as completely as you can. Pushing these disturbing thoughts away can actually make them worse, so try to really let yourself go. Bring your mindfulness practice to the exercise so that you can accept and allow any reactions you have and continue to clarify what matters to you most. If you cannot think of what to write next, repeat the same thing over and over until something new comes to you. Be sure to write for the entire 20 minutes. Don't be concerned with spelling, punctuation, or grammar; just write whatever comes to mind.
- You may notice that you often have thoughts about why you cannot be the way you would like to be in your relationships. This is natural and we will explore these obstacles at other times. So, for this particular exercise, see if you can notice these thoughts as they arise and gently turn your attention back to how you would like to be, if you were not experiencing the obstacle, so that you can really explore what matters to you.
- Choose two or three relationships that are important to you. You can either pick actual relationships (e.g., "my relationship with my brother") or relationships you would like to have (e.g., "I would like to be part of a couple," "I would like to make more friends"). Briefly write about how you would like to be in those relationships. Think about how you would like to *communicate with others* (e.g., how open vs. private you would like to be, how direct vs. passive you would like to be in asking for what you need and in giving feedback to others). Think about *what sort of*

support you would like from other people and *what sort of support you can give* without sacrificing your self-care. Write about anything else that matters to you in your relationships with others.

Working with clients to cultivate wisdom and compassion requires that we cultivate wisdom and compassion (toward self and other) in ourselves as well. We are engaged in a constant practice of observing our reactions and our clients' reactions with compassion and curiosity, and seeing our humanness reflected in one another. By sharing this process with our clients, we can learn from their wisdom, just as they can learn from ours.

ACKNOWLEDGMENTS

We are grateful to the National Institute of Mental Health for supporting our work and this chapter through Grant No. MH074589. We also thank the clients, therapists, colleagues, and loved ones who constantly deepen and expand our understanding of anxiety, compassion, and how to live a meaningful life.

CHAPTER 18

Depression
Suffering in the Flow of Life

Paul Gilbert

> If we have a realistic attitude and understand that problems are naturally bound to arise in one form or another, it's a simple fact of life, we will be more effective in coping with the problems when they arise.
> —TENZIN GYATSO, the 14th Dalai Lama (2009a, p. 196)

Although depression can take many different forms and vary in severity, chronicity, and age of onset, its symptoms are all too familiar. They include a loss of motivation, the inability to experience pleasure, and a sense of being wrapped in a cloud of hopelessness and pessimism. One feels physically tired, on edge, racked with feelings of dread, permeated by a sense of being inadequate. The darkness of depression can engulf us in such despair and entrapment that suicide seems the only release. The experience of depression is sadly very common; the World Health Organization (2011) estimates that the world prevalence could be 121 million people or more. Population prevalence rates vary between 3 and 10% depending on the exact definition of depression and the social contexts in which it is measured. Not surprisingly, communities enmeshed in poverty tend to have much higher rates of depression than wealthy ones.

We also know that depression is not a creation of modern life, although modern life may increase the rates of depression and other mental health problems (Twenge et al., 2010). Indeed, tales of depression stretch back to our earliest records (Jackson, 1990). Biblical characters such as King Solomon suffered black moods, linked to his belief that he had angered God and was no longer favored. We should also not be too species-centric in our notions about depression because it is likely that many animals are also afflicted. They can certainly behave as if they are depressed, and animals have been used in a vast number of research studies on depression.

Depression can be understood from many points of view (e.g., genetic, biochemical, brain state, psychological, and social) (Power, 2004), but none elucidates exactly how to develop the necessary wisdom for engaging and connecting with this deep darkness of the mind. In this endeavor we can use our evolved ability for thinking, reasoning, intuiting; we can even use objective science. Wisdom with compassion is not an abstract metaphysical set of beliefs, aspirations, or personal orientations, but emerges from careful study, analysis, and reflection. We treat physical diseases by studying them in detail, discovering their nature and what heals them. Countless diseases and conditions—from smallpox to malaria, diabetes to brain tumors—have revealed their secrets after centuries of medical inquiry. Similarly, the basis for wise compassion is understanding and using our human brain—a unique organ that can grow to understand ourselves and our world; to build on the thoughts, knowledge, discoveries, and experiences of those long dead; is *willing* to learn; and *desires* to heal.

So wisdom is more than knowledge—it is how we build knowledge over generations and integrate it into a set of values and a way of being in the world. As Monika Ardelt (2003) suggests, wisdom is a multifaceted concept linked to cognitive, reflective, and emotion-related elements (see Chapter 1). First, there is a facet of *motivation* to understand, an openness to the new—seeking knowledge rather than relying on tradition or superstition. Second, wisdom involves the ability to *reflect* on the human condition, on human nature, and to grapple with complexity and paradox (e.g., death, decay, and suffering). Third, *wise reasoning* enables us to think about situations from different points of view and to cultivate a calm mind (mindfulness), minimizing projection and emotional reasoning and allowing us to learn from experience. Fourth, *emotions* underpinning wisdom are based on compassion and caring, on the wish to relieve suffering and promote prosperity for ourselves and others. Meeks and Jeste (2009) suggest that wisdom involves a range of prosocial attitudes and behaviors together with reflective and informed decision making, and that these qualities are underpinned by a number of neurotransmitters such as dopamine, serotonoin, vasopressin, and oxytocin (see Chapter 14). Understanding the nature and functions of wisdom is particularly important to both Buddhist psychology and evolutionary approaches to mental suffering as outlined in this chapter.

THE EVOLUTION OF MIND

While depression has many roots, it usually touches our search for meaning. Descent into the darkness of depression may begin with the loss of a loved one, a personal defeat, trauma, abuse, or the onset of a painful and crippling illness. We seek to understand "Why *this*, why *now*, why *me*?" The meanings we give to pain, trauma, and tragedy are important in how we deal with them in ourselves and in our patients. For many depressed people the answers to these questions tend to be self-focused—it is something about the self rather than "the nature of things" that resulted in loss or failure. In contrast, Buddhist and evolutionary approaches emphasize the development of more objective insight, a standing back from the personal to recognize and understand the universal roots of suffering (see Chapters 4 and 8).

An important biological discovery from the past that can contribute to human wisdom is the concept of *evolution*. Evolution provides a key insight that we are all products of the *flow of life*—genetically designed beings that exist in this universe, at this point in evolutionary time. We can enjoy the benefits of a flexible, nonreified sense of self (Chapter 13) or an interconnected, less individualized self (Chapter 12) from the perspective of biological evolution.

Human beings evolved out of the struggles of millions of other life forms, most now extinct. Our gene-built brains and bodies reflect variations in the basic mammalian blueprint. Our genes are built on primate motivational systems, supplying desires to form attachments to our parents and peers; to want to love, be loved and valued; to desire sexual relationships that are not necessarily monogamous; to want to protect and promote our own survival and that of our kin; and to want to belong to and be accepted by groups (which in turn feeds the dark side of tribalism and hatred of the out-group). We see these social motives and desires acted out in many species all over the world. Carl Jung (1981) used the word *archetypes* to describe the psychological experience of these universal dispositions that evolved in the flow of life.

Our genetic endowment builds brains and bodies that can detect and react to threats with alarm, anxiety, or anger; to good things with pleasure; and to setbacks with disappointment and a dip in mood. So, as in many other animals, anger and aggression can flare up when we're faced with conflicts and obstacles; anxiety can cause flight and avoidance when dangers arise; and the loss of positive feelings and abilities to engage in the world (depression) can pattern our minds when we are confronted by major losses and stresses we feel unable to control. Depression has thus haunted the mind of many living things—it is the brain's way of defensively shutting down under conditions of adversity to maintain attention on threats and losses (Gilbert, 1984, 1992, 2005, 2007b; Nesse, 2000). So as a basic defensive strategy, the capacity for "depression" long preceded the emergence of humanity.

A second insight that grows out of this fundamental understanding of "how we are built" is that much of what goes on in our minds—the urgency of our desires, the power of our emotions, and depth of our moods—is not of our personal design nor of our choosing *and therefore is not our fault.* Depression is something we would never choose, and it is only made possible because evolution has designed it within us as a potential strategy. My experience is that when depressed people really understand the evolution of mind, and why depression is not their fault, it can help cut through the deep-rooted shame and self-criticism associated with feelings of weakness, inadequacy, or worthlessness. These dark states arise because depression often carries with it the feeling that there's something wrong with ourselves—we are failures, inadequate losers, unwanted, trapped in pain, and a burden to others.

A third insight is that evolution itself is immensely painful. We all just find ourselves here with our genetic orientations and guidance, susceptible to multiple diseases from genetic vulnerabilities, viruses, bacteria, parasites, and injuries to our frighteningly fragile bodies. Indeed, evidence suggests that viruses have been very important to the evolutionary process itself because of their ability to create genetic mutations, but the diseases they cause can inflict severe pain and dysfunction to us and to those we love. The bottom line is, we evolved for, and by, reproduction—the replication of genes through generations. We did not evolve *for* happiness as such but to navigate the challenges of survival and reproduction (Buss, 2000).

Even if things go relatively well, we will grow, blossom, and then slowly decay and die, as will everything and everyone we love. We hope that our decay will not be prolonged in the clutches of a dementia or some other wasting disease, but decay we will because this is the nature and destiny of all biological beings—a life process we never chose. Like the characters in films such as *Blade Runner* and *Moon*, we come to realize that although we feel unique and individual, actually we are clones of our parents, patterned from their genetic sharing and shaped by our social experiences. We have to make sense of this extraordinarily short, painful reality of being born from genetic material that has evolved over millions of years, with a brain capable of creating a sense of self with a desperate wish to continue to live free of suffering and to find meaning—yet knowing we are destined to decay and die.

Many have come to believe that happiness is not for this life but for the next (McMahon, 2006). Many have argued too that the reality of the pain, tragedies, impermanence, and fragility of existence can be so difficult to bear that we constantly turn away from them. So we focus on achievements—to secure our careers and those of our children; to make money and not have to worry about our next meal; to live in comfortable, warm, watertight houses; to afford medical insurance to protect us (at least sometimes) from the pain of disease and injury. We also know that as an evolved social species we can take great comfort from relationships with others (Cozolino, 2007). In fact, from the day we are born to the day we die, the love, kindness, and support we receive from others will have a huge impact on our physical and mental health in the face of life's painful realities (see Chapters 1 and 8). However, at other times we will feel unable to achieve our goals, feel misunderstood, criticized, or socially isolated. Within our own heads we will be self-critical or even self-loathing rather than self-compassionate. Under these conditions we can easily slip into depressed states.

THREE EMOTION REGULATION SYSTEMS

Depression is a brain state (Gilbert, 1984, 1989, 1992, 2007b) and knowing how brain states are generated neurophysiologically can help us better understand them and develop ways of cultivating the healing qualities of compassion and wisdom that can be such powerful antidotes for depression. Three emotion regulation systems play important roles in both positive and negative brains states (Depue & Morrone-Strupinsky, 2005). Each system has a specific function, with specific triggers and outputs. The three emotion regulation systems (depicted in Figure 18.1) are:

1. Threat detection and response system
2. Drive, resource-seeking, achieving, activating system
3. Contentment, soothing, affiliative system

Each system is described below. Of course, the systems are more complex than this and constantly interacting to create blends of feelings and even conflicts between feelings. For example, one might be very motivated to approach and meet a potential sexual partner but also anxious about being rejected. The balance of these emotions will determine the emotional color of the mating game, or whether we even bother to give it a try.

The Threat System

The most basic system, "our factory setting," so to speak, is our threat system, whose purpose is to protect us. With various modifications we can plot its basic design and structures back through evolutionary time,

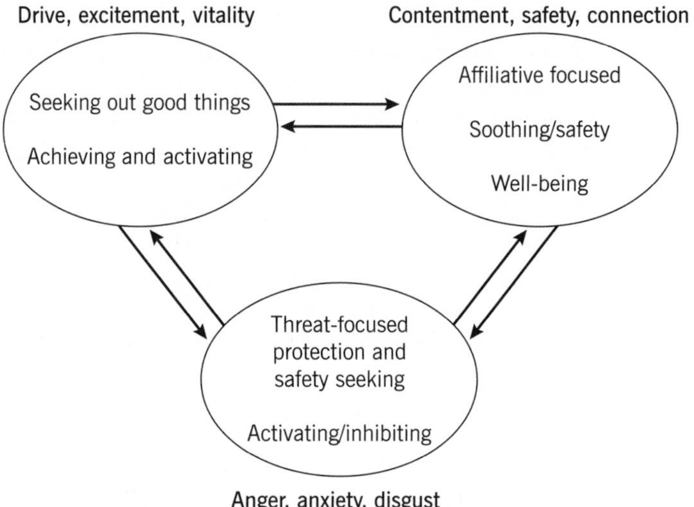

FIGURE 18.1. The interaction among our three major emotion regulation systems. From Gilbert (2009c, p. 22). Copyright 2009 by Paul Gilbert. Adapted with permission from Constable & Robinson Ltd.

recognizing similar brain mechanisms for dealing with threats in the rat, rabbit, and monkey (LeDoux, 1998; Panksepp, 1998). One of the major areas of this system is the amygdala, which responds very rapidly to signals indicating threat or disappointment—often before conscious thinking arises. The threat system can bias and focus attention, activate defensive emotions (e.g., anxiety, anger), and generate defensive behaviors (e.g., fight, freeze, or flight) (LeDoux, 1998). We detect and respond to threats faster than we do to positive stimuli, and we remember painful events more easily than we remember positive ones (Baumeister, Bratslavsky, Finkenauer, & Vohs, 2001). If you go to a shopping mall and nine shop assistants are kind to you but one is rude, chances are you will remember, talk to your partner about, and ruminate on the rude one—and not the fact that you encountered nine (90%) kind shop assistants! That is the nature of a threat system—it is remarkably easy to focus on what threatens us and get caught in spirals of threat-focused thinking and ruminating.

It is the threat system that is typically involved in mental health difficulties (Gilbert, 1989, 1993), and depressed people have elevated sensitivities here. Early frightening experiences, particularly those related to abuse, can have a permanent impact on threat processing systems, with increased risk of depression later in life (Bale et al., 2010). We also know that depression is linked to rumination on threat-focused themes that constantly stimulate the threat system (Cheung, Gilbert, & Irons, 2004; Watkins, 2008). So, a combination of genes and early learning can give us a brain that, through no fault of our own, is highly focused on possible threat and easily stressed and depressed.

The Drive and Achievement System

Depression is not just about feeling threatened and stressed–it is also about the loss of positive emotion and hope, sometimes referred to as *anhedonia*. This state is more complex than commonly thought for two reasons. Not only can anhedonia relate to different concepts (e.g., loss of drive and motivation, which is different from loss of positive feeling [e.g., joy]), but we also have two different types positive feeling and emotion systems. The distinction between these two systems is very important for working with depressed people and for understanding the alleviating power of compassion.

Depue and Morrone-Strupinsky (2005) distinguished a drive, resource-seeking, achievement, and activating system from a contentment, safeness, affiliation, and soothing system. The drive system is especially linked to dopamine and can be triggered by anticipation of, or actual, rewards. For example, if we win the lottery and become millionaires, chances are that we will have a mild hypomania, associated with dopamine activation, racing thoughts, excitement states, and difficulty sleeping–at least for a day or two. In contrast, defeats, setbacks, and uncontrollable stress can deplete dopamine, leaving us feeling exhausted and unable to feel or anticipate pleasure (see Gilbert, 1992, 2005, 2007b, for evolutionary explanations).

Much has been written on whether Western society seriously overstimulates this dopaminergic system, with its constant focus on needing to achieve and own more and more, media that glorifies celebrity, and materialistic, competitive computer games–all leading to increased stress and exhaustion (Pani, 2000). Western society appears to be promoting extrinsic goals of self-promotion, self-fulfillment, and achievement at the expense of intrinsic goals of cooporation and community building, with clear indications of deteriorating mental health consequences in the last 30 years (Twenge & Campbell, 2009). These findings make very plain that individual mental states are linked to social and cultural values, discourses, and structures.

Depression becomes more serious when individuals *identify* with the state and *see themselves* as worthless, personally inadequate, or failures. It is one thing to feel one has failed in a situation but quite another to see *oneself* as a failure. The state may unlock memories of feeling defeated or powerless, perhaps from abuse or being labeled as inadequate, useless, or bad.

The Contentment, Safeness, and Affiliation System

The contentment system is subjectively quite different than the drive system. It gives rise to positive emotions associated with well-being, peacefulness, and calmness. The neurochemistry of this system is linked to neuropeptides, especially oxytocin and the endorphins (Carter, 1998; Depue & Morrone-Strupinsky, 2005). Many wisdom traditions focus on developing a *contented* and *compassionate* mind (Hofmann, Grossman, & Hinton, 2011). This focus is in complete contrast to Western competitive values of striving and achieving, followed by judging, rating, and ranking self and others. This is not a mind without ambition (e.g., the Dalai Lama travels the world keen to enhance spiritual values), but it is a mind that is cautious about, and aware of, how it engages the seeking and ambitious drive system.

Recent research has shown that the endorphin and oxytocin systems, which seem to underpin feelings of contentment, safeness, and well-being, were adapted during the evolution of mammalian attachment and social affiliation (Bell, 2001; Depue & Morrone-Strupinsky, 2005; Wang, 2005). In fact, feeling loved, cared for, and supported is probably one of our most of important sources of contentment and well-being (Mikulincer & Shaver, 2007). In addition, these social affiliative experiences can play a fundamental role in regulating our sense of threat. It is also the case that the evolution of mammalian infant attachment, whereby the infant stays close to the parent and the parent protects and regulates the needs and physical state of the infant, was marked by major changes in the regulation of the sympathetic and parasympathetic nervous system (Porges, 2007)—along with an important evolving role for the neurohormone *oxytocin*.

There is now good evidence that oxytocin facilitates attachment behavior and opens individuals to trusting, affiliative possibilities (Carter, 1998; MacDonald & MacDonald, 2010). When an infant, child, or adult is distressed, physical affection (in voice tones and with holding and cuddling) stimulates the oxytocin and endorphin system, calming distress. Repeated throughout childhood, this process of affection leading to calm stimulates the growth of neurophysiological pathways that have major effects on our ability to regulate emotions and moods and to develop a positive sense of self that does not collapse under the weight of setbacks or failure (Cozolino, 2007; Siegel, 2001). The endorphin–oxytocin system, associated with feelings of well-being and connectedness that help us feel safe (Carter, 1998; Wang, 2005), may also underpin feelings of bliss and connectedness associated with meditative or transcendental states (Coxhead, 1985). Affiliative experiences may exert their powerful effect on threat and stress states through oxytocin receptors in the amygdala, which down-regulate threat responses (Kirsch et al., 2005). So from the day we are born to the day we die, the kindness of others will have major physiological impacts on our brains and bodies (Cozolino, 2007, 2008). The same is true for *self*-kindness, in contrast to self-criticism or self-hatred (Neff, 2003a, 2003b, 2011b).

Although humans have understood the importance of kindness for thousands of years, it's only recently that we have begun to see that our brains *are biologically set up* to need kindness to function optimally. We are a species whose bodies and brains are designed to detect and physiologically respond to kindness (Gilbert, 2009a; Mikulincer & Shaver 2007; Wang, 2005). It is *completely unscientific* and certainly unwise to dismiss compassion and kindness as nice but "soft and fluffy." Although people have a variety of fears about showing and experiencing compassion (Gilbert, McEwan, Matos, & Rivis, 2011), the scientific evidence from physiological, psychological, and social research is that compassion has powerful effects on our bodies, minds, and relationships (Carter, 1998; Cozolino, 2007; Wang, 2005).

Depression

Looking at depression in terms of our three affect regulation systems, we know that depressed people have increased threat processing (i.e., they are more prone to experience anxiety, anger, irritability, and dread) *and* reductions in the two types of positive affect. When the drive system is toned down, we may experience an inner deadening, a loss of motivation, and decreased ability to enjoy, look forward to, or feel excited about things. Food, sex, and holidays can seem pointless or just too much effort. The world is gray, black, and lifeless. When in a deep depression, we can feel full of dread, regretting each morning we wake up. We may feel like inadequate, defeated failures.

When the soothing and affiliative systems are toned down, we experience ourselves as cut off from others, disconnected, alone, isolated, unloved, and unwanted. It is difficult to feel affection or understanding. It is as though there's a kind of barrier between us and others. There may even be types of depression that are slightly more oriented to one system or another (defeat or loss of connectedness) and, of course, the blends of these systems can be very subtle.

The potential for depressed brain states has been built into us via evolution. That is not our fault—and by becoming compassionately mindful of this blamelessness, we can learn to not identify with these states of mind. It's like water that can be dyed blue, yellow, or green—the water is not the color. So it is with depressed brain states, with all of the bodily feelings and self-evaluative systems that are part of it. These can be separated from the essence of the self—the experiencer can be separated from the experience.

The Ruminative Mind

A biological view of how the mind evolved and how the nervous system functions allows us to become wise—to see our mental processes in perspective—when we are depressed. A depressed brain state includes a human capacity for rumination, pessimistic projection into the future, and self-judgment. These processes constantly activate the threat system by holding in mind stressful events or engaging in self-critical and self-deprecating evaluations. Our self-aware mind can activate, maintain, and even accentuate and amplify the basic defenses of anxiety, anger, and/or depression. Just as our fantasies of sexual scenes can stimulate pituitary-mediated physiological arousal, causing changes in our bodies, so our own focus on self-critical or hopeless thinking stimulates our brains in certain ways. Our thinking, fantasizing, and ruminating affect the balance and relationship between our three affect regulation systems. Uniquely for humans, the world we create in our heads—in which we live—can trap our minds in suffering by stimulating basic evolved physiological systems (Gilbert, 2009a, 2010c; Siegel, 2010a, 2010b).

DEVELOPING COMPASSION AND WISDOM IN THERAPY

Compassion can emerge from the insight that we are all caught up in the flow of life with brains that we didn't choose and that are capable of some very painful mental states. This is absolutely not our fault—we're hardwired to feel bad at times. When a patient really understands this basic fact at a deep level (and this can be promoted by the therapist gently repeating in a soft, slow voice "This is not your fault" at appropriate moments), it is not uncommon for the patient to become tearful as he or she lets go of struggle and blaming.

Wisdom can also develop from the insight that we're part of an evolutionary process; we are creatures with inbuilt programming and social conditioning. Each of us could be different versions of ourselves had we grown in different environments. I often say the following to my patients: "If I had been adopted at birth into a Mexican drug cartel, chances are I would either be dead by now, could have killed other people, could be in prison, or could be rich. These are the likely paths for young males in those environments. Paul Gilbert, a professor of psychology interested in compassion-focused therapy, would never have existed."

Compassion-Focused Therapy

It is against this background that compassion-focused therapy (CFT; Gilbert, 2000, 2009b, 2010a, 2010b) teaches people about the three affect regulation systems. The first task in this approach is to understand current problems by building a narrative of life history to develop a formulation. Next, we work with key external (e.g., social relationships) and/or internal threats (unhelpful, intrusive, or ruminative thoughts or feared feelings and memories). In addition, the therapist tries to stimulate the drive system, helping people become more engaged and active in their lives. However, from a CFT point of view, because the soothing affiliation system is so fundamental, all interventions need to be experienced in the spirit of compassion, kindness, encouragement, and support–and it is here that many depressed people, especially those high in self-criticism and shame, may particularly struggle (Gilbert, 2007a, 2010b).

CFT focuses specifically on the *feeling tone* of an individual's efforts to recover. Those who use cognitive approaches might advise patients that negative thoughts are only theories and can be tested by thinking of alternatives, considering different perspectives, or imagining what they would say to a friend in a similar circumstance. Attention-focused therapies might take a more Buddhist position of cultivating mindfulness–teaching us how to be more observant without judging our thoughts, not overly identifying with their content or emotional textures (Allen & Knight, 2005; Williams, Teasdale, Segal, & Kabat-Zinn, 2007). In CFT, however, more attention is given to the *emotional experience* of, say, considering the alternative thoughts. For example, having the thought that "It's understandable why I'm lying in bed because I'm depressed, but getting up might help me feel a little better and might help me get going" can be heard in one's head in a neutral, matter-of-fact way, in a fairly aggressive way ("Come on, get up, you lazy so-and-so!"), or with a real warmth and compassionate understanding for the difficulty of depression and the kind encouragement needed to act against it. In CFT the focus is on *kind* and helpful attention, thinking, feeling, imagery, sensory focusing, motivations, and behavior; the emphasis is on *feeling the kindness* and the caring intent in any intervention (Gilbert, 2000, 2009a, 2009b, 2010a, 2010b).

CFT is rooted in evolved attachment and affiliative processes whereby a compassionate "other" can provide a safe base for soothing and calming threat and distress responses (as a mother might provide for her child) and that facilitate exploration and engagement with both the outer world and the inner world of feelings (Feeney & Thrush, 2008). Similarly, creating an inner compassionate sense of self can create a safe base for working on painful feelings and memories. This is especially important for people who are avoidant of emotion in general (e.g., suffer from alexithymia) and find it hard to think about feelings without being overwhelmed or frightened of them. This difficulty is associated with problems in empathy (understanding one's own feelings and those of others) and mentalizing/ metacognition (being able to think about one's own and other people's actions as linked to intentions, desires, and beliefs) (see Allen, Fonagy, & Bateman, 2008; Lysaker, Gumley, & Dimaggio, 2011). Clearly such difficulties may interfere with mindfulness and developing compassionate insight and wisdom.

WORKING COMPASSIONATELY WITH A DEPRESSED MIND

Exercises in CFT are designed to (1) create an inner "safe base" that links to the soothing system, (2) enhance our ability to mentalize, and (3) help us to engage difficult feelings. We primarily use compassionate imagery and focused attention. Imagery can have a powerful effect on our physiology, perhaps even more than the use of words (Stopa, 2009). In CFT, imagery is focused on a number of different domains, described below. Detailed descriptions of these and many other imagery exercises can be found in Gilbert (2009a, 2009c, 2010c) and in training materials at *www.compassionatemind.co.uk*.

Developing the Inner Compassionate Self

The aim of this category of exercises is to create a sense of a "compassionate self," just as actors do when they are trying to get into a role. Here the individual focuses on the qualities of compassionate attention, thinking, feeling, and behavior. This focus provides a new perspective for considering emotional challenges–a perspective that is quite different from that of, say, the "angry self" or the "anxious self." One way of developing the compassionate self is as follows:

- Assume a relaxed posture and begin breathing in a soothing, rhythmic manner, focusing a little longer than usual on the out-breath, allowing your body to slow down.
- Now imagine yourself to be a deeply compassionate person. Think about all the qualities you would have if you are a deeply compassionate person—then imagine having them. Like an actor, recall when you were kind to someone and let yourself become that person in posture, facial expression, and mood.

- Next, imagine yourself as wise; feel that focus in your body—given that you know that all people are struggling to be happy, that we are not in control of everything that happens to us, that we are not to blame for our human frailty, and that "we all just find ourselves here" by the tide of evolution.
- Imagine yourself with the confidence, strength, and authority that arise from this understanding. Focus on that sense of authority and confidence and your natural wish to relieve suffering and promote well-being in yourself and others.
- Reflect on this state of mind and sense of self.
- Put time aside to connect with and try to sense and become your compassionate self.

Compassion Flowing Out *to Others*

This category of exercises follows the practice above–after we have learned to evoke a compassionate self. The focus here is on experiencing compassion for others and how that feeling can lead to feeling connected and safe. For example:

- Bring to mind a living being who naturally makes you smile. This could be, for example, a beloved child, a pet, or dear friend.
- Remember how we are all vulnerable beings—all in this life together—subject to stress, injury, and misfortune.
- Connect with your compassionate self and direct warm feelings toward a loved person, wishing him or her to be happy and free of suffering. Focus on the positive feelings that arise if this occurs—the joy of others' happiness.
- When the feeling of warmth and goodwill is flowing through your body and mind, extend your goodwill to other people whom you know and love.
- If you wish, you can even begin to include other people in your circle of compassion, including those you might have seen but don't know.
- Enjoy the experience of feeling compassionate toward others.

You might eventually want to send good wishes to people who are challenging in some way. This is an advanced practice and is used less often in the early stages of CFT. It's similar to but also different from traditional Buddhist loving-kindness meditation (Germer, 2009; Salzberg, 1997). However you want to practice, try to create a compassionate state of mind. Keep in mind that it is the focusing and intentions that are important; the feeling states may come and go.

Compassion Flowing into *the Self*

Here we focus the mind on receiving the kindness of others, attuning to the relief and sense of safety that arise when we are the receivers of compassion. We may recall *specific episodes* or *events* when people have been kind to us. In another set of exercises we may focus on creating and imagining an *ideal compassionate being*, one who has your best interest at heart.

- Create in your mind an image of an *ideally* caring and compassionate figure, someone who embodies the qualities of unconditional acceptance, warmth, quiet strength, and wisdom. Evoke an image beyond human fallibility, just right for you in terms of age, gender, parental qualities, and so forth. The key is to evoke a *sense* of the compassionate figure—the exact physical characteristics are less essential.
- Now direct your attention to the inner wisdom that your compassionate ideal embodies—sensing his or her strength, kindness, and complete commitment to your well-being. What might your compassionate ideal say to you, or how might this being relate to you, knowing the challenges that you are facing in your life right now?

This exercise is similar to the Tibetan Buddhist practice of using compassionate Buddha images (*avalokitesvara*; also known as *chenrezig* in Tibetan traditions) in a prescribed manner (Vessantara, 1993; Choden, personal communication). There are also important female figures such as Kuan Yin–"she who hears the cries of the world"–that can be used for visualizations (Karcher, 2001). While there is increasing evidence that meditating on loving-kindness and compassion (including compassionate images) can exert powerful psychological (Fredrickson, Cohn, Coffey, Pek, & Finkel, 2008; see Chapter 3) and neurophysiological (Lutz, Brefczynski-Lewis, Johnstone, & Davidson, 2008; see Chapter 8) effects, research is yet to explore how creating one's *own* image of compassion might compare to traditionally prescribed images that are laden with cultural importance and meaning.

Many imagery-based therapies use exercises similar to the one given above (Frederick & McNeal, 1999). In CFT, the point of working with a compassionate image is to stimulate the brain system related to the image. In this case, it's the safeness/soothing system. Other types of images affect the brain and body in their own unique ways, such as imagining a sexual image or a frightening image. Where and how we choose to direct our attention can have an important impact on our well-being.

Compassion toward Oneself

One of the key challenges in overcoming depression is switching from self-criticism (even self-hatred) to self-understanding and self-compassion. One way to practice this new relationship with oneself is to first evoke the "compassionate self," and then imagine looking at oneself in the mind's eye and try to develop a sense of compassion for being depressed. Then as you do this, say, "May you be happy, [say your name]; may you be free from suffering, [say your name]; may you flourish, [say your name]."

We can also use the compassionate self to work with *parts* of ourselves that are troubling, such as the "angry self," "anxious self," "self-critical self," or with difficult memories and situations with other people (see also Chapter 13). Here's an example:

- Engage your compassionate self (as above) for a few minutes.
- Now focus on a challenging aspect of yourself or of a situation. For example, it might be when you feel anxious or angry and in conflict with someone. For a moment picture yourself in your mind's eye as anxious, angry, or in conflict; note how you look and the expressions on your face, how you talk and how you want to act.
- Now, looking as this aspect of self though the eyes of your compassionate self, direct compassion toward the troubled part of yourself. With your compassionate sense of authority, wisdom, and care, just focus on sending compassion to help that anxious, angry part of you or your conflict.
- Note how that part of you responds to your holding it compassionately.
- If you become entangled in difficult emotions, you just return to slow, rhythmic breathing, and refocus yourself on your compassionate self for a while.

Self-compassion exercises such as this one can be rather difficult to do, especially for depressed patients. Feelings of unworthiness and fear are likely to emerge, often negative core beliefs that were internalized to maintain connection with primary caregivers in childhood (see Chapter 7). However, through gradual exposure to genuine compassionate intentions and desires, these emotional obstacles can be recognized and transformed.

CFT uses the "safe base" of a compassionate mind state from which to experience and desensitize difficult emotions. Otherwise, powerful emotions or traumatic memories can be overwhelming or traumatizing. Compassion is not so much about *soothing away* difficult experience as about developing the courage and support to *engage* what is frightening or overwhelming. This is similar to the ancient Buddhist practice of "feeding your demons" (Allione, 2008). Germer (2009) provides an excellent range of exercises for the development of self-compassion in the therapy context, first using mindfulness to safely anchor awareness and then moving into loving-kindness practices (see also Allen & Knight, 2005).

WISDOM AND COMPASSION REVISITED

Today we know that our feelings and moods are rooted in our evolved brains—that our brains were designed not by us but within the flow of life. Our tendency to think and feel as we do evolved for purposes of survival and gene replication, not for happiness. Through the lens of wisdom, we can see that anger, anxiety, and depression are related to our basic brain design, but they are not "us." Our capacity to generate these emotions and moods is absolutely not our fault. Indeed, some of us even have built-in genetic biases toward depression. We are not helpless, however. As this book well attests, wisdom and compassion practices gleaned from both the East and West can help us effectively engage our evolved, socially shaped minds to enhance our well-being.

With insight and practice we can influence our mental patterns. Wise compassion allows us to fully engage with both positive and negative experiences, yet not identify with them. Sometimes our courage and ability to feel connected to others fails and the candle of hope flickers, but fortunately we can *practice* compassion for ourselves and others and thereby stimulate the emotional systems that can counteract our loss of positive feeling. Nature, it seems, has made loving-kindness a powerful healing agent (Hofmann et al., 2011).

CHAPTER 19

Working with Trauma
Mindfulness and Compassion

John Briere

The past is never dead. It's not even past.
—WILLIAM FAULKNER (1951/1975, p. 80)

As the Buddha taught, the joyful and fulfilling aspects of life are inextricably intertwined with experiences of pain and loss. Some people's adversities are especially hurtful and destabilizing: Many children are abused, unloved, or abandoned, and many adults endure disasters, war, assaults, torture, or traumatic deaths of loved ones. In fact, more than half of people in North America will undergo one or more major adverse events in their lives (Kessler, Sonnega, Bromet, Hughes, & Nelson, 1995). Although the dividing line is somewhat arbitrary, these more extreme experiences are referred to as *psychological trauma*.

TRAUMATIC REACTIONS

When a traumatic event or loss is of sufficient magnitude, it pushes the individual into an emergency state, activates biological systems associated with survival, produces great anxiety, and usually narrows awareness to immediate survival (Charney, Friedman, & Deutch, 1995; Siegel, 2005). Memories are formed, carrying with them emotions, cognitions, and sensations that become associated with the trauma and that can be triggered and relived as flashbacks, intrusive thoughts, painful feelings, and other aspects of posttraumatic stress (Briere, 2004). In some cases, these memories may be continuously activated, leading to chronic anxiety, depression, or anger. Trauma can also breach the assumptions most of us carry about ourselves, our safety, the future, and sometimes the goodness of other people (Foa, Ehlers, Clark, Tolin, & Orsillo, 1999; McCann & Pearlman, 1990). Finally, trauma can involve existential confrontation. A rape, heart attack, or traumatic loss can rip the fabric of consensual reality, leaving the affected person feeling entirely alone, irrevocably changed, and flooded with awareness of the fragility of life and well-being.

Faced with overwhelming experience, many trauma survivors are understandably motivated to avoid thoughts, feelings, and memories about what happened to them. This may be especially true in Western cultures, with their tendency to pathologize extended sadness or fear, blame the victim, and encourage emotional numbing and externalization in response to painful experience. As a result, a traumatized person may engage in chronic suppression of thoughts, feelings, and memories, or behavior such as substance abuse or harmful acts toward self and others (e.g., Briere, Hodges, & Godbout, 2010). These responses are often associated with further suffering, since they not only produce additional problems but decrease the extent to which pain is processed and/or accommodated.

Human compassion, which is as ancient as trauma itself, can help address these issues. In this chapter, I explore the role of compassion in treating trauma. I suggest that unconditional caring, attunement, and acceptance, in combination with the therapist's overall mindfulness of self and the client, can provide new experiences that support both emotional and cognitive trauma processing.

Therapeutic Approaches to Trauma

Western clinicians generally view trauma-related memories and emotions, negative self attributions, and defensive avoidance strategies as symptoms of psychiatric disorders, for which a range of therapeutic interventions have been developed. These include exposure therapy (Foa & Rothbaum, 1998), cognitive therapy (Resick & Schnicke, 1993), and relational psychotherapy (Pearlman & Courtois, 2005). The first two of these include techniques that have been shown to increase the client's emotional and cognitive processing of trauma memories, thereby reducing their intrusive and painful qualities and diminishing their capacity to motivate problematic avoidance responses. The latter intervention, relational psychotherapy, stresses the importance of the therapeutic relationship, especially therapeutic attunement and nonjudgment, in addressing posttraumatic difficulties. All three of these approaches typically overlap: exposure therapy usually includes cognitive processing (Foa & Rothbaum,

1998), cognitive therapy usually involves exposure (Resick & Schnicke, 1993), both exposure and cognitive therapy may work best within a positive therapeutic relationship (Cloitre et al., 2010), and relational therapies implicitly include emotional and cognitive processing (Briere & Scott, in press; Fulton & Siegel, 2005).

Interestingly, a major finding of the psychotherapy outcome literature is that a positive therapeutic relationship and an attuned therapist may be the most helpful components of treatment—often exceeding the effects of specific interventions (Lambert & Barley, 2001; Martin, Garske, & Davis, 2000). In fact, it appears that these therapist attitudes and qualities—first described decades ago by Rogers (1957)—have special ameliorative qualities in the treatment of traumatized individuals (Cloitre, Stovall-McClough, Miranda, & Chemtob, 2004).

COMPASSION

The value of a compassionate and nonjudgmental attitude has been described from at least two different perspectives: in the context of relational psychotherapy (as described above) and in the spiritual or contemplative domain, including (but not limited to) Buddhist psychology.[1] These approaches have been combined in the last several decades, especially as Buddhist principles and practices have been integrated into secular psychological interventions ranging from psychoanalysis (e.g., Bobrow, 2010; Epstein, 2007) to cognitive-behavioral therapy (e.g., Hayes, Follette, & Linehan, 2004; Segal, Williams, & Teasdale, 2002).

Compassion can be defined from a Buddhist perspective as nonjudgmental awareness and appreciation of the predicament and suffering of others (and oneself), with the felt desire to relieve that suffering and increase well-being. Although a similar construct, *empathy*, entails expressed understanding and appreciation of the client's experience and difficulties, compassion includes a positive emotional state involving feelings of unconditional caring, kindness, and warmth that are directed to others regardless of their actual or presumed qualities or "lovability" (see also Chapter 1).

When adopted into Western forms of psychotherapy, compassion is often seen as grounded in *mindfulness*: the capacity to sustain moment-by-moment focused awareness of—and openness to—one's internal experience and immediate environment, without judgment and with acceptance

---

[1]Themes of compassion and nonjudgmental love, although sometimes intermingled with their opposites, can be found in many other traditions as well, including Christian, Judaic, Hindu, and Islamic faiths.

(see Chapter 2). Mindful awareness helps the clinician maintain an unusual level of attunement to the client (Germer, 2005c; Morgan & Morgan, 2005), as well as allowing him or her to better understand the subjective nature of his or her own thoughts, feelings, and reactions, so that they can be placed in proper perspective before they result in significant countertransferential judgments or behaviors (Briere & Scott, in press; Shapiro & Carlson, 2009). In combination, these learnable capacities to focus benign, loving, and noncountertransferential attention on the client, while feeling and communicating acceptance and nonjudgment, may be critically important–if not essential–for the trauma survivor to fully engage his or her history and pain, while, at the same time, appreciating his or her own innate value and abilities.

Benefits for Trauma Survivors

Although compassionate attention surely has positive effects on everyone, anecdotal experience suggests that its impact on trauma survivors is particularly noteworthy. Trauma, especially interpersonal victimization, often results in alienation from others and oneself, expectations of further maltreatment, and other lasting breaches in the normal connections and relationships between people. Because compassionate attention encourages the redevelopment of these connections, it may be of great benefit, even if it is sometimes hard for the survivor to accept (Gilbert, 2009b).

There is relatively little empirical literature regarding the effects of compassion on traumatized people, nor do most discussions of compassion refer to the specific concerns of trauma survivors (Gilbert, 2009a, 2009c). The remainder of this chapter draws on the general compassion literature, and on my (and others') clinical experience, to discuss the often observed, but not well-documented, relationship between caring, attuned therapist responses and increased well-being for those exposed to adversity. I'll try to show how the therapist's compassionate attitude may have both direct effects on the traumatized client and indirect effects arising from the therapist's increased clinical effectiveness.

Direct Effects

As noted earlier, trauma survivors have experienced one or more events that have altered their subsequent experience of self, others, and the world at large. Such events typically produce terror, horror, or helplessness at a level rarely encountered by nontraumatized individuals (American Psychiatric Association, 2000). The horror associated with, for example, torture or rape can dramatically change the survivor's experience of reality, propelling him or her into a state of consciousness characterized by extreme fear, uncontrollably painful memories, and radically altered expectations of people and the future. The distress and pain associated with extreme trauma may or may not diminish with time, but typically is reexperienced when the survivor is reminded of the trauma by similar phenomena in his or her current environment. In this way, the hyper-accessibility of horrific memories means that, as Faulkner (1951/1975) noted in a different context, "The past is never dead. It's not even past" (p.80).

Although the sustained anguish associated with trauma can be seen as evidence of psychological disorder, in some ways the survivor suffers not from a distorted sense of reality as much as an unwanted awareness of what, in fact, can happen. The torture victim knows what authority figures can do, the rape victim cannot forget some people's capacity to violate and destroy, and the incest survivor or battered woman has intimate knowledge of how badly one can be hurt in a supposedly loving relationship. Thus, trauma-related perspectives and expectations are not always distorted understandings; they can be more accurate—although often overgeneralized—revisions of previous beliefs about the intrinsically benign nature of the world. Furthermore, the survivor's insufficient and temporary solutions to trauma-related distress, such as denial, substance abuse, or self-injurious behavior, make good sense to him or her; they are not illogical, and perhaps not even pathological, but rather coping responses to externally invisible but internally overwhelming experiences (Briere, 2002). This is good news, as it suggests that the survivor's "maladaptive" behaviors are reality-based, reflecting problem solving and adaptation, and therefore potentially responsive to new learning.

Emotional Processing. The powerful emotional effects of a caring, trauma-antithetic relationship have been discussed by many theoreticians and practitioners, both in psychodynamic contexts (e.g., Fonagy, Gergely, Jurist, & Target, 2002) and by trauma specialists (e.g., Courtois, 2010; Dalenberg, 2000). Generally, it is suggested that the therapeutic relationship, by virtue of its superficial similarity to aspects of the original trauma (e.g., the client–therapist power imbalance, the therapist's characteristics, or the likelihood of vulnerability), activates the client's trauma-related memories, relational schema, and conditioned emotional responses.

Once these phenomena are evoked, disparate experiences of compassion and safety in the current relationship can serve to weaken painful emotional associations to previous trauma. Such emotional processing may occur through a multistep process: The therapist's visible, sustained, noncontingent caring (1) engages the client's inborn attachment system, which is sensitive to, and triggered by, loving attention from important relational figures (Bowlby, 1988); (2) activates biological self-soothing circuitry that down-regulates the activity of threat recognition systems (Gilbert, 2009b; see Chapter 18); and (3) leads to the eventual counterconditioning and extinction of classically conditioned anxiety associated with trauma-reminiscent stimuli. The anxiety/stress-reducing effects of compassion, in fact, may extend beyond trauma processing to include positive impacts on neurobiology (e.g., Lutz, Brefczynski-Lewis, Johnstone, & Davidson, 2008).

Cognitive Processing. Compassion also appears to work on a cognitive level, providing the trauma survivor with new information that can update his or her assumptions and subsequent behavior. By offering unconditional caring, acceptance, mindful awareness, and attunement, the compassionate clinician becomes the antithesis of, if not the antidote to, the client's initial traumatization, providing input for changes in the survivor's perception and response systems. The therapeutic relationship itself becomes a nonverbal cognitive therapy instrument, heightening awareness of the disparity between then and now. Whereas others have hurt, violated, or rejected, the therapist actively supports, cares for, and accepts; where once there was danger and violence, now there is safety; where the survivor was exposed to chaos and powerful negative emotions, the therapist projects stability, calm, and nonegocentric loving attention.

Although the survivor's tendency may be to avoid interpersonal attachments,[2] he or she inevitably needs them due to our evolutionary heritage as social beings (Gilbert, 2009b; Schore, 1994) and as a result of previous personal deprivation (Bowlby, 1988). The survivor is caught in a predicament: Avoidance and isolation are protective against being hurt in intimate contexts, yet such behaviors are associated with emptiness, loneliness, and depression, and interfere with the self-esteem and well-being associated with relatedness (Cacioppo & Patrick, 2008; Chapter 12). By demonstrating caring, positive regard, and a willingness to connect at whatever level the client can tolerate, the compassionate therapist becomes an exception to trauma's lessons. For example, in contrast to a woman's sexually abusive father or violent spouse, a male therapist might be regarded as someone who likes and cares about her, will not exploit

---

[2]Although attachment is problematic in the Buddhist sense, the current use of this word reflects the notion of interpersonal relatedness in the context of intimacy, which is a positive phenomenon. The specific point at which relational attachment can become what Buddhists refer to as attachment (e.g., involving grasping, obsession, or possessiveness) is a subject of some debate. I believe they are separate phenomena.

or transgress, and is, in fact, not dangerous. And if such exceptions exist, then all men are not necessarily perpetrators, and conclusions drawn from earlier horrors can be tentatively revised or limited.

Many survivors of interpersonal traumas were devalued, rejected, or shamed in the context of victimization and, as a result, have come to believe that they must be unacceptable or deserving of maltreatment (Briere, 1992; McCann & Pearlman, 1990). The survivor's trauma-related responses (e.g., posttraumatic stress, depression, or relationship issues) and coping strategies (e.g., substance abuse or dissociation) are also typically stigmatized by society, with the result that he or she is seen as pathological or bad. Fortunately, the therapist's noncontingent acceptance of the trauma survivor can significantly impact these difficulties. As the therapist conveys by behavior and words his or her unconditional positive regard and caring, the survivor has the opportunity to undergo trauma-disparate experiences that gradually undercut negative conclusions about him- or herself associated with victimization. Shame, for example, involves assumptions about personal badness that must be kept from others—a response that tends to decrease in the context of therapeutic compassion and acceptance (Gilbert, 2009b). As the survivor's history and posttraumatic responses are gradually expressed, normalized, and accepted, there is less for him or her to judge as unacceptable, and thus less to keep secret and avoid—ultimately leading to greater cognitive and emotional processing.

Acceptance, in this context, may involve two components: the therapist's visible noncontingent acceptance of the client as a person, entitled to happiness and well-being (although the therapist may not necessarily accept the client's self- or other-destructive behavior), and the client's therapist-supported integration of especially overwhelming and potentially stigmatizing traumatic material into "mere" or "just" painful memory. This unencumbered recollection of painful events of the past (i.e., with less activation of associated cognitions and emotions), occurs as trauma is remembered and recounted in the context of the therapist's willingness to share—and bear nonjudgmental witness to—the survivor's experience. As therapeutic compassion and acceptance reduce the stigma and personal badness associated with trauma memory, such recollections slowly lose their power to shame and motivate avoidance, thereby facilitating further processing and integration.

Indirect Effects

Compassion also assists trauma survivors by creating conditions that support the therapist's effectiveness in his or her work. As the clinician extends loving-kindness toward the survivor, he or she engages warm and positive feelings that, especially in the context of mindfulness, allow him or her to be exposed to considerable pain and suffering without being disarmed, distracted, or personally activated. Since trauma therapy often is most effective when it facilitates the client's direct, verbalized, experience of distress, the therapist's ability to be less reactive while hearing otherwise painful and upsetting things increases the client's opportunity to process emotional pain in the context of more complete attunement. A mindful stance also allows the therapist to more clearly view expressed emotional pain as just emotional pain—not as intrinsically negative, nor as a trigger for countertransference, but rather as a process wherein the client can metabolize his or her history and ultimately experience reduced suffering (Briere & Scott, in press). In this sense, the client's pain is not perceived as "bad," and therefore the clinician is not impacted in the same way, nor is he or she as likely to be vicariously traumatized.

The effects of compassion are not limited to the client. Engendering this relational state produces real benefits for the therapist, allowing him or her not only to become a better therapist, but also to grow as a person and experience increased well-being (Gilbert, 2009a; Salzberg, 1997; D. J. Siegel, 2010a). His Holiness the 14th Dalai Lama notes, "If you want others to be happy, practice compassion. If you want to be happy, practice compassion" (Dalai Lama & Cutler, 2009). As many have described, compassion involves not only a felt experience of love and acceptance toward others when they are in pain, but also similar feelings toward oneself. So what goes around does appear to come around, and the compassionate practitioner may come to experience a sense of peace and (seemingly paradoxical) nonegocentric appreciation of self. The nonselfish aspect of this experience appears to involve the slow remission of the perceived duality of self versus others as individual objects of caring, such that self is valued in the same way that others are. However accomplished, and from whatever tradition, noncontingent, nonegocentric caring for others may have the side effect of grounding the clinician and increasing his or her well-being in a way that, reciprocally, may then allow the helper to help all the more.

FINDING THE CENTER

As many have noted, writing or reading about mindfulness and compassion is quite different from experiencing it directly. The following brief section describes my personal experience of trying to cultivate these qualities as a trauma specialist and teacher in a large public health care system.

Most of the people my colleagues and I encounter are struggling with some combination of poverty, homelessness, drug addiction, or severe mental illness. Many present to emergency services following sexual or physical assaults, major losses, overdoses, or suicide attempts. Some are dealing with HIV/AIDS, are patients in burn units, or come with histories of political oppression or torture. Others are described as prostitutes, gang members, or criminals.

The clinical and spiritual issues in this work often converge: Can we inhabit a mode that allows objective assessment and intervention, yet, at the same time, supports compassion and receptive attention? And, how do we address or relate to our own experience in the face of such suffering?

I seem to be more helpful when I am able to access a state in which empathic connection with a hurt person is possible, even desirable–partially because the presenting issue has been reinterpreted. From this position, I am less likely to view the client's pain as intrinsically negative, but instead as an objective fact–in some cases, even as an opportunity for recovery or growth. This does not mean that the trauma survivor's distress should be dismissed in any way. Yet, rarely is it helpful to accept–and therefore reinforce–the stigmatization, hopelessness, and demoralization that people can infer from horrible things. Instead, the challenge is to acknowledge the sometimes incredible hurt that has occurred, while, at the same time, communicating that the individual's ongoing presence signals implicit strength, adaptive capacity, and hopefulness for the future. In this way, his or her difficulties and suffering are "just" that, not evidence for the labels that he or she may collect (and that I, ironically, may later write in a chart). The survivor becomes more than the sum of his or her wounds, and I cease to be a detached clinician, but rather someone who's job is to provide a space and context for the client's immediate experience and future recovery–a process that may require the client (and me) to sit with the fragility and impermanence of life.

When possible, I try to spend a few early minutes not only evaluating the immediate needs of the person in front of me, but also checking my own internal experience, noting feelings, thoughts, and impulses that arise and seek to dominate. I hope to see the person as he or she actually is: someone who, at this point in time, is in trouble or in pain–a scenario that, but for random circumstance, might be true for me as well. Were things to have gone differently, I could be my most injured or "disturbed" client–or even the person who may have hurt him or her. This reflection helps break the delusion that, as a therapist, I am essentially different from, or somehow better than, the person I am trying to help.

From one perspective, the trauma, psychosis, or substance abuse is the problem. But the problem is not the person, and the pain, in one way or another, will eventually change or depart. In fact, the experience of the pain often turns out to be the route out of pain. When I am able to engage that view, I can intentionally focus on caring in a way that is both involved and not. I do not want the person to suffer (although I may have little impact on that), and I know that we are all ultimately in the same boat around this "feeling bad and hurting" business.

Compassion grows if one pays attention to it. As it expands, it allows the client (and me) to increasingly confront, engage, and accept upsetting feelings and thoughts, until, slowly, the painful aspects change and hopefully diminish from lack of sustenance.

CULTIVATING COMPASSION

Since compassion seems to have significant positive effects on the trauma survivor, as well as the clinician, how can it be developed?

Western clinical training programs expect that therapists should be objective, empathically attuned, and to the extent possible, unconditionally positive in their regard for clients–yet they usually do little to help trainees to accomplish these goals (Fulton, 2005). It seems that the assumption is often that (1) the clinician can learn, intellectually, how to do these things, such that merely being told to do so will suffice; or (2) nonjudgment and attunement are natural characteristics of some therapists, and only they should practice psychotherapy; or (3) if one doesn't feel compassionate, accepting, and nonjudgmental, one should learn how to fake it. Unfortunately, none of these approaches is necessarily correct or effective. Although there appear to be "natural therapists," clearly many other practitioners cannot immediately access these psychological capacities merely by being told that they should do so, and yet may have the potential to be effective clinicians with sufficient training. And, it is often the case that clients (perhaps especially trauma survivors, given their interpersonal hypervigilance) can detect inauthentic caring or attention in others, leading to further distrust of the therapist rather than reassurance. Finally, misrepresenting one's caring on a regular basis requires unusual effort and energy and is likely to have negative emotional impacts on the therapist.

Fortunately, the insights and methodologies of Buddhist and other spiritual traditions can be helpful here, since the development of compassion and mindfulness are common themes in those literatures. Most suggest that although some degree of compassion probably exists as part of the human condition, its expansion is a learned skill that can arise in the context of extended introspection, discussion, and discernment.

Meditation and Mindfulness Training

From most Buddhist perspectives, the primary pathway to the development of compassion and unconditional regard is through meditation. As described in other chapters of this book, a regular meditation practice and exposure to a teacher or books and CDs on meditation can accomplish several things for those who are able to sustain this approach. First, mindfulness is a common outgrowth of meditation, since the latter typically includes learning how to concentrate on a single process (often one's breath), paying attention to the present moment, and allowing thoughts and feelings to come and go without attachment to them (see Germer, 2005c; Chapter 2; and for another perspective on this process, see Siff, 2010). Among those things allowed to arise and fall away are judgments about oneself and one's internal experiences, such that the meditator becomes increasingly able to attend to ongoing experience without viewing it as good or bad.

As described by Teasdale, Segal, and Williams (1995), and others, an emergent phenomenon during this process is *metacognitive awareness*: the growing ability to observe and reflect upon one's thoughts and feelings and to learn that such internal processes are, most immediately, products of the mind and not necessarily evidence about the true state of reality. As metacognitive awareness grows, the individual begins to discern the transient nature of even very compelling cognitive and emotional processes, and discover that emotional reactions, intrusive experiences, and cognitions or beliefs are not necessarily "real": They may be more relevant to the past than the present. From the meditating therapist's perspective, the result is increased attunement to the client's experience, as the clinician is better able to pay attention with less internal distraction and less interference from his or her own history.

Together, these components of meditation-based mindfulness allow the therapist to perceive and respond to the client in a more attuned and nonreactive way, producing many of the requirements of an optimal therapeutic relationship. These outcomes are largely in the cognitive and attentional domains, however. They reduce distraction and judgments; they do not specifically engender the caring associated with compassion. Fortunately, meditation can be of use here as well. First, it is the experience of many meditators that, as mindfulness grows, compassion arises as well (Shapiro & Carlson, 2009). The nature of this often co-emergent process is unclear. However, the capacity to experience caring for others and oneself appears to be naturally existent, probably as a function of psychobiological attachment processes, whereas the full expression of this response may require reduced interference from personal history and cultural training–including the need to judge experience and imbue it with egocentric needs and concerns. Some suggest that mindful awareness brings to the forefront a realization of the nondual nature of reality, such that one's own happiness and the happiness of others are viewed as inextricably coexistent (e.g., Dalai Lama, 1995; see Chapter 4). Although this insight may not engender caring, per se, it supports the intention to transfer feelings from self to others and the reverse.

Finally, some meditation practices are specifically targeted toward the development of nonegocentric love and positive regard for others. For example, the Theravadin practice of *metta bhavana*, or loving-kindness (Germer, 2009; Salzberg, 1997) and the Tibetan practice of *tonglen* ("sending and taking"; Chödrön, 2000; Chapter 7) are centered around the meditational cultivation of compassion. In *metta* meditations, the practitioner locates and intensifies loving feelings toward him- or herself (although Westerners seemingly have more difficulty accessing self-love than individuals in some other cultures) and then applies these feelings, sequentially, toward a valued other, then more neutrally valued people (e.g., acquaintances or coworkers), then difficult people or enemies, and, finally, all sentient beings (see Chapter 3). In *tonglen* and its Western variations, the meditator "breathes in" pain and suffering from the world and specific people and "breathes out" love, compassion, and happiness back to them (see Chapter 7). From an experiential perspective, such exercises allow the practitioner to locate, identify, and "grow" loving feelings, which are then applied to self and others. With practice, this exercise of focusing and encouraging loving affects–even independent of its spiritual or religious intention–appears to make such feelings more experientially salient and easily generated, perhaps especially when mindfulness is also present.

REFLECTIONS FOR THE HELPER

- Sit for a minute or two with your eyes closed. Allow your mind to settle down a bit. Focus on the breath, letting your tasks and concerns fall away for just a little while.
- Bring your attention to what you do for a living. Consider all the people you see who suffer and the work you do to help them, whether through psychotherapy, medicine, spiritual guidance, or being a parent or friend to someone struggling with life. Reflect on your intentions for these people: that they suffer less, that they be happy, that they have some sense of peace in their lives.
- Allow your compassion to grow—all these beings, caught in painful circumstance, in one way or another doing the best they can. Send caring feelings to them, and to yourself, as someone not that different, although perhaps more fortunate at this specific moment.
- Bring one of these people to mind—someone whose difficulties are especially significant to you right now. Let yourself feel what he or she feels, see what he or she sees. Try not to get lost in this person's suffering; watch it from the grounded, caring place that you have established. Allow yourself to feel the pain but not get caught in it.

- Reflect on this person's experience. Note that it is not a bad thing to hurt when you have been hurt. This person's distress may be part of recovery, certainly part of being alive. It is ultimately transient; it will, inevitably, change or depart. Feel the honor that you can be present with this person at this moment in time, in all the complexity of pain and caring.
- Embrace any gratitude that arises. How lucky you are to be where you are, doing what you are doing. Your occupation or relationship is a special gift, although it may not always seem that way. See if you can directly experience the honor of being able to intervene in the suffering of others. It could have gone differently. You might have ended up doing something less meaningful or beneficial. Remember how you've always wanted to help, how lucky you are that you can.

Nonmeditative Compassion Training

Outside of (or in addition to) meditation, certain aspects of compassion can be learned more didactically. In compassion-focused therapy (CFT; Gilbert, 2009a, 2009b), for example, an entire therapeutic philosophy and intervention approach has been developed to treat clients who suffer from significant shame, self-criticism, and depression (see Chapter 18 for a detailed description of CFT). Gilbert contends that compassion is a learnable skill set that provides the clinician with ways to foster a range of compassionate attributes (e.g., caring for well-being, empathy, and nonjudgment) and skills (e.g., compassionate attention, compassionate reasoning, and compassionate behavior). It is likely that these attitudes and skills may be especially helpful in work with trauma survivors—especially in light of CFT's attention to adults with childhood maltreatment experiences (Gilbert, 2009b).

In a less structured way, compassion also may be increased by helping clinicians to appreciate the existential validity of phenomena such as suffering, impermanence, interdependence, and nonegocentric love. In many Buddhist traditions, this insight develops as the student interacts with his or her teacher and studies, reflects, and meditates on various aspects of *dharma* (i.e., the true nature of reality/existence, typically as explicated by the Buddha). In our culture, this may also take place within the context of books, CDs, and DVDs offered by traditional teachers such as His Holiness the 14th Dalai Lama (1998) or Western writers such as Tara Brach (2003; see also Chapter 2), Pema Chödrön (2000), Jon Kabat-Zinn (1994), and Jack Kornfield (2008b).

Such didactic and exploratory exercises are often especially helpful in explicating *dependent arising*, the notion that experience and behavior arise from concrete conditions and causes (Bodhi, 2005), as opposed to doing so independent of causality (e.g., through an act of a deity, or the Aristotelian notion of a spontaneous "First Cause"). This exploration frequently leads to the realization that people are the way they are because of prior causes and influences, as opposed to inherent psychopathology or evil. As the conditioned and etiological aspects of previously unacceptable or "sick" behaviors are examined, it becomes harder to blame (and, perhaps, to label) individuals, leading to less judgment of them. This insight often is not that difficult for the clinician to appreciate, at least intellectually, since the science of psychology assumes that there are specific reasons why people behave the way they do. Especially in trauma, the conversation between the teacher/consultant and therapist often highlights the notion that "disordered," "acting-out," "dysfunctional," or "bad" client behaviors arise from predispositions, coping responses to trauma-related pain and suffering, and lack of information or options regarding better ways of seeing or doing things—much as Buddhist psychology suggests. Such discussions also facilitate the notion that individuals who commit violence against others, ranging from abusive parents to rapists to murderers, are not intrinsically evil, but rather are responding to causalities and vagaries of the human condition—including, in some cases, trauma[3] (Briere, in press).

In more directly clinical contexts, the teacher, consultant, or supervisor may use the therapist's reports or videotapes of sessions to continue this discussion. As the clinician explores his or her inevitable (dependently arising) countertransferential responses to the client, there are multiple opportunities for the teacher to point out the conditioned/historical aspects of the client's behavior and the therapist's reactions, hopefully increasing the clinician's metacognitive awareness and decreasing his or her judgments. In many cases, there will be opportunities for the teacher to give permission for the clinician to care about the client, perhaps in ways that existed when the therapist began his or her career, but that lost their power through clinical training to be "objective." Therapists are sometimes able to rekindle their compassion when compassion is considered a valid clinical goal rather than an expression of naiveté or lack of clinical sophistication. This rekindling is more likely to occur when the consultant or supervisor models the same attitudes and responses that the clinician is encouraged to apply to the client.

Some therapists grow in compassion during the course of their careers because of an implicit aspect of their work—the voluntary decision to be

[3]This perspective may be especially helpful on occasions when the therapist discovers that his or her survivor client is also a perpetrator of abuse or violence against others.

with people who are undergoing especially difficult times. By working with individuals who are greatly challenged or *in extremis*—for example those who are confronting impending death or who have been traumatized in major ways—the clinician may come to see more clearly the components and etiologies of suffering, as well as the subtle opportunities that can arise from chaos and crisis. Such work exposes him or her to impermanence in a real way and can engender a growing realization that we are not only fragile, but also worthy of appreciation and love; that we are not here long, yet we are involved in a compelling and, in some ways, awe-inspiring process. As we assist and accompany people who are experiencing what we, in our culture, tend to deny or discount, there is the chance to access deepening levels of caring for others and ourselves, as we realize that we are all in this together.

CHAPTER 20

The Heart of Couple Therapy

Richard Borofsky
Antra K. Borofsky

> For one human being to love another: that is perhaps the most difficult of all our tasks, the ultimate, the last test and proof, the work for which all other work is but preparation.
> —RAINER MARIA RILKE (1954, p. 41)

Intimate couple relationships awaken us to both the fullness and the difficulty of loving one another. On the one hand, love illuminates and animates the best in us. Through love, we are able to enlarge the span of our compassion and caring, and to deepen our faith in our own and each other's essential goodness. Together, we are able to find fulfillment simply in our being present and find the courage to face our future, whatever it may bring.

On the other hand, intimate relationships reveal everything that limits our capacity to love and be loved. These limitations are often the result of painful experiences with significant others—partners, parents, siblings—which have left unhealed emotional injuries. Painful disconnections, collisions of differences, imbalances of power, and experiences of emotional deprivation, shaming, abandonment, violation, and betrayal are among the many wounding experiences that may be evoked in intimate relationships. Often these experiences are repeated until they can be integrated and transformed in the context of a present relationship.

Love also pushes the limits of our emotional development. For an intimate relationship to be sustainable, partners must become *both* more differentiated *and* more connected. "Secure dependence and autonomy are two sides of the same coin, rather than dichotomies" (Johnson, 2009, p. 263). Potentially, both can be challenging. The experience of differentiation is inherently uncomfortable and often painful because it can threaten our sense of a safe and secure attachment. The experience of a deeper connection can likewise be frightening and painful, since it can threaten our sense of a separate, autonomous self. Over time, love stretches our capacity for being one and being two.

Love relationships can confound us for other reasons as well. As Bowlby (1980) points out, "The most intense emotions arise during the formation, the maintenance, the disruption and the renewal of attachment relationships" (p. 60). Because they often evoke our contradictory longings for safety and excitement, connection and autonomy, or freedom and commitment, intimate partnerships are fertile ground for intrapersonal and interpersonal conflicts. In addition, they often challenge our cherished self-images as well as our idealized expectations about what love is, how it should feel, and what it should look like. Lastly, because it is in the nature of love to expand endlessly, love relationships eventually expose our deepest vulnerabilities, along with everything in us that is exiled, orphaned, or unloved.

For all these reasons, intimate couple relationships can be daunting and difficult. For all the same reasons, couple relationships and couple therapy can be an extraordinary context for the cultivation of compassion and wisdom.

COMPASSION

> Before you know kindness as the deepest thing inside,
> you must know sorrow as the other deepest thing.
>
> —NAOMI SHIHAB NYE (1995, p. 42)

An important part of couple therapy is helping both partners manage their vulnerabilities. We assume that whatever a couple's presenting problem may be, both partners in the couple are having difficulty acknowledging, accepting, balancing, and sharing their respective vulnerabilities. *Vulnerabilities*, as we are using the word here, includes a wide range of experiences, all of which have in common a sense of feeling helpless or diminished. Couples who come to therapy may be contending with any number of vulnerabilities—ranging from physical handicaps, illnesses, or injuries to fears, needs, losses, feelings of failure and inadequacy, shame and humiliation, rejection, loneliness, hurt, disappointment, confusion, and helplessness. Our aim is to help couples manage their vulnerabilities in such a way that they become a vehicle for cultivating compassion. We do this by helping partners hold *together* whatever vulnerabilities appear in the crucible of their two-person intimate partnership, and share them in such a way that loving-kindness arises.

The word *compassion* means literally "to suffer together." *Passion* here has its original meaning of pain or suffering, as in the "Passion of Christ." The prefix *com* means "together" (see also Chapter 1). So, compassion is the capacity for sharing painful and vulnerable experiences in both meanings of the word *share*—to talk and listen to each other, as well as to hold each other's vulnerabilities collectively. When a couple can do this, there is a kind of alchemical transmutation that can happen. Rather than feeling burdened by each other's vulnerabilities or suffering, both can feel uplifted. An old Jewish proverb advises, "A sorrow kept to oneself is a sorrow that is doubled. A sorrow that is shared is a sorrow that is divided." Through the paradoxical math of compassion, vulnerabilities that are added together reduce the overall level of vulnerability in a couple and deepen the bond between them—a bond of compassion.

Compassion happens because vulnerabilities are at the deepest level a call for connection. That is, each vulnerability naturally gives rise to a relational need, a need to be helped or attended to by ourselves or another in some way. As Rainer Maria Rilke wrote in one of his letters to a young poet, "Perhaps everything that frightens us is, in its deepest essence, something helpless that wants our love" (1984, p. 92). The love that is wanted and needed appears spontaneously when a vulnerability and its attendant need can be shared without defensiveness, fear, or shame. In this way, compassion—which is a mix of love and vulnerability—arises.

Just as vulnerability is a call for loving connection and attention, love needs vulnerability to grow. The openhearted sharing of vulnerability and need is one of the principal ways that love is renewed and sustained. Often partners are surprised to discover that the love they have been longing for or demanding from each other can appear quite genuinely and spontaneously in response to the mutual revelation of their vulnerabilities.

Learning how to foster compassion in this way can be transforming for both partners and for their relationship. Feeling that one's partner is able to accept and hold one's deepest vulnerabilities creates a profound experience of safety and connection. This in turn makes it possible to unlock a couple's repetitive negative patterns of relating as well as neurotic individual patterns—many of which have their origin in relational wounds. Also, an increase in compassion for one's partner can often transform one's resistance to the other into a heartfelt willingness to help or a willingness to change in ways that the other has wanted for a long time. Once evoked, compassion is a profound and powerful motivator of change.

WISDOM

> There is no Paradise, no place of true completion,
> that does not include within its walls the unknown.
> —JANE HIRSHFIELD (2008, p. 23)

Wisdom implies an openness to not knowing (see Chapters 1 and 10). This openness and humility make it possible to learn and to become more aware. Wisdom, in the context of a couple relationship, involves accepting that we all have blind spots, that our awareness is limited, and that these limitations of awareness can be disturbing and even hurtful to our partners. Most complaints that relationship partners have about each other distill down to wanting to raise the other's awareness—or at least wanting the other to acknowledge that he or she has been unaware in some way.

Unless they are able to acknowledge the limits of their own awareness and their own knowing, intimate partners are like the blind men in the Indian parable, who are feeling different parts of an elephant and mistake the part they are touching for the whole. The one who is feeling the elephant's leg concludes that an elephant is a kind of tree. Another who is feeling the elephant's tail says that an elephant is really a rope. And so on. They argue, but their argument cannot be resolved because they lack the vision that would enable them to see a bigger picture. That is, they lack the awareness and wisdom that would enable them to know that their personal, partial understanding of an elephant is incomplete.

Couple therapy is akin to helping the blind men in the parable speak to one another, mindfully describing what they are aware of and what they are experiencing at each moment as they feel their way toward each other, leading eventually to a more complete understanding of themselves and their relationship—or what Mary Catherine Bateson calls "insight." "Insight," she writes, "refers to the depth of understanding that comes by setting experiences, yours and mine, familiar and exotic, new and old, side by side, learning from letting them speak to one another" (1994, p. 14). Our goal in couple therapy is to help both partners set their individual truths side by side and to enable them to speak to each other—as well as to listen—so that a bigger picture, a fuller awareness, and a deeper understanding can emerge, along with an increased humility about the limits of their knowing and their awareness.

Wisdom also implies seeing clearly into the nature of reality and an acceptance of difficult truths about the human condition—such as the truth of our mortality or the truth that life is a mix of positive and negative experience. Intimate partnerships—despite our wish that it be otherwise—are a mix of inspiration and difficulty, possibility and limitation, safety and vulnerability, fulfillment and disappointment, pleasure and pain. In a bigger and wiser vision of love and relationship, all these pairings and polarities can coexist peacefully. In this bigger and wiser vision, love has no opposite—because it includes everything.

COUPLE THERAPY

There are two goals that we are trying to accomplish in couple therapy. The first is to offer a steady, aware presence in which both partners can safely be themselves and see each other clearly, without defensiveness or fear. This is the presence of mindfulness, the impartial light of awareness. As described by Irish poet William Butler Yeats, this mindful presence can have a powerful and empowering effect. "We can," he wrote, "make our minds so like still water that beings gather about us that they may see, it may be, their own images, and so live for a moment with a clearer, perhaps even with a fiercer life because of our quiet" (1902/2004, p. 69). We hope that our stilled attention will provide a container or crucible in which love and vulnerability can meet and mix, and that our mindful presence will serve as a catalyst, which—nonreactive itself—will facilitate the transmutation of love and vulnerability into compassion. We also hope that we can inspire both partners to learn over time how to be a still mirror of mindfulness for themselves and for each other—even when they are hurting or frightened or angry. This will increase their capacity for "empathic concern" and "perspective-taking" (Block-Lerner, Adair, Plumb, Rhatigan, & Orsillo, 2007).

Our second aim is to facilitate a deepening emotional exchange between partners in which they mindfully share whatever they are feeling *right now.* This exchange requires that they have a "felt sense" of themselves (Gendlin, 1981, p. 32) and that they learn how to give and receive their feelings mindfully and trustingly—no matter how painful they may be. This is what Naranjo (1970) describes as "a verbalized meditation . . . a meditation carried into the interpersonal situation as an act of self-disclosure" (p. 54; see also Kramer, 2007). We assume that change will happen through this process of emotional exchange (Borofsky & Borofsky, 1994; Johnson, 2004) and that these exchanges are a powerful means by which compassion and wisdom can deepen through relationship.

CARL AND PATRICIA, PART I

Carl and Patricia have been married for 6 years and have two children—a son who is 2 and a daughter who is 4 years old. The younger child has developmental difficulties and is suspected of having autism. Patricia is a full-time mother; Carl is a salesman for a technology company and travels 2–4 days a week. The couple has not had a sexual relationship for over 2 years, since their son was conceived. The strain and disconnection between them are painfully apparent.

After gathering some background information, we ask them to turn their attention directly to each other.

RICH: I would like to ask you to please look at each other for a moment. (*pause*) Please look for a few seconds and notice how this feels.

CARL: (*to us*) It feels uncomfortable.

ANTRA: Could you please tell this to Patricia?

CARL: (*after a short pause, looking nervously and hesitantly at her*) I feel awkward looking at you. It's uncomfortable.

RICH: Where in your body do you feel the awkwardness?

CARL: (*to Rich, looking confused*) What do you mean?

RICH: Do you feel the awkwardness in your face, in your chest, or somewhere else? (*slowly, compassionately*) Showing her, letting her *see* how you feel uncomfortable, will help her start to understand and care about what it's like for you.

CARL: (*to Patricia, looking vulnerable*) I'm feeling how painful it is that we've become such strangers. (*Looks away for a few seconds and then looks back at Patricia.*) My face feels all stiff. Kind of like a mask. (*pause*) Now I'm feeling a lump in my throat.

PATRICIA: (*beginning to tear up*) I have been so angry at you because I have needed you and you haven't been there.

ANTRA: (*kindly*) Patricia, are you feeling angry right now?

PATRICIA: (*slowly to Antra*) No, not right now. (*pause*) No . . . right now, I'm feeling sad.

ANTRA: Please let him see your sadness. (*pause*) Can you see him seeing how you are sad right now?

PATRICIA: (*looking at Carl while crying softly*) I miss you. I really miss you.

CARL: (*Silently and slowly reaches over to hold Patricia's hand.*)

THE COMPASSIONATE TRUTH

In the above exchange, we are trying to help Carl and Patricia have an experience of directly meeting each other in the present moment. To facilitate this, we focus on what is personal, present, and palpable. We call this "the compassionate truth" because these three qualities increase the likelihood that compassion will result from any verbal exchange.

First, talking about one's own personal experience rather than talking about the other reduces defensiveness. When both partners take responsibility for their perceptions, interpretations, feelings, and reactions, and acknowledge them as their own, it makes it easier to hold their two different realities side by side so they can listen to each other.

Second, we are trying to help both partners focus on what is actually occurring in the present moment. Antra asks Patricia to be aware that she is not angry now, but is actually sad, and that Carl is seeing her sadness—*right now.* This emphasis on the present moment makes it more likely that what happens between them will be grounded in their current actuality, rather than being a reaction to memories of past happenings or to generalizations about each other. Partners who are unable to be present with each other inevitably repeat the past and stay stuck longing for a future that they can't find. By helping both partners enter into whatever experience they are presently having—pleasant or unpleasant or mixed—and by mindfully bringing these experiences into direct contact with each other in the present, it is more likely that something new will emerge and that this new something will be in the service of deepening compassion and wisdom.

Lastly, we are asking Carl and Patricia to focus on their bodily sensations and feelings. We focus on sensations because a compassionate response is more likely to occur when we can sense or see the palpable, physical experience of the other, rather than hearing a report *about* it. For this reason, Rich asks Carl to notice the specific sensations in his body and to describe these for Patricia so that she can sense directly how he feels awkward and pained, and she can begin to care about how he feels.

All these interventions are intended to help Carl and Patricia move toward an undefended, openhearted meeting with each other's vulnerability in the present moment. We are trying to help them palpably sense that they are both hurting, and to make it safe for them to begin holding their suffering together.

At the same time we want to help them become witnesses to their own and the other's experience. Wisdom requires the capacity to witness mindfully without automatically reacting and an openness to seeing a bigger picture—one that includes the other's pain as well as one's own (see Chapters 1 and 10). As it becomes apparent to each of them that they are *both* suffering, and as they can begin to share their suffering with each other, the healing of their disconnection can start to happen.

CARL AND PATRICIA, PART II

ANTRA: I can sense that both of you have been hurting and there is mistrust between you. (*pause*) I would like to ask you to try something that I think may help you learn how to restore a sense of trust. (*picks up a stone egg from the table in front of her*) I would like you to take this stone egg and take turns giving it to the other.

(*Patricia looks puzzled; Carl looks skeptical.*)

ANTRA: Trust is communicated by how we give to and receive from each other. So I would like you to pass this stone back and forth *very slowly* without saying anything, as if you are entrusting something of importance to the other. As you do this, try to stay aware of both yourself and the other.

Antra demonstrates with Rich by first holding the egg for a moment, closing her eyes, taking a deep breath, and concentrating her attention. She then opens her eyes, reaches out for Rich's hand, puts the stone egg gently in his palm, and holds her hand on his for just a moment. She then releases his hand. Rich acknowledges that he has received the egg by carefully holding it in his hand, looking at it, then looking directly at Antra and saying, "Thank you" *He closes his eyes, takes a deep breath, gathers his attention before he is ready to open his eyes, and then he offers her the stone.*

Hesitantly and awkwardly at first, Carl and Patricia pass the stone back and forth, but after a few exchanges they settle into a more concentrated silence, each starting to sense more clearly how they are giving and receiving.

RICH: I would like to ask you now to tell each other something about how you have been struggling. Each time you put the stone in the other's hand, please tell the other something about you that's been hard for you to share, something that you really would like the other to understand. The only thing we ask is that you try to talk about yourself and not blame each other.

PATRICIA: (*After thinking for a moment, carefully puts the egg in Carl's hand.*) I resent that so much of the burden of caring for our children falls on me.

RICH: (*to Carl*) See if you can open yourself to receiving this. Even if this is painful to hear, see if you can hold this with her. If you are willing, please say, "yes." This "yes" lets her know your willingness to hear and let in how it is for her and to let it sit side by side with how it is for you. This doesn't mean that you agree or see the situation the same way she does.

CARL: (*Looking cautiously at Patricia and, accepting the egg from her, responds hesitantly.*) Well . . . Maybe . . . (*pause*) well, OK . . . yes . . . I can hear this. I can hold this with you. (*Closes his eyes, takes a deep breath, and after a long pause looks at Patricia and reaches for her hand, gently putting the egg in her palm.*) I am afraid that no matter what I do, it won't be enough. I feel like a failure.

ANTRA (*to Patricia*) Please let him know if you're willing to hold this feeling of being a failure with him.

PATRICIA: (*letting this sink in*) Yes. I'm willing to hear this. (*pause*) As long as you aren't blaming me. So, yes, I'm willing to hold this with you. (*Now holds the stone that Carl gave her in both her hands, next to her chest.*)

CARL: Thank you. I appreciate that.

PATRICIA: (*beginning to cry, and reaching for Carl's hand to give the stone back to him*) It's been very hard for me to go alone to all the doctor's appointments. I've felt so scared and confused.

CARL: (*tenderly*) Yes, I'm willing to hold this with you, right now.

PATRICIA: Thank you. Thank you (*crying some more*).

CARL: (*passing the stone back to Patricia*) I feel so guilty about not being able to find a job that lets me be at home more, so I could go with you. I really hate my job. I feel really trapped.

PATRICIA: (*as both of them are holding the stone together, with four hands, while looking deeply into Carl's eyes*) I know. I'm sorry that I've been so angry. I know it's not your fault. I can feel that you have been doing your best. We both have.

GIVING AND RECEIVING

Our interventions with Carl and Patricia are intended to structure and facilitate an exchange between them. This exchange is happening on several levels. First of all, it is an exchange of words describing what is most upsetting to each of them. For example, Patricia tells Carl that she has resented carrying the burden of caring for their children alone, and he tells her how he feels trapped in his job. But they are also giving and receiving their *feelings*, the actual, palpable experience of their pain. Lastly, they are learning how to give and receive a quality of attention to their painful feelings that is open, steady, focused, and trusting. In our experience, it is this quality of attention that is the most important feature of successful exchanges.

The simple structure of passing a stone between them helps make the process of exchange more mindful or conscious. This structure helps them learn how to mindfully execute the essential elements in a successful exchange. In our model of couple therapy (Borofsky & Borofsky, 1994), we have identified four parts of giving and four parts of receiving that are all necessary for a successful exchange to occur. Each of these parts has a distinctive quality of attention.

Giving

Gathering

Holding our attention inside to become aware of and gather a sense of our personal, present, palpable experience—the alive, authentic, immediate inner experience that we have to give—makes it more likely that what is exchanged will be fresh and authentic and will lead to a compassionate connection.

Offering

Slowly moving our attention from a felt sense of what is inside and extending this to the other requires courage—especially if we are feeling vulnerable. Whether we are offering our words, our touch, or an object, it is the steadiness of the offering that communicates our willingness to place our trust in the other's kindness.

Aiming

For an offering to touch the other, we must precisely aim what is being given. We must sharpen the focus of our attention on the other, aiming precisely where our attention is going—for example, the pupil of one eye, or the hand that we want to touch—without losing a sense of our self. Aiming gives a sense of direction, intention, and commitment. It gives the receiver the experience that he or she is being met, being seen, and given to *personally*. This focused, simultaneous awareness of self and other creates a synapse of contact, a moment of direct connection.

Releasing

For an exchange to be complete, we must completely release whatever is being given to the other. Releasing involves letting go of the need to control the receiver's response. Relaxing our attention back inside our self communicates that the receiver is free to respond in whatever way is authentic for him or her. This communicates respect—the awareness of the true otherness of the receiver. If the letting go is complete, there is a sense of satisfaction and completion.

Receiving

Needing

In order to receive, we must first sense and acknowledge that we need something. By sensing and accepting the relational need inside each vulnerability, reaching from this need with our attention toward our partner, and offering the need trustingly, it becomes possible for compassion to be awakened in the other.

Opening

To receive what we need, our attention must be open and receptive. Having reached toward the other, our attention must now relax back inside ourself, opening an inner space to receive what is needed. This requires letting go of past disappointments and resentments and expanding to the possibility of receiving something new—right now.

Welcoming

Welcoming involves letting what is outside ourself come in, and experiencing the full contact and aliveness as this influx is received. To fully welcome what is available in the present moment, we must let go of all thinking, expectations, and preferences. This involves noticing, trusting, and savoring what is actually here.

Gratitude

Feeling appreciation and gratitude completes the process of receiving. This involves letting go of the connection with the other and bringing the energy of the contact into ourself, where we can assimilate what has been given and make it our own. This creates a feeling of fulfillment and satisfaction that makes it possible to offer a deeply felt sense of gratitude.

When all of these eight elements are present, the likelihood that an exchange will lead to greater compassion and wisdom is enormously increased. When any of these elements is missing, the likelihood of a positive outcome is diminished. By looking at the process of giving and receiving in detail, we are able to precisely identify how an exchange is being interrupted and how to intervene. We are mindfully attending to the *process* of giving and receiving, rather than to the *content* of the exchange per se. Whether the content is a positive feeling such as love or a negative feeling such as anger, we are primarily focused on *how* the feeling is communicated.

SHARING VULNERABILITIES WITH AN INTIMATE PARTNER

- Take a small object that is precious to you both (e.g., a stone from a special place, a wedding ring) and take turns mindfully giving it to each other. As you give this object to each other, pay close attention to the four aspects of giving—gathering, offering, aiming, releasing—described above. Practice giving and receiving this object in a way that creates a sense of trust.
- Both of you then close your eyes and take a minute to think of some of your deepest vulnerabilities that you have not shared with your partner recently—or perhaps ever.
- One of you begins by reaching out for the other's hand and slowly, mindfully puts the object in the other's palm. While holding the object together, the giver verbally offers a vulnerability to the receiver.
- When the vulnerability has been shared, the receiving partner simply says, "I am willing to hold this with you." After that, the giver releases the object to the receiver.
- Both of you then close your eyes for several breaths, absorbing the impact of what was shared, until the receiver is ready to offer one of his or her vulnerabilities.
- Continue slowly taking turns until you both sense a deepening of compassion between you.

CONCLUSION

> The Zen student, the poet, the husband and the wife–none knows with certainty what he or she is staying for, but all know the likelihood that they will be staying "a while": to find out what they are staying for. And it is the faith of all of these disciplines that they will not stay to find out that they should not have stayed.
>
> That faith has nothing to do with what is usually called optimism. As the traditional marriage ceremony insists, not everything that we stay to find out will make us happy. The faith, rather, is that by staying, and only by staying, we will learn something of the truth, that the truth is good to know, and that it is always both different and larger than we thought.
>
> –WENDELL BERRY (2005, p. 98)

By helping intimate partners stay with whatever is happening in the present and by helping them share this together, couple therapy can strengthen a couple's faith that all their respective and collective experiences are in the service of learning how to become more compassionate, wise, loving, and whole human beings (Borofsky, 2011).

The Roman playwright Terence (2001) famously wrote, "I am a human being, and I hold nothing human alien to me" (p. 186). When nothing human is alien to us, then the entire human condition becomes our curriculum. Sorrow, for example, teaches us the poignant truth of loss and opens us to receiving others' comfort and kindness. Joy renews our faith in the possibility of fulfillment and freedom. Fear confronts us with our fragility and insists that we learn how to live with it courageously and compassionately. Love reassures us that we are deeply, indelibly connected to one another as well as to something larger than ourselves. And our capacity for mindfully witnessing whatever is happening moment by moment enables us to learn that we are more than our thoughts, our feelings, and our conditioned habits of acting and reacting. Ultimately, mindfulness reveals that we are free and unassailably safe.

By learning to mindfully share the full breadth and depth of their experience, couples can keep extending the horizon of their humanity. This inclusive, wholehearted openness to the human condition is the hallmark of both compassion and wisdom.

PART V

In and Around the Consultation Room

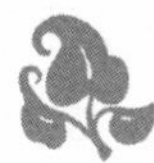

Compassion and wisdom allow us to fully engage the myriad joys and sorrows of ordinary life without layering additional stress upon ourselves or others. They can develop into personality traits–ways of being–with consistent practice over time. This practice requires that we exercise these virtues not only in therapy but also in daily life.

Chapter 21 describes how parenting can be used as an opportunity to practice mindful presence with children, progressing into compassion (and self-compassion) and wisdom (especially equanimity). The following chapter reminds therapists that the world's religions are repositories of great wisdom and compassion for many people, including our clients, and are a resource that can be tapped in therapy and in daily life. Finally, Chapter 23 points toward ethical behavior as an important means to alleviating individual and collective suffering, and as a way of practicing compassion and wisdom during the therapy hour itself.

CHAPTER 21

Mindful Parenting as a Path to Wisdom and Compassion

Trudy Goodman
Susan Kaiser Greenland
Daniel J. Siegel

> In my case also, the seeds for compassion were sown by my mother.
>
> —TENZIN GYATSO, the 14th Dalai Lama (2010a)

Integrating compassion and wisdom into the fabric of our daily lives takes time, patience, creativity, and a lot of practice. So does raising children.

Recent research demonstrates that purposefully creating a particular mental state, such as being mindful or compassionate, can develop over time into an enduring personality trait (see Chapters 3 and 8). Furthermore, when we examine how two brains interact, we see that the mind state of one person can induce a similar frame of mind in others nearby (Rizzolatti, Fadiga, Gallese, & Fogassi, 1996). It follows that parents' efforts to be more compassionate, wise, and mindful could therefore have a significant impact on their children's ability to know and to manage their own emotions, thinking, and behavior (Bluth & Wahler, 2011; van der Oord, Bögels, & Peijnenburg, 2011).

Our assumption in this chapter is that practicing mindfulness cultivates a way of being that is suffused with compassion toward oneself and others, and that creates a foundation for wisdom by opening space around our moment-to-moment experience—space in which we can more wisely choose how to respond to everyday events. And there is no better training ground for cultivating mindfulness than parenting. Indeed, Jack

Kornfield (2008a), a pioneering American meditation teacher, often calls family life "advanced practice." Raising children brings parents into a direct relationship with some of the most profound and poignant emotional experiences in life—selfless love, profound attachment, grievous loss. These experiences create a need for, and a perfect opportunity to cultivate, mindfulness, compassion, and wisdom. But what should parents know in order to make these qualities an everyday part of their interactions with children? This chapter offers some suggestions.

CHALLENGE AND OPPORTUNITY

The practice of mindfulness (on the cushion or in daily life) involves bringing kindly and refined awareness to our moment-to-moment experience (see Chapter 2). Any experience will do—internal experiences such as sensations and feelings or external perceptions such as sights and sounds—but in every case we intentionally *choose* the focus of awareness and then *stay with* the chosen object for a specified period of time. The Dalai Lama considers mindfulness to be a mental faculty that helps us maintain concentration: "of course, there needs to be a presence of mindfulness . . . and that way, the mind is able to stay focused on the chosen object" (2009b). Also, mindfulness allows us to make conscious, compassionate choices about how to behave. *Moments* of mindfulness are quite common but *continuity* of this quality of compassionate awareness is rare indeed. We see this rarity no more clearly than in caring for children.

> "Initially, the most challenging aspect of parenting was the utter and complete shock of having a small creature attached to me, completely reliant on me for his entire existence and survival, 24 hours a day, 7 days a week, from the day he was born. I was completely unprepared and overwhelmed by the loss of freedom and the loss of my identity. Before he was born I was sure of who I was . . . now I have no idea!"[1]

Parenting is as rigorous and intense a mindfulness training program as any. Relentless day and night caregiving responsibilities give rise to a

[1]This and subsequent parenting anecdotes are drawn from comments made in response to an inquiry we posted on an online community/social network comprised of those who practice mindfulness with kids and families (*www.mindfulnesstogether.net*). We asked two questions: "What have been the most challenging aspects of parenting for you?" and "What helps you to be a wise parent?"

seemingly endless parade of emotional and physical demands. Parents of young children carry on through exhaustion, stress, and strain, 24 hours a day, 7 days a week, no matter what.

Mindfulness supports parenting in many important ways (Bögels, Lehtonen, & Restifo, 2010). The challenges we face as parents inevitably sweep us out of the present moment and into "mindless" rumination—concerns about my teenage daughter's moods, my son's rough friends, my baby's skin rash. But by choosing to carefully refocus, calmly staying with what's happening in the present moment, we can steady our hearts and minds.

Understanding parenting as an opportunity for training the mind can reframe and ennoble the work of endless laundry, lunches, and little ones calling for attention. As Myla Kabat-Zinn (1998) wrote:

> Attentive parenting requires the desire to really examine the fabric of your life. If we look at our family life, and we ask ourselves, "Is this really working for all of us?" that may mean making choices. . . . We all need support in this. In some ways due to the pressures on us, we are becoming managers of our children's lives rather than really loving, connected human beings in relationship to our children.
>
> One mom struggled with being a young, single mom; she grieved that she couldn't possibly be the loving mother she envisioned herself to be while she was feeling so lonely and depressed. "After touching my profound sadness in mindfulness meditation, I started to recognize something similar in the eyes of other moms I met on the playground and in the grocery store," she recalled. "I started to feel less alone, like I was sharing a common experience of motherhood. With that, my sense of myself as a person slowly expanded: 'Oh, this is how it is to be a human being who is lonely, this is simply how it is, it's like this . . . and it's not just *my* problem.'" That's one way that mindful parenting gives birth to wisdom and compassion. We see the commonality of suffering—helping us to no longer identify with every experience as a personal possession ("This is me, this is mine alone").

The progression from mindful awareness to compassion and wisdom has been repeated an infinite number of times by parents throughout millennia. We begin simply by accepting our moment-to-moment experience, with open eyes and open hearts. When our sense of self is under siege—"I'm no good at parenting!" "I can't cope!"—we extend compassion to ourselves. That compassion then extends to others. We can teach our children what we know, both through example and by wisely (when we're lucky!) guiding our children through problems that arise in their lives.

INTERNAL AND EXTERNAL MINDFULNESS

The core mindfulness meditation text, "Discourse on the Establishment of Mindfulness" (*satipatthana-sutta*) recommends "contemplating with mindfulness internally and externally" (Analayo, 2003, pp. 94–95). *Internal* mindfulness is generally associated with sitting on a cushion or chair, feeling the movement of the breath in the body, and gradually expanding our field of awareness to include other body sensations, feelings, and thoughts. For young parents, internal mindfulness is hard to come by:

> "I didn't realize it at the time, but before I had children it came much more naturally for me to be present in the moment. If I was skiing, I was one hundred percent skiing. If I was working, I was one hundred percent working. If I was out with my husband . . . you get the picture.
>
> "Something happens when you have children that changes the ease with which we can be present in the moment. It is as if our multitasking brain kicks into high gear. For example, I might find myself at the park with my 2-year-old on a beautiful sunny afternoon. I run into a neighbor with whom I have a half-sentenced piecemeal conversation because we are both making sure our little ones don't fall off the monkey bars. At the same time I am checking my cell phone to see when my husband will be home and if he is picking my 4-year-old up from school. Meanwhile, in my head I am planning dinner, wondering if I need to go to the store and what other groceries we need, thinking about a meeting I have at work tomorrow, feeling guilty because I didn't exercise today, and wondering if I remembered to pay the phone bill last month. I may as well not be at the park with my 2-year-old at all!
>
> "It has taken a lot of time, practice, and persistence, but I have realized that I need to be intentional about being present with my children. I almost have to schedule it. When we wake up in the morning I tell myself I am going to be completely present with them until they go to school. No computer, no phone calls, no laundry. In a busy world with a busy life this is far from easy, but that time in the morning sets the tone for our day together. It goes a long way for all of us!"

External mindfulness, especially relational mindfulness (see Chapter 12), may be easier and even more useful for parents to practice. Too often this sort of mindfulness is overlooked, yet it is an essential skill. Learning how to focus on being present, aware, and attuned to what is occurring in the environment (knowing where the body is located in space, or observing closely how children may be feeling by noticing their facial expressions and body language) complements and enhances the experience of internal mindfulness. In fact, the very circuits of the brain we use to attune to ourselves during internal mindfulness practice are what we use to attune interpersonally with others (Siegel, 2007). So by attuning ourselves to the internal environment, whether in sitting meditation or going about our daily lives, we increase our capacity to be attuned interpersonally. How does this happen?

When our mindfulness practice is limited to internal mindfulness, a child's request for help or attention may feel like an unwelcome intrusion, requiring us to shift gears in order to respond. But another way for us to view the demands of children on our time and presence is as a chance to practice external mindfulness. For example, if we are mindfully slicing carrots and a child calls for our attention, our awareness can shift from inner personal carrot-focused experience to the external interpersonal environment (attending to the child), and our child's request simply becomes another expression of the way life is, endlessly changing its shape and appearance.

When parents commit themselves not only to be mindful of their inner experience (internal mindfulness) but also of the people around them (external mindfulness), they are more likely to slow down, to pause before reacting, and to see clearly whatever is happening right in the moment. A mindful pause in the rush of getting a child off to school, for example, allows us to notice what is arising inside as well as what's going on outside with our kids. This does *not* mean observing with eyes unclouded by the exhaustion of caring for young children or unruffled by emotional reactivity. If exhaustion or reactivity arises, we simply notice it. Strong emotions are inevitably part of our experience—but they need not obscure our vision. In the practice of mindful parenting, whatever is most salient and alive in our experience is a worthy object of awareness, including intense and uncomfortable mind states. "Oh, that's confusion." "That's despair." "That's rage at the child I love."

This practice is called *looking deeply* (Hanh, 1999). The process of resting in present-moment experience, just as it is, putting aside judgments of self and other if only for a moment, helps us remember what is most important and enables us to ride the sometimes turbulent waves of parenting from a place of inner clarity. We can remind ourselves of who we truly are, and we can be increasingly competent, caring adults.

The following visual experiment provides a nice metaphor for the effects of mindfulness, and it can also be demonstrated to children:

CLEAR MIND ACTIVITY

- Take a clear glass cylinder full of water, put it on a table, and ask your children to look through and see what's on the other side. They'll probably see you or whatever's sitting on the tabletop.
- Pour a cupful of baking soda in the water and shake the cylinder. What does it look like now? Can they still see through to the other side? Probably not: The baking soda clouds the water and obscures their vision. Just like baking soda in water, thoughts, emotions, and stressful life events can cloud our perspectives.
- After a minute or two, take another look at the water. What happens when you leave it alone? Sure enough, the more the water rests, the more the baking soda settles and the clearer the water becomes. Soon all of the baking soda will settle to the bottom of the cylinder and your children will be able to see through the glass again. Does the baking soda disappear entirely? No, but it has settled to the bottom of the cylinder and no longer clouds the water.

Just as the baking soda doesn't disappear in the cylinder, all of life's challenges don't disappear if you practice mindfulness. But mindfulness does give us a way to maneuver the challenges of daily life. By resting in the steady rhythm of our breathing, the thoughts, emotions, stresses, and strains of daily life settle and our perspectives become clearer (Kaiser Greenland, 2010).

BUILDING OUR CAPACITY TO TOLERATE DISCOMFORT

Paul Russell (as cited in Pizer, 2006) refers to "the crunch" in psychotherapy, which applies equally well to parenting. The crunch refers to emotional crises generated when our capacities are tested, perhaps by the discomfort of our children's painful emotions or by our own intense emotions. We have so much love for our children and such intense longing for their happiness that when they are challenged, or they challenge us, sometimes we feel that our hearts will break. Given the ferocity of our feelings, it can seem almost too much to bear. Love of children fills our hearts, but along with fulfillment comes an awareness of human vulnerability and a deep yearning to protect our children. Should our child face a life-threatening crisis, we would do anything to magically trade places with him or her.

"One of my greatest challenges as a parent has been managing the almost omnipresent anxiety that I feel being so responsible for the well-being of my children, who are dearer to me than life itself. Sometimes the anxiety is background noise ('What if the lunch lady is mean to him again and he has a meltdown in the cafeteria? What if he falls off the monkey bars? What if he has a cavity? What if the other children tease him?'). Other times, the anxiety is front and center and very hard to shake ('What if something terrible happens to them? What if something terrible happens to me? What if any one of us dies?'). My love is so deep for these little lives, and I want so much for them to be happy and healthy and vibrant and loving and loved, and I worry so much about my wishes for their well-being being thwarted in some way by life's unpredictabilities."

Receptive versus Reactive Modes of Being

If we want to provide a safe and protected space for our children, where they can play outside the shadow of our "omnipresent anxiety," we first have to find a way to feel safe within ourselves.

Our brains have two fundamental states or modes of being: receptive and reactive. When we are operating in a receptive mode, our nervous system relaxes and we become open to what is happening; it is a mindful and compassionate state (see Chapters 14 and 18). When we are operating in reactive mode, without mindfulness, our emotions stream too fast and strong for us to reflect upon them. We enter the fight–flight–freeze response as we prepare for danger and our openness shuts down. In contrast, the receptive state of mindful awareness provides emotional safety, moments of refuge where we can stop, take a deep breath, become internally and externally mindful, and self-soothe enough to be able to bear our own discomfort as well as soothe a distressed child. We open to whatever is happening right now.

To illustrate the contrast between a reactive versus receptive mode, you can try the following brief exercise:

YES OR NO

Notice what you feel when you imagine hearing the following words spoken:

- First, harshly and quickly, imagine hearing: "No. No. No. No. No. No. No!"
  [Stay with this feeling for a few moments.]
- Now, calmly, sweetly, and slowly, imagine hearing: "Yes. Yes. Yes. Yes. Yes. Yes. Yes!"
  [Stay with this feeling for a few moments.]

Many people find that "no" puts them into a reactive state of fight–flight–freeze and "yes" invites a shift to a receptive sense of openness, calm, and clarity.

Parenting from the Inside Out

Becoming a parent exposes us to some of the most intense possible human emotions, often inducing strong reactivity. Patterns of reactivity engrained in our brains from childhood are reactivated when we become parents (Siegel & Hartzell, 2003). We relive our own growing up and do our best to rework it in the fervent hope that we won't repeat our parents' mistakes. Remaining receptive through training the mind to be more mindful and compassionate, moment by moment, helps us parent our children in a less stressful, less reactive, and thus wiser way (Bögels, Hoogstad, van Dun, de Schutter, & Restifo, 2008).

As our children grow up, we recapitulate our own developmental stages. We were all children once, and we carry memories of how we were treated as children. These memories either support or undermine our ability to parent wisely (and all too often cause us to lose our emotional cool). Research in the field of parent–child relationships suggests, in fact, that our ability to understand how our own childhoods influenced our development as adults is the best predictor of how securely our children will become attached to us (Cassidy & Shaver, 2010). Recent studies also reveal that this "adult security of attachment," which occurs when we've made sense of our own childhoods, is related to how often we are mindful (DiNoble, 2009). Our "leftover issues" or "unresolved traumas or losses" from childhood put us at risk of becoming reactive too frequently or too intensely. They impel us to react automatically, triggered by conscious or unconscious memories, and to do or say things we swore we never would. This is also where mindfulness practice can gracefully help us out.

> "The hardest part for me has been the self-disappointment that I feel when I know I haven't handled a situation as kindly, patiently, or lovingly as I could have. And then doing it again the next day,

> even though I know better. I said I would never act the same as my own mom (critical, impatient, short-fused), and I don't act like her for the most part. But sometimes I do and then I wake up at 3:00 A.M. wishing I didn't (. . . which makes me tired the next day, and even more likely to repeat myself). NOTHING is more important to me than being a good mother (. . . I never felt this way at my old job, so this feeling of inadequacy is new to me).
>
> "As my children are either in or approaching adolescence, I am working on letting go of my own experiences at the same ages. I find myself reexperiencing my own adolescence at times, and it's not pretty. I'm left without a template to draw from, except from the negative. So, I return, over and over again, to wanting to impart to them the idea that my love is constant, my trust and admiration for them are real, and that I will try my best to support their search for themselves."

This "return, over and over again" is remembering to be mindful, remembering we know a way to calm and soothe the difficult emotions. It is the counterinstinctive act of mindfully turning toward our pain with the intention to hold the experience with kindness and compassion. It is paradoxical, but clinicians and mindfulness practitioners know that the most effective way to meet discomfort is to face it with the intention to understand rather than to judge (Leyro, Zvolensky, & Bernstein, 2010).

Learning to be receptive is the key to the journey of both healing and being fully present. Studies of mindfulness training reveal that a "left-shift" in baseline frontal brain activity is created even after 8 weeks of practice. This brain shift suggests that the mindfulness practitioner has become more likely to approach rather than withdraw from challenging situations (Davidson & Kabat-Zinn, 2004; D. J. Siegel, 2010b), which is also a "neurosignature" of psychological resilience.

Through the practice of turning toward discomfort, our mindfulness and compassion become *an embodied experience, a way to live from our heart*. Instead of being swept up in our internal struggles or running away from them, we learn to be more fully present with our own emotions and memories. Facing them directly, receptively, within awareness becomes a gateway to change.

We can model for our children how to engage discomfort safely and effectively. A child's neural system resonates with our own receptive states, we believe mediated in part by mirror neurons. Beyond mere behavioral imitation, mirror neurons are a proposed mechanism that, in theory, enable one person to simulate the internal state of the other. There is a suggestion of their importance in both adults and children. Children learn from us not just what to *do*, but how to *be* (Iacoboni, 2008).

A parent's willingness to be present with his or her child, over and over again (even when we don't succeed!), creates what pediatrician and psychoanalyst D. W. Winnicott (1960) described as "the good enough parental environment"—that is, an environment that allows children to bear their own discomfort, to be who they are, and to grow. Parents can take heart from what Korean Zen Master Dae Soen Su Nim (1987) taught: "to fall down 100 times, get up 101 times." Eventually, the "good enough" parental environment is internalized as a place of refuge within the child's own mind.

WISE STANCE: EQUANIMITY FOR PARENTS

In Buddhist psychology, one of the factors traditionally allied with mindfulness is equanimity. The root of the Pali term for equanimity, *upekkha*, means "taking a close look." Another translation is "considering mind," defined as "pliable," "stable," "flexible," and "not fluttering" (Mu Soeng, 2010, p. 82). How can parents develop this "considering" stance, especially in the face of their children's pain?

Once parents' mindfulness becomes strong, they have the capacity to pause and feel safe enough to be more aware internally and externally. Then they can tolerate their own emotional discomfort without acting on it, and they are able to take the next step—to "consider" it with compassionate curiosity.

A young mother took up mindfulness practice. She typically felt very badly about herself when she yelled at her kids. Lately, however, instead of sinking into shame or blame, she became curious about what she's feeling. Recognizing and naming her experience allows her to be more compassionate with herself, and to watch out for her triggers:

"1. *Sleep deprivation.* It affects my ability to drive safely, be safe in the kitchen, avoid heat and sharp objects, be kind with responses, not be irritable, not feel overwhelmed, etc. Meditation has given me some skills to manage my mind and discipline my attention, even in the face of extreme exhaustion.

"2. *Powerlessness.* When my kids don't do what I want them to do (sit in the stroller, put on shoes, stop whining/complaining), I feel powerless. After trying and trying to coax, threaten, wheedle, redirect, cajole, make fun, talk gently, etc., I sometimes have just flat out yelled—which is effective but feels terrible for all of us. Then, I went to a talk by Sharon Salzberg and something she said caught my ear: 'Underneath anger is powerlessness.' Now I see that I am angriest when I have

> completely lost any power in the situation, and so when I see powerlessness I think, 'OK now, watch out, you're about to get super angry!' "

Another parent wrote:

> "I have three children–two active boys ages 10 and 7, and a daughter age 4. Mindfulness practice is very important to me and builds my relationship with my children in so many positive ways. My challenging moments are all the calls to my attention. Here I am, noticing the beautiful colors of a carrot as I wash it, feeling the texture, present with my breath, and then SPLASH–I'm thrown into the middle of a Calgon commercial with three children with crisis in their voices, all needing me RIGHT NOW. Frankly, I find the immediacy of my children's needs (including serious medical needs) the most challenging part of parenting."

As parents we wonder, "How do I wade through the emotional muck to find a considered, benevolent response?" "How do I sustain a friendly middle stance, a way of being close without getting flooded with my own reactions or pushing my child away to get some distance from my reactivity?" This challenge is not new. Thousands of years ago, the Buddha was asked a similar question about how to navigate a flood of emotion without getting stuck in a polarized response: "But how, dear sir, did you cross over the flood without pushing forward, without staying in place?" He replied: "When I pushed forward, I was whirled about, exhausted. When I hesitated and stayed back, I sank. And so I crossed over the flood without pushing forward, and without hesitating, staying in place" (Thanissaro Bhikku, 2011).

The Buddha found a wise pace by being present–neither lingering in the past nor rushing toward the future. We can do this by practicing being patient, calm, and mindful, one step at a time.

> "The most challenging aspect of parenting my 8-year-old son and 6-year-old daughter is finding both the patience and the confidence that the job requires on a daily basis. My son, especially, is an extreme, strong personality with strong emotions to match. I am always trying to stay centered enough to parent in a way that is not simply reactive, and it is so very hard. My fear of failure kicks in and my emotions follow suit. So often I am asking him to 'calm down' and 'get control' of himself as my own control and calm slip away."

With unflinching honesty, this parent describes how she asks her child to behave in the very way that eludes her.

It's all too easy to blame children for pushing our buttons when we don't know how to turn toward their pain without getting entangled in it. In the search for perspective, we may move back too far and abandon the child—becoming too detached in a way that leaves him or her feeling all alone. Or instead we might move in too close, wanting to fix the pain:

> "It continues to be hard to listen, just listen, without responding to the intense desire to fix things for them, the desire to take their pain, their suffering, so that they don't have to be in it."

TRUSTING IN IMPERFECTION

> Every moment of mindfulness is also a moment of confidence or trust, it is not a shaky or tentative state of mind. . . . It is all at once a peaceful, buoyant, flexible, capable, and morally upright state of mind.
>
> —ANDREW OLENDZKI (2010, p. 173)

In Buddhist psychology, mindfulness is accompanied by supporting mental factors that include kindness, equanimity, and *trust*. In Pali, *saddha*, or trust, means "to place the heart upon." It is also translated as *faith* or *confidence*. Without *saddha*, self-compassion is impossible, and self-compassion is a vital antidote to the guilt and shame people feel when they inevitably fail or feel inadequate (see Chapter 6).

The Dalai Lama (2009b) suggests that beneath self-criticism, blame, and shame lies an expectation of perfection, and when we fail to be perfect, we get angry with ourselves:

> In order to develop a genuine sense of concern of others' well-being, firstly, concern of self well-being, one's own well-being must be there. Although on the conscious level, the mental state is that of criticism and hatred toward one's self. Underlying that, there must be some kind of expectation or ideal for perfection. Then when you see yourself failing, you're overly critical, and being angry toward yourself, hateful toward yourself.

The pressure parents feel to measure up to some ideal of perfection pulls them away from trusting themselves. Winnicott's notion of the "good enough" parent, mentioned above, helps to put the demands of parenting into positive perspective and relieve parental guilt. He talked about the "ordinary devotion" of mothers (Phillips, 1989, p. 140); the daily extraordinary dedication we only call ordinary because it's the common experience—changing diaper after diaper when you'd rather do anything else, making meal after meal when all you want to do is curl up on the couch and read. By relating to oneself with kindly awareness and compassion, parents find that the attitudes that get in the way of accepting themselves for who they are ("I'm selfish," "I'm no good at this!") tend to naturally dissolve. We avoid the familiar trap eloquently described by Katie Sanford (2010), a Jungian analyst: "Driven by what we should be, we miss the chance to be what we could be."

Parents can overcome the cycle of perfectionism, expectation, and self-criticism by trusting in the value of self-compassion and self-forgiveness. This is how we release the all-too-common habit of "should-ing" ourselves. As one parent put it:

> "I just choose to trust that doing my best and loving them for who they truly are will be enough to keep them on a mostly mindful path that suits them just perfectly. (Oh and I pray, a lot.)"

Another parent speaks of the perfection of imperfection, at least when we can accept ourselves more fully:

> "I have a 12-year-old and a 9-year-old. One of the most challenging things about parenting . . . is helping my children find their true inner compass—their own motivation for personal freedom/success/enlightenment. I find it hard to find a balance between letting them figure things out on their own and guiding them through healthy, mindful practices. In a perfect world I would be always consistent, serenely mindful, and they would be magically at peace, motivated, and on their path. The reality is, we're human and I guess there's an ironic perfection to our imperfection."

Letting go of the pressure to be perfect is both wise and uplifting. It is a way of creating a receptive state of mind that enables us to attune to ourselves and our children. We feel freer to appreciate and be grateful for the blessings of our lives. As we stop struggling against the realities of life, we enjoy times of ease and grace. We can invite our children to come rest with us in the cool shade of our own peaceful heart.

> "I find it so critical to anchor myself in the present moment and be mindful of what I am telling myself and believing, and being mindful of what it creates in my body–mind, as compared to what I aspire for us as a parent–child connection at the heart

> level. The other thing is when there are challenging emotions around—in me, in my 5-year-old son, in my spouse—resisting the temptation to want to make them go away. . . . How to be there, present in a moment-to-moment awareness with them, free from judging what is there, just allowing for the beauty of needs that are unfolding, free from a desire to change them or make them better . . . free of an agenda that things be any different than how they are, and trusting in the beauty of what is happening, even if it is at a deeper level than can easily be grasped."

The wise-enough parent also trusts that children will find their way. Trusting the momentum of healthy development gives parents both courage and freedom.

> "I guess the theme here is letting go because in my son's case, I struggled to trust that he would learn to overcome his struggles with peer relationships. He was very small for his age until his second year in high school and was often a target of unkind remarks and a few times of bullies. I needed to learn to trust in his ability to handle himself and find his path, which happily he has. But we had a few very painful years."

Parents can tolerate discomfort as they learn to trust the messy, arduous, beautiful path of living with children. Wisdom will come as parents learn to turn toward discomfort with compassionate curiosity, not taking it on as their own. We who step onto this path of mindful living stumble and muddle through, learning when to hold on and when to let go. We trust that things will usually work out—never perfectly—but well enough. Given sunlight, soil, and water, a plant will find a way to grow.

INTEGRATING THE CHILD'S BRAIN

As the psychotherapy profession embraces the ancient wisdom of Buddhist meditation practice and blends it with neuroscience (see Chapters 8 and 14), our understanding of parenting is also being enriched. The parent–child relationship is being studied using the tools of "interpersonal neurobiology" or "social neuroscience." Within this approach, emotional well-being is seen as the outcome of a process of *integration* (Siegel, 2007). Through the linkage of different elements of a system, integration enables us to function flexibly and adaptively in the world.

Through the scientific study of parenting, we see that when a caregiver honors the unique self of the child and connects with the child through kind, compassionate communication, a secure attachment results (Bretherton & Beeghly, 1982; Fonagy & Target, 1997; Grienenberger, Slade, & Kelly, 2005; Meins et al., 2002). This integrative relationship in childhood is associated with a wealth of positive outcomes in social, emotional, and cognitive development (Siegel, 1999; Siegel & Hartzell, 2003). Secure attachment creates a resilient child.

When we turn to the brain, we find that the integrative fibers that appear to be involved in secure attachment are also involved in mindfulness meditation. These are fibers that link differentiated neural regions to one another. One of the most integrative brain areas rests just behind the forehead, in the middle. Nine functions that are relevant to both mindfulness and to parenting occur in this middle prefrontal region: (1) regulating the body; (2) attuning to others; (3) balancing emotions; (4) soothing fear; (5) being flexible; (6) insightful linking of past, present, and future; (7) experiencing empathy for another's mental experience; (8) behaving/feeling morally—behaving/thinking of the larger social good, even when alone; and (9) accessing intuition or being open to the wisdom of the body.

Interestingly, these same nine functions of the integrative middle prefrontal region are all outcomes of mindfulness practice. Jon Kabat-Zinn, a pioneer in introducing mindfulness practice to the medical community, remarked that these functions are also the "way of being mindful" (Ackerman, Kabat-Zinn, & Siegel, 2005). The first eight functions are also proven outcomes of secure parent–child relationships (Cassidy & Shaver, 2010; Siegel, 2007). (The ninth function—intuition—has just not yet been studied.) Many mental health practitioners view this list as a good description of the components of well-being. In recent times, a number of practitioners of various wisdom traditions (Inuit, Lakota, Polynesian, Hindu) have remarked that this list also describes the essence of the teachings of their elders for how to live a wise and kind life (D. J. Siegel, personal communication, 2011).

Children not only receive their formative experiences within their families; their brains are growing when they are with friends, in school, while watching TV, and everywhere else. We look forward to a future in which mindful reflection, emotional resilience, and healing relationships—a new set of R's—can be a foundation for parents, teachers, and everyone who interacts with children. As we learn to understand and embrace our deeply interconnected biopsychosocial selves, perhaps the next generation will be better prepared to take loving responsibility for themselves and for one another—to grow in compassion and wisdom.

Cultivating the wisdom and compassion that we need to raise children well requires continual and committed practice. Although almost all parents want to succeed at this undertaking, many lack good maps or guidelines. Mindfulness practice, and the insights that derive from it, can help. The joys and challenges of parenting bring forth daily opportunities to be present, to let go, to not take things personally, to see our children clearly, and to open our hearts—practices that can bring rich rewards in both our own satisfaction and in the success and emotional well-being of the children we love.

CHAPTER 22

Drawing on the Wisdom of Religious Traditions in Psychotherapy

Kenneth I. Pargament
Carol Ann Faigin

Dear God, help me get up. I can fall down by myself.
—JEWISH SAYING

PRELUDE

"You're the best therapist I've ever worked with."

I didn't take my client's words as a compliment. Instead, I knew I was in trouble.[1] I had been working with Mary for a few months. She had been referred to me by a colleague, a female Christian therapist, who felt that she had gone as far as she could in treatment with Mary, and thought that Mary needed to work with a male. Mary was aware that she was coming to see a male Jewish therapist with interests in spiritually integrated psychotherapy.

First impressions can be deceiving, but Mary looked like a 19th-century school marm, and the impression stuck with me. With blond hair pulled back severely off an angular face devoid of makeup, she appeared older than her 35 years. And she spoke in tightly clipped sentences and an edgy tone that left me feeling uneasy, as if she would snap at me at any moment.

[1]Mary was seen in psychotherapy by K. I. P.

Mary introduced herself as a devout Catholic, but she presented with a problem that had no immediate connection to religion. For the past 15 years she had been trying to find herself a suitable husband, settle down, and have a family. But she had been repeatedly frustrated. At the age of 35, Mary was desperate, with her days marked by sharp anger, moments of despair, and panic attacks. Her "biological clock was ticking," and she didn't have a clue what the problem was. At one point in the first session, she proclaimed "All men are scum" and at another point she described herself as "fatally flawed."

I spent a few sessions with Mary exploring her romantic history. Although she had dated a variety of men, the pattern of her relationships was consistent. Within a date or two, she became infatuated with her new partner. He was the "perfect guy," the man sent to her from heaven. She would begin to fantasize about their future lives together–engagement, wedding, and children–all of this unbeknown to her "soul mate." Within a few months, her boyfriend would do something stupid–show up late for a date, make an insensitive remark, glance at another woman in the room. Invariably, Mary would react by storming off, repeating her mantra "All men are scum," and ending the brief relationship. Mary would spend the next several months in depressed seclusion, "licking her wounds" as she described it, until the fear of spinsterhood and the sound of her biological clock ticking forced her back into the world of dating. This had been the pattern for 15 years.

And now Mary was telling me that I was the best therapist with whom she'd ever worked. It didn't take extraordinary clinical insight to realize that I had become the latest man in Mary's life to be placed on the altar of worshipful devotion. But I knew that my time on the pedestal would be as brief as that of her many spurned suitors. I had to do something and do it quickly.

I chose to intervene by drawing on the wisdom and resources within Mary's own religious tradition.

INTERLUDE

Helping clients access their own religious resources is unfamiliar territory for most psychotherapists. For example, as a group, psychologists are considerably less religious than the general population (Shafranske, 2001), and therefore often unaware of the wealth of resources that are contained in the world's religions. This problem is compounded by the fact that only a small percentage of graduate programs in clinical psychology provide students with any training in religion and spirituality (Brawer, Handal, Fabricatore, Roberts, & Wajda-Johnston, 2002). But the problem may go beyond unfamiliarity. From Freud to Skinner to Ellis, there is a long tradition of religious antipathy in the field, perhaps growing out of its efforts to establish itself as a "hard science" and distinguish itself from its disciplinary kin—philosophy and theology. Stereotypic notions of religion as a pacifier, a defense, or a form of denial are still commonplace among mental health professionals, even though these stereotypes are not empirically supported (Pargament, 1997). It would be more accurate to describe religion as a potential resource for many people.

Organized religion provides its members with models of exemplary behavior, morals and ethics, virtues, spiritual coping methods, connection with others, systems of belief, rituals, and methods for communicating with a higher power through prayer and meditation. These beliefs and practices serve a number of critical functions by providing emotional comfort, meaning and purpose, protection, intimacy with others, identity, healing, self-regulation, and connectedness with the sacred. For example, spiritual purification rituals are a powerful resource for forgiveness and healing from even the deepest wounds of guilt, sin, doubt, and self-condemnation. Judaism offers the Ten Days of Repentance, Native American spirituality offers the healing powers of the sweat lodge, Catholicism provides confession through a priest, Islam provides personal prayer for forgiveness from Allah as one of the Five Pillars of their faith, Buddhism teaches compassionate mind training, and Protestantism offers confession through private prayer. It is important to add that religious beliefs and practices can also be spiritually individualized and expressed outside established religious structures.

A large body of empirical research has pointed to the benefits of religious resources for the health and well-being of people facing a variety of major psychological and physical challenges (for a review, see Ano & Vasconcelles, 2005; Pargament, 1997). These resources include meditation, prayer, positive religious reframing, religious and spiritual support, ritual practices, and forgiveness. Consider one striking study conducted by Janine Jones (2007), which describes the power of religious coping for 71 African American children (ages 7–9) living in the high-poverty and high-crime community of an inner-city project. A large percentage of these children had seen strangers or someone they knew being assaulted with a weapon, and many of these young children had already witnessed the murder of a stranger or someone they knew. They themselves had also been victims of violent crimes, such as being chased or threatened, being beaten or assaulted with a weapon. As Jones notes, these experiences are severe enough to cause complex posttraumatic stress disorder (PTSD). Despite these risk factors, however, in children who drew upon their spirituality (spiritual beliefs, church attendance, prayer, use of spiritual support and coping), exposure to severe violence in the community was *unrelated* to developing complex PTSD. However, children with low spirituality who were exposed to the same community violence were more likely to develop complex PTSD. This notable study underscores the protective role of spiritual beliefs, religious practices, and spiritual coping.

It could be argued that religion does not add anything distinctive to the mix of coping resources people can draw on when they encounter major life stressors. After all, religious and spiritual support could be viewed as merely examples of more general support. Transcendent meaning systems could be understood as simply one subset of secular meaning systems. Yet, several empirical studies suggest that religious resources make unique contributions to health and well-being, even after accounting for the effects of secular coping resources. For instance, working with a national sample of elders, Krause (2006) compared the role of emotional support received from church members with the emotional support received from nonchurch members as buffers of the effects of financial strain on self-rated health. Whereas church-based emotional support emerged as a buffer, secular support did not. Interpreting these findings, Krause emphasized the distinctive character of church-based support: It is particularly helpful because it is enacted in a group that shares a spiritual worldview and commitment to God, a common set of sacred beliefs, values, and coping methods, shared religious principles, rituals, and memories, and a support that is "imbued with the mantle of religious authority" (p. S36).

Important as religious resources may be, questions could be raised about whether clients, in fact, want to have the topics of religion and spirituality broached in treatment. Perhaps they prefer to separate matters of faith from psychological problems and treatment, just as church is separated from state in the political system in the United States. Empirical studies have addressed this question and their findings suggest that most people in the United States would prefer a spiritually sensitive approach to treatment. For example, in one study of clients seeking psychological treatment, over half (55%) reported a desire to talk about religious and spiritual matters in counseling (Rose, Westefeld, & Ansley, 2001). Similarly, Lindgren and Coursey (1995) found that two-thirds of a sample of clients struggling with serious mental illness were interested in speaking with their therapist about religious and spiritual matters affecting their lives and recovery.

Evidence is also accumulating that by integrating spirituality into treatment, practitioners may enhance the effectiveness of psychotherapy (for a review, see Pargament, 2007). In a recent meta-analysis of 31 outcome studies, Smith, Bartz, and Richards (2007) found that spiritually integrated therapies were beneficial to clients coping with anxiety, depression, stress, and eating disorders.

One such example is a new cognitive-behavioral therapy, developed by Avants, Beitel, and Margolin (2005), that highlights how spirituality can add an important dimension in treating drug use and HIV risk-taking behavior. This 8-week treatment, called spiritual self-schema (3-S) therapy, is spiritually flexible and can be used for people of any—or no—religious tradition. Drawing upon the Buddhist philosophy of "do no harm," 3-S therapy teaches that addiction is not one's true nature and that each person contains an inherent wisdom. By shifting in self-concept from an "addict" to a "spiritual self," the individual is taught to tap into a source of personal healing. The spiritual self is promoted through the development of 10 spiritual and socially desirable qualities based on Buddhist tradition: morality, loving-kindness, equanimity, strong determination, truth, tolerance, effort, renunciation, generosity, and wisdom. Mastery of these spiritual qualities is developed through participation in self-awareness exercises, daily meditation, mindfulness practices, and self-generated affirmations and prayers (see Chapter 16 for a related addictions treatment approach). A majority of participants in the 3-S therapy significantly decreased their drug use (cocaine or heroin), experienced less craving for drugs, and manifested increased motivation for abstinence and HIV prevention. When asked how this spiritually integrated therapy was helpful, one client responded, "The freedom. The freedom of knowing that my true self is spiritual not the addict. That's freedom itself" (Avants et al., 2005, p. 176).

Despite these encouraging findings, there are challenges involved in helping clients draw on spiritual resources in treatment. Perhaps the greatest obstacle is that spiritual resources are less than fully developed for many clients, including those who are ostensibly religious or spiritual. Commenting ruefully on the results of a national survey pointing to the prevalence of spirituality in the United States, George Gallup, Jr., and D. Michael Lindsay (1999) said: "Spirituality in the United States may be three thousand miles wide, but it remains only three inches deep" (p. 45). The American culture of independence and cafeteria-style spirituality leads many people to pick and choose their personal beliefs in isolation from the wisdom and support of religious communities. As a result, they may be left with a religious framework or "orienting system" that lacks the breadth, depth, and integration necessary to respond effectively to the full range of life's challenges (Pargament, 2007). Consider two examples, one involving the limited capacity for religious meaning making and the other involving limited understandings of God or higher powers.

Many combat veterans exposed to the traumatic experiences of war grapple with profound spiritual questions (Tick, 2005), such as "Why did I survive?", "How can God allow such human suffering?", "How can I reconcile my own behavior or that of others with my religious commitments?"

Without a religious frame of reference capable of providing meaningful answers to these terribly difficult questions, the individual may find that his or her psychological, social, and physical struggles are compounded by religious struggle and strain. In fact, mental health professionals are beginning to expand services to help soldiers and veterans anticipate and address these religious struggles (Pargament & Sweeney, 2011) and "moral injuries" (Litz et al., 2009).

Another problem arises when people ascribe to narrow views of a higher power or what they hold divine. Phillips (1997) offers several illustrations of "small gods" that are incapable of helping individuals deal effectively with the multitude of dilemmas of life. There is the image of God as a Heavenly Bosom who provides limitless comfort and solace without asking for anything in return; the God of Absolute Perfection who insists upon complete flawlessness; the Grand Old Man who is relatively disengaged from modern life; and the Resident Policeman who serves as the critical, negative, internal voice that consistently threatens ultimate punishment. Small gods of these kinds cannot provide people with a strong, reliable resource in coping with life's demands.

Because spiritual resources are less than fully developed for many clients, it takes skill on the part of therapists and work or "spiritual discipline" on the part of clients to draw successfully on the wisdom of religious traditions in treatment. However, this undertaking is no different than what is required in helping clients access other resources, such as developing a social support network, physical fitness, or self-confidence. The wisdom of religious traditions simply represents one more potentially valuable pathway to greater health and well-being.

FINALE

Interaction 1

Shortly after Mary announced that I was the best therapist with whom she had ever worked, I said, "I notice that you seem to have two categories for describing people; you've got your saints and you've got your sinners."

Mary thought for a moment and then said, "Not really. I think of people as angels and demons."

Close enough, I thought. I went on: "Well, from my point of view, I think you're missing a third category of people.

"Who's that," she asked?

"Human beings," I responded. "I have to say that I personally haven't come across too many angels or demons, but I've met a lot of human beings who seem to have a bit of the angelic and a bit of the demonic inside."

Mary sat quietly with that idea. It was a new one for her. She had a long history of splitting people into good and bad. Her father had been such a black-and-white figure. He could be distant and uninvolved with Mary for weeks at a time. At other times, he would be angry and critical. And yet, Mary also recalled moments of warmth and closeness with her father when she felt loved and protected. "I kept trying to be the perfect girl, but I was never good enough for him." At an intellectual level, Mary had some recognition that she was pursuing an impossible dream—an attempt to find "the perfect father" she'd never had—through her romantic relations. The insight, however, hadn't touched her at a deeper emotional level.

By raising the notion of a third category of people, human beings, I was trying to encourage Mary to move to a more differentiated perspective of people, not just her father but potential romantic partners too. But I knew she'd need some help in the process.

Interaction 2

"I know you're a devout person, Mary," I said, "and it seems to me that you have a wonderful resource from your religious tradition that could help you deal with people as human beings—you know, people with a bit of the angelic and demonic in them."

"OK, I'll bite," Mary said semijokingly. "What's that?"

"Forgiveness," I said.

Mary paused again and then remarked, "I've never been very good at that."

Even though forgiveness is a cornerstone of Christian theology, Mary was unfamiliar with this religious resource. A part of her had resonated with the ideas of compassion, mercy, and grace she had read about in catechism classes and heard in her Roman Catholic parish. But these concepts were distant and removed from her own personal experiences and understanding of God. In fact, her view of God was not unlike that of the darker side of her father: a critical being who was waiting to pounce should she make a mistake.

Mary was showing many of the signs of a religious orienting system that lacked breadth, depth, and integration. Her understanding of Catholicism was narrow and shallow. Her experience of the transcendent was constricted. Hers was a "small god," a god who could demand, oversee, and punish without the possibility of compassion, concern, and forgiveness.

I asked Mary if she might be willing to look further into this idea of forgiveness. She agreed.

Focus on Forgiveness

Over the next few months, Mary and I spent much of our time together talking about forgiveness. I recommended some readings on the topic, which she eagerly studied, such as *To Forgive Is Human* (McCullough, Sandage, & Worthington, 1997). We talked about forgiveness as a process that involves a transformation from a focus on anger, resentment, and retribution to acceptance, compassion, and letting go. Mary struggled with these ideas. She had spent her life trying to perfect herself in the hopes of winning the love of her father, God, and other men. To give up that pursuit left her feeling confused and disoriented. In place of striving for perfection to find the love she had been missing, I drew her attention to the wisdom in her religious tradition of being loved in spite of being human and flawed. As we discussed concepts of compassion, love, and forgiveness, we found that they applied as much to the way Mary treated herself as to the way she treated other people. We talked about the periods of unrelenting criticism Mary had experienced from her father and from her punitive representation of God, and then considered those times when she had felt a sense of forgiveness from others when she had made a mistake. Mary teared up when she recalled a few instances in which other people had responded to her errors with compassion rather than criticism (a process similar to the compassionate letter exercise in Chapter 6).

"That's forgiveness," I said.

As we moved through these conversations, Mary began to change physically. She removed the rubber band holding her hair back so tautly off of her face and let her hair fall naturally on to her shoulders. She began to wear makeup that softened her sharper edges. And she was smiling more often and speaking more easily.

Our conversation shifted back to romantic relationships. Mary still hoped to meet an eligible man, marry and have a family. This time, though, she seemed better prepared. I talked with Mary about what she might expect when she met a guy.

Interaction 3

"OK, you're going to meet this great guy, you're going to think he's perfect, and then you know he's going to go ahead and do something bonehead dumb. What are you going to do then," I asked?

"Well, I know my first reaction will be to go into my 'All men are scum' routine and then go into the corner to eat worms, but I think I know better now," she said.

"So what will you do," I pushed?

"I'm going to try to remember that he's not an angel or a demon, that he's a human being, and I'm going to try to treat him with some understanding and compassion as a human being and one of God's children," she said.

"You might even be able to talk things out or talk things through—kind of like we do in here," I suggested.

"You know, if you had said that to me a few months ago, I would have laughed at you, but now it's something I might actually like to try to do."

"And I've got a hunch you'd do pretty well," I responded.

I have always been suspicious of writers or speakers who present "fast or miraculous" cures. I have rarely experienced them myself. Change tends to take time, with starts and stops, like an engine that needs to be primed several times before it catches. Mary was an exception, however. The week after my interaction with her, Mary met a man at a concert. He had been attracted to Mary's smile, gotten up the nerve to start a conversation, and asked her out on a date. The two dated for several months, and as we had anticipated, experienced some ups and downs. This time, however, Mary stayed in the relationship and put the lessons of compassion and forgiveness into practice. The two were able to resolve their differences and were engaged a year later. By that time, Mary had terminated therapy. Occasionally, I receive a family portrait in a seasons greeting card—Mary with a warm smile, her husband, and their two rambunctious children.

CONCLUSIONS

Clients don't come to psychotherapy empty-handed. They bring their own resources as well as resources embedded in their larger social and cultural contexts. Religion is one such repository of wisdom for many people. However, many clients do not fully access their own religious resources. Therapists can play a valuable role here by helping clients develop more accessible and integrated religious frameworks.

If there is resistance to this process, it is more likely to come from therapists than clients, but as we have noted here, there are a number of good reasons why mental health professionals should integrate religious and spiritual issues in treatment. The bottom line is that drawing on the religious wisdom traditions in psychotherapy makes good sense.

Though there is now a developing literature in this area, we have a great deal more to learn about religious integration in treatment. Specific questions include how to educate ourselves more fully about matters of religion and spirituality, how to assess religious resources and problems, how to relate to a client's religious community, how to address religious resources and problems while remaining respectful of the client's autonomy in this domain, how to avoid both the danger of imposing a religious or secular perspective on clients and the danger of neglecting the topic altogether, and how to identify and deal with the therapist's own biases in the religious domain and their potential impact on the treatment process.

Made manifest in psychotherapy, wisdom and compassion are grounded in appreciation for the full range of human nature—biological, psychological, social, *and* spiritual.

CHAPTER 23

Compassion and Wisdom

Growing through Ethics

Stephanie P. Morgan

> The really important kind of freedom involves attention, and awareness, and discipline, and effort, and being able to truly care about other people. . . . over and over, in myriad pretty little unsexy ways, every day.
>
> —DAVID FOSTER WALLACE (2008, p. W14)

Compassion and wisdom, the two unifying threads woven throughout this book, are often expressed in ethical behavior. This final chapter focuses on the power of ethical training for us as therapists in the development and expression of wise, compassionate action. Although teachings on compassion are remarkably consistent across the world's major religious traditions (Dalai Lama, 2010b), ethical training in Buddhism is unusual in that the teachings are not passed down from a divine source, but rather derive from direct exploration of internal and external experience. They are thus readily applicable to secular, empirical, psychotherapy. In all traditions, ethical behavior is valued because it alleviates suffering, within us and in others. This chapter introduces Buddhist ethical practices to serve as a kind of high-powered lens that can add aliveness, growth, and integrity to clinical work—helping us become wiser, more compassionate psychotherapists.

Western psychotherapeutic traditions have historically steered clear of integrating ethics into mental health treatment (beyond restraining clinicians from gross misconduct). While this distance may be attributable to many factors, two concerns seem to be central: (1) the need to legitimize psychology and psychiatry as sciences, leaving morality within the purview of religion; and (2) concern that a psychotherapeutic approach emphasizing values might constrain individual freedom. However, in the last decade, research from the field of positive psychology points to the relevance of ethical considerations for happiness and well-being (Dahlsgaard, Peterson, & Seligman, 2005; Peterson & Seligman, 2004). More recently, ethical training has been introduced as critical to developing mindfulness in therapy (Monteiro, Nuttall, & Musten, 2010). This chapter builds on these trends to demonstrate the value and relevance of ethical training for the psychotherapist.

GUIDELINES FOR SKILLFUL BEHAVIOR

In Buddhist practice, moral action is cultivated by observing five basic precepts (Hanh, 1998). Rather than prohibitions, precepts are guidelines for living skillfully. Traditionally, the five precepts have been framed as restraint from (1) killing, (2) stealing, (3) sexual misconduct, (4) lying, and (5) using intoxicants. In the last few decades, Zen master and teacher Thich Nhat Hanh (2007) has offered a reformulation of these five basic precepts to address the realities and challenges of contemporary living. In this reformulation, the guidelines for skillful behavior include acts of commission as well as acts of restraint:

1. Restraint from killing—compassionate action, reverence for life
2. Restraint from stealing—concern for equity, generosity
3. Restraint from sexual misconduct—skillfulness with sexual energy
4. Restraint from lying—honest, skillful speech
5. Restraint from using intoxicants—awareness of consumption

From a Buddhist psychological perspective, the cultivation of wisdom and compassion—developing an awakened mind and heart—necessitates training in three dimensions: concentration (*samadhi*), insight (*prajna*), and moral action (*sila*). Traditionally referred to as the "threefold training," these dimensions are interdependent—each one potentiates the other two. In undertaking the precepts, there is a calming, settling effect in one's life that aids in concentration. Greater concentration leads to more insight, and insight in turn deepens and refines our understanding of, and ability to embody, the precepts. Thich Nhat Hanh refers to this mutually reinforcing interaction by saying that these three dimensions of practice "inter-are" (Hanh, 2007, p. 2). *Sila* or morality practice pushes and develops our understanding, while it is also an expression of our understanding (Fischer, Drolma, & Olendzki, 2010). We *work it*, so to speak, and *it works us*. Additionally, each of the precepts is understood to represent a continuum, offering the opportunity to attend, practice, and learn with increasing refinement in wisdom and skillful means. Practicing with the precepts involves reflection, intentionality with one's behavior, and awareness of cause and effect.

This practice involves taking care with a light touch. In understanding that the precepts are actually impossible to keep, we cultivate genuine humility and an absence of self-righteousness. We undertake the five precepts knowing that we will fail, and knowing that as our understanding deepens, we will more often act skillfully. Precept practice opens us increasingly to what we might call our "practice edges." On these edges, we hone our discernment. We understand more about the causes, conditions, and outcomes of our behavior. We express our willingness to begin again, time after time—much as one does when trying to simply be with the breath in meditation practice.

A simple exercise can help us begin.

BEGINNING PRECEPT PRACTICE

- Take a moment to breathe and check into your present-moment experience.
- Now ask yourself the question: *"What is my intention in doing psychotherapy?"* Give yourself some time to inquire deeply and to rest with this reflection.
- As you emerge with awareness of your intention, appreciate it.

Precept practice is best understood as a day-to-day way to live in increased alignment with our heartfelt intention to alleviate suffering—in ourselves, in our clients, in all beings. In the following pages, we focus on ways in which working with each of the five precepts can help us cultivate wisdom and compassion while refreshing and illuminating our clinical work.

FIRST PRECEPT: REVERENCE FOR LIFE

The Hippocratic oath states "First, do no harm." While this is certainly our intention as psychotherapists, looking more closely, we see that this precept is impossible to keep. We become aware that in taking one footstep on the earth, we kill life. As we take each breath, we kill microorganisms in the air. My colleague, Ed Yeats, wisely warns, "We are most dangerous when we are unaware of our capacity for harm" (personal communication, 1995). Working with this precept clinically, we investigate those ways in which our actions can be unintentionally harmful.

Working with Anger

How do we deal with our own anger when it arises in a session? Noticing that anger is present is the first step. If we repudiate this aspect of our experience, we are more likely to be driven by the anger in some way–be it a reduction in empathy, an unskillful response, or a distancing from the client. In working with a client who had a pattern of cancellations, I found that I became slower than usual in returning his phone calls for rescheduling. In becoming aware of my own enactment, it became possible to bring the issue into the treatment for mutual exploration.

At times our anger can be important information to share with a patient because it may shed light on a relevant interpersonal issue–but we need to take utmost care when conveying it. A client, Ali, owed me a large amount of money. We had made an agreement that when her financial situation changed, she would settle the debt. When she commenced repayment with a significant installment, she spoke of it much as if she was giving me a gift. Initially, I found this attitude irksome and did not address it, but when the attitude persisted, I raised the issue. I acknowledged that I was feeling put off by the spirit that colored the repayment process. Although awkward and bumpy initially, this mutual conversation led to a productive investigation of Ali's sense of entitlement and the way in which it had caused her difficulties in many of her relationships.

Subtle Forms of Mistreatment

It can be useful to step back from our caseload and examine the quality of care that we are bringing to each of our clients. We all have our own standards with regard to punctuality, responsiveness to phone calls, how we end sessions. Wherever your bar is set, are there any clients with whom the bar is a bit lower? Becoming aware of those individuals whose appointment time we might more readily shift, or with whom we're comfortable being a few minutes late, focuses our awareness on these less-than-caring behaviors, enabling us to bring more wholehearted attention. In our sloppiness, we may be taking advantage of a client's goodwill or reenacting a subtle form of neglect familiar to him or her. Again, the wonderful aspect of working with this first precept is that it invites us to examine our behaviors on this subtler level, increasing coherence between our intentions and our behaviors.

After Therapy Ends

We continue to exist for our clients in many ways after therapy ends. The healing power of a positive connection far outlives the formal treatment episode. If a former client makes contact again, for whatever reason, unresponsiveness on our part can leave him or her questioning the genuineness of the relationship and our regard. This is the harm. It's not just the former client's disappointment with whatever does or doesn't unfold. It's that our unresponsiveness can cast a shadow back on the treatment and make him or her question whether it was real.

Over the holidays one year, I received a long and lovely letter from a former client who had ended therapy years before and subsequently moved out of state. Enclosed with the letter was a novel that she had written. I spent over a year not responding to her in any way, all the while feeling quite guilty about my inaction. My delay was not motivated by disregard. Rather, I felt that I couldn't get back to her until I had read her novel. Finally, I became aware that in requiring this of myself, I was doing both of us a disservice. I was able to write a note addressing my delayed response, thanking her for the book and wishing her well. Ironically, we are sometimes unskillful because we have been unfair and unrealistic in our expectations of ourselves. Our lives are often dense with demands. Modesty about what we can offer and do is important. The practice of nonharming applies to ourselves as well.

SECOND PRECEPT: MONEY AND EQUITY

For What Are We Being Paid?

In attempting to be fair to both our clients and ourselves in the treatment enterprise, we might ask, "What are they paying us for?" Perhaps we can all agree that one thing our clients are paying us for is skillful attention. We intend to provide our attention, yet we have, as Joan Halifax (1993) says, "wayward minds and forgetful hearts" (p. 144). Although harshly stated, when we work with this precept, we undertake not to rob our clients through our inattention. Time is precious. Think of your hourly rate and divide by 50, if you do the 50-minute hour. So if your fee is $100.00, a client is paying $2.00 a minute. If we're off doing our grocery list, our client is not getting full value. While our inattention might also be pointing to other factors in the treatment, this reflection adds another dimension to our awareness. Again, working the precept is not about indicting ourselves; it is about looking carefully at our motivations, our behaviors, and cause and effect.

There are other ways that we can exploit our clients' time. I once worked with Jim, a landscaper, in my home office. While walking in, Jim would often make comments about the yard. I remember on one occasion exercising inordinate restraint not to ask his advice about the wooly adelgids that were decimating a hemlock. This can sometimes be a nuanced issue; conversation that is validating a person's identity is different than appropriating someone's expertise and time for our own ends.

A similar issue arises with gratifying content. When a client is entertaining or funny, we love to sit back and enjoy the ride. When someone falls in love, we delight in hearing all of the intoxicating details. Again, these are delicate and nuanced issues for our discernment. Our delight isn't necessarily problematic, and people so want to be enjoyed. Both of these dynamics can be just the right medicine. But we also want to be tracking what is going on within ourselves and our motives in the moment. We can bring mindful attention to the questions that we ask and why we ask them. If we are asking out of idle curiosity or to satisfy a particular interest of ours, it might be more equitable to exercise restraint. A colleague told me he once asked his therapist, a well-known analyst, "Is that question for me or for you?"

Fees

This second precept concerning equity also provides a lens we can bring to our fees. Getting paid for the work we do is essential and appropriate. Payment and the boundaries around time enable us to sit with clients in a way that is, as Paul Russell (1996, p. 202) said, "free of need." The value of this can't be overestimated. A person is paying to be in a relationship where we need nothing of him or her and have no need for our patient to be anything for us. Yet within the complicated territory of fees and payment, working with this second precept involves the following:

- Viewing our work as an ecological system, wherein higher fees can enable us to provide some services for lower fees. In social work training, the tradition of pro bono work is a hallmark of the profession. Working with this precept involves the practice of generosity with our time and effort.
- Knowing what side of the road we're on and our leanings and vulnerabilities with regard to money. Are we too concerned with money? Are we insufficiently attentive to these issues? If we are unaware of our tendencies, they will play out in the treatment.
- Awareness of when we make special arrangements with regard to fees. We need to be very clear that realities might change. It is skillful to establish at the outset of the arrangement a future time for review.
- Noticing when we are either overly eager to collect a bill or reluctant to issue a one. Each posture can indicate unexamined feelings

with regard to the client or the treatment. I've noticed that at times when I am reluctant to give someone a bill, it is the first sign that I feel the treatment is stuck—and a signal to look at that issue more directly either in supervision or with the client.

THIRD PRECEPT: SKILLFULNESS WITH SEXUALITY

This precept refers to restraint from any sexual involvement with our patients. Bringing more refinement to this area of investigation and practice involves recognizing the power of sexual energy and our commitment to the development of compassion and wisdom in this arena. As therapists, it is a great gift to our clients to be loving and safe to love. By "safe to love" I mean that our clients can have their full range of feeling, which might include love and desire. Awareness helps us stay steady and receptive to this full range of expression, while at the same time not leaving our seat.

In working this precept, we attempt to refrain from using our clients for our own gratification. If we find ourselves doing something unusual with our apparel or in any other way in anticipation of seeing a particular client, it might indicate the need for further attention to our internal process. Does our behavior point to some hunger, absence, or dimension of feeling in our own life that merits attention?

Flirtatious Energy

Working with this precept also raises the question of how we relate to flirtatious energy. Flirtatious energy can represent so many different things, in and out of the therapy hour. Is it a celebration of life and vitality? Is it a deadened and habitual way of relating? Is it an avoidance of pain that deserves attention? Is it a veiled form of aggression? For many of us, our reflexive comfort or discomfort with sexual energy can inhibit our awareness and investigation. We might disengage by either reflexively shutting down or participating with less awareness. Navigating these waters wisely takes attention and practice.

Playfulness can be life-affirming. I've noticed that there are instances when I've been working with someone over time and then one day I simply see him in a fresh way, as more attractive. Becoming aware of this new energy is often a harbinger of the person feeling better—less depressed, or less anxious.

If the flirtatious energy feels like a defense against underlying vulnerability, a gracious acknowledgment can be skillful. For example, "While I am complimented that you are flirting with me, perhaps your heart needs a different kind of attention." When the flirtation feels deadened or deadening, there might be underlying hostility. In trying to effectively respond to this form of flirtation, we often feel tied up and uncomfortable. At such times, the introduction of an existential perspective can be helpful. I sometimes find a way to bring up aging or death. Working with a powerful CEO in his 60s, I was repeatedly struggling, feeling powerless and ineffective in the face of his antics. One day, I simply stated, "You know, we're both growing old." This existential truth had a great settling effect and grounded our connection in something real.

FOURTH PRECEPT: SKILLFUL SPEECH

The fourth precept pertaining to skillful speech probably has the most ramifications for psychotherapy. What we say or don't say is a central feature of the therapy encounter. Most importantly, our trustworthiness is paramount to the therapeutic power of the relationship.

Honesty

Joseph Goldstein, a wise and senior *vipassana* meditation teacher, once said that if we undertook this precept completely, it would be a full practice, meaning that it would cultivate sufficient awareness and discernment to bring enlightenment. We lie in little ways all the time. Precept practice directs us to look in the mirror. What do we rationalize on a tax return or how impeccable are we in our dealings with insurers? When we are less than honest with our clients, what are the implications?

Bare honesty advances our work. I remember a moment from my own treatment. I was looking down, talking about something, and happened to look up and sensed that my therapist's attention had wandered. I asked, "Where'd you go?" She responded, "Not far." I loved her response because I felt fully met in that moment. Her honesty enriched the texture of intimacy and authenticity in our relationship.

At times, we are less than honest about things that we haven't done, but said that we would do. This might come up in areas of collateral contact, referral information, insurance business, etc. Perhaps we said that we would do something and the week goes by and we haven't done it. In the session, we might be asked, or we might bring it up ourselves, saying, "We're playing phone tag" or "We haven't yet spoken directly," implying that we've made efforts we haven't yet actually made. We ask our clients to be truthful, and yet we are not necessarily so forthcoming. At such times, we experience a decrease in contact and intimacy, becoming less present and available.

Lack of truthfulness may also constrain our clients' freedom. In psychotherapy, we are trying to foster an accepting environment in which our clients can think, feel, and express themselves freely. Perhaps they sense that we are fudging, but they may also sense that we don't want to be challenged. We bid them to collude with protecting us. I've observed that it is easy to invite negative feelings about something we feel fine about, such as going on vacation. But when we ourselves feel badly about something, it's harder to be open to hearing what our client feels about it.

When we can step up and acknowledge our missteps, it often brings both discomfort *and greater intimacy*. Months ago, I had a phone appointment set up at a time when I don't usually work. I remembered hours later. As I prepared to call my client, I considered the multiple ways I could put a spin on what had occurred. Of course, none felt very satisfactory because none was true. I called her and said, "Jean, I completely forgot." We make our very best attempts and when we fall short, this precept invites us to be truthful about things, just as they are. In the context of responsible treatment, people can usually forgive our fallibility. Certainly there are times in which bare honesty is not appropriate and can be hurtful. But the motivation for our little white lies is more often reflective of what Steven Pinker (2008) describes as "a nasty tendency to put self on the side of the angels" (p. 58).

Restraint from Frivolous Speech

Working with the precept of skillful speech also includes an examination of frivolous speech—talking that is unnecessary and can diminish the richness of a moment. At times, the texture of a silence is best left undisturbed, as a shared silence can give birth to a deepening of expression. When we are fully available to accompany a patient in silence we might be helping him or her find freedom in just simply being.

At the beginning and end of the hour, we are more prone to fall into reflexive patterns of speech. We want to convey warmth, yet this might be more effectively conveyed in eye contact, fully taking the person in as we greet him or her, rather than through a more socially conventional "chatty" greeting. Although a person is sometimes freed to ease into the session via a friendly greeting, we want to be conscious of what motivates our talking. Similarly, the end of a session can be an occasion for more care with speech. There are times when I've gotten up and seen the person to the door in a manner that isn't in keeping with the affect of the session we've just had, when I've fallen into a less present, socially conditioned way of saying goodbye. Practicing skillful speech supports us in extending our attention to the transitional interactions that are part of the therapy encounter.

When Clients Speak about Others

How do we sit, listen, and respond to our clients when they are complaining about other people? We often walk a fine line. On the one hand, we sometimes fall into a superficial form of empathy that not only honors our client's subjectivity but goes further and aligns with him or her in blaming or condemning someone else. We all can become sensitive to such moments. It cheapens the bond at someone else's expense.

On the other hand, we can do others a grave disservice if we don't step up and name things. If someone has been mistreated, our willingness to speak is critical. To shy away or adopt a quiet stance may reflect resistance to engaging with the suffering. At times, our voice is necessary to help a client find his or her own voice. We are called upon to be the first to say "This is harmful" or "That should never have happened." The following questions can be helpful in refining our awareness in this arena:

- What is the person's leaning or inclination? Does he or she tend to blame others and avoid responsibility? Or conversely, does he or she lean toward self-blame and taking too much responsibility?
- What is the pulse of the exchange? Is it alive and moving toward life and discovery, or does it have a static, deadened quality?
- Are we remembering as we sit with one person, that he or she lives within the context of a greater web of multiple interacting subjectivities? If we keep this wider truth in our awareness, we bring this understanding forward in implicit ways in our responses.

When we become aware that we feel pulled off our seats, either through overidentification or through inhibited empathy with our client's experience, wise action may reside in speaking directly to the issue. If we feel complicit in an unproductive blaming session, we might ask, "Are you feeling that you need agreement from me to accept how you are feeling about this?" Conversely, if we feel that our client has given insufficient voice to something, we can inquire, "I have the sense that I am feeling more about this than you are. What is your experience of what you are saying?"

Disclosure

Meditation teachers often advise that skillful speech requires that we ask two questions: (1) Is it honest? and (2) is it skillful? We've been looking at honesty. Exploring disclosure takes us into the question of skillfulness. Will the information be helpful and is it a good use of the client's limited time with us?

Recently, I was working with a man who started the session by saying that he had just heard Mary Oliver, the wonderful poet, read her poems. My client went on to say that when she was about to read "Wild Geese," the crowd exploded in applause, like at a rock concert. By coincidence, that very day, my son was going to recite the same poem in school. I watched the desire rise up to tell him about this coincidence. I didn't speak. I let the urge arise and pass. I could have told myself that it was about joining with him, but we were already joined. It would have been more about my pride in my son. And in fact, soon after he shifted gears and spoke about a matter of current distress.

Just to be truthful in my "disclosure about disclosure," I should add the companion example to this story: A client was happily telling me about his son's trip to a beautiful area of southern Spain and the slides he had just seen. Having just been there myself, I blurted out, "I've been there. It is so beautiful." So often, when we disclose in this unbidden way, it reflects what Joseph Goldstein (2010) refers to as "the irresistible, pregnant-with-conceit desire to say, 'Here I am.' " Such comments rarely add to our client's experience.

Although there are no hard and fast recipes with regard to disclosure, leaning toward restraint gives us space and time to be aware of our motivations and to consider consequences. Certainly, when an absence of disclosure contributes to a lack of reality testing, it may be harmful to be silent. In addition, there are times when someone asks us a question and a straightforward answer helps him or her experience mutuality and respect in the relationship. When we are in doubt about whether to disclose, we also have a third option, which is to share our process of consideration.

FIFTH PRECEPT: MINDFUL CONSUMPTION

This precept is about restraining from the use of any substances that cloud the mind and, I might add, *heart*. Clearly, if we are struggling with substance abuse, there is a level of pain in our lives that will hamper our capacity to sit fully with someone else.

More broadly, and framed according to Thich Nhat Hanh's formulation, this precept pertains to all that we consume. It opens us to examine what we ingest with each of our senses. As the adage goes, "We are what we eat." We do our best work when we take care of ourselves. In addition to the healthfulness of the food we eat, we can investigate the material we read, the media we take in, the degree to which we are nurturing our full selves. As we look closely in this area, we can see the impact that mindful consumption can have on our clinical work as well as our overall well-being.

We all have times when we are struggling with life's circumstances and feel depleted. We notice that we are not as fully present or that we are seeking something to provide additional stimulation within the therapy hour. We might find ourselves asking more questions or becoming overly active in a manner that isn't responsive to our client, but rather an attempt to rouse our own energy. Or we might look to our clients for that which we should seek elsewhere. As Warkentin (1972) commented, "If we are not taking care of our hearts, we offer our patients but an empty hand" (p. 254). With mindfulness, we recognize that this heart care is not always the yummy romantic fulfillment of the movies. It might be that we need to feed on rejuvenating music, quiet time in nature, or nurturing friendship. In working with this precept, we look at cause and effect, both when we are taking care of ourselves and when we are not. Years ago, a colleague was back at work after having been away for a weeklong meditation retreat. He reported that one of his clients (who didn't know about the retreat) looked at him in the middle of the session and said, "You're listening differently."

With clients who are very difficult, we might need to take extra care, such as having some free time available before or after the session. Having a wise and inspiring book available in our offices to read in between sessions can also be nurturing. In working with one particularly challenging client, I found it helpful to take a walk outside before our sessions. The walking enabled me to feel more grounded and aware of a fuller sense of embodiment that was helpful as I sat with her. Walking can also be a powerful reminder of our basic humanity, something we share with whomever we sit.

Andrea was a client in her 40s who was terrified by a recent diagnosis of breast cancer. She felt as if she could barely breathe, let alone continue to live her life fully as she was dealing with the uncertainties of her illness and her future. Early on, when her prognosis was looking grim, she was working with Narayan Liebenson-Grady, a *vipassana* meditation teacher. She recounted that Narayan said, "Whatever happens, you can take care of your heart." This fifth precept on mindful consumption invites us to examine whether the choices we are making in our lives moment-by-moment are nurturing our hearts and minds.

WORKING WITH THE FIVE PRECEPTS

How can we make precept practice part of our personal and professional lives? Many people find that a structure, such as the following exercise, can help:

FIVE-IN-FIVE

- Choose one precept to focus on each week for 5 weeks, for both your private life and your clinical practice.
- For the first week, choose a precept with which you feel most aligned. In the last week, work with the precept that you find most challenging. Arrange them accordingly for the 5 weeks.
- Start each day refreshing your intention to work with the precept. Reflect at day's end, "What causes and conditions made it more or less difficult to practice with the precept?"
- Keep a light touch.

We have looked at specific ways in which the consideration and practice of the five ethical precepts can inform our clinical practice. There are broader and deeper implications as well. As we actively engage this lens of examination and practice, a growing integrity informs how we sit with someone. Precept practice . . .

- Supports us in the development of trustworthiness—we trust ourselves more and are less afraid, more fully available to engage with our clients.
- Cultivates genuine humility because we are intimately aware of our own failings, our own practice edges.
- Grounds our interventions in respect and mutuality; while we are aware that our client is walking a different path, we are also aware of our own daily footsteps and the fact that the same earth is under our feet.
- Fosters fuller presence, less encumbered by anxiety and concerns—we are freer to attend to the person in front of us.
- Nurtures confidence in our capacity to grow in wisdom and compassion—the more we practice, the more we notice, the more we understand.

The five precepts can offer valuable support to us in the psychotherapy trenches and in our lives. In the words of the Dalai Lama (2001a), "It is these seemingly elementary meditation practices that are, I believe, the most effective way of bringing about the fundamental changes necessary in our quest for happiness" (p. 35).

References

Abercrombie, H. C., Glese-Davis, J., Sephton, S., Epel, E., Turner-Cobb, J. M., & Spiegel, D. (2004). Flattened cortisol rhythms in metastatic breast cancer patients. *Psychoneuroenocrinology, 29*(8), 1082–1092.

Aberson, C. L., Healy, M., & Romero, V. (2000). Ingroup bias and self-esteem: A meta-analysis. *Personality and Social Psychology Review, 4,* 157–173.

Ackerman, D., Kabat-Zinn, J., & Siegel, D. J. (2005, March 19). Panel discussion at the Psychotherapy Networker Symposium, Washington DC.

Adams, C. E., & Leary, M. R. (2007). Promoting self-compassionate attitudes toward eating among restrictive and guilty eaters. *Journal of Social and Clinical Psychology, 26,* 1120–1144.

Adyashanti. (2006). *True meditation.* Boulder: Sounds True.

Aimone, J., Deng, W., & Gage, R. (2010). Adult neurogenesis: Integrating theories and separating functions. *Trends in Cognitive Sciences, 14*(7), 325–337.

Ainsworth, M., Blehar, M., Waters, E., & Wall, S. (1978). *Patterns of attachment: A psychological study of the strange situation.* Mahwah, NJ: Erlbaum.

Aitken, R. (1982). *Taking the path of Zen.* San Francisco: North Point Press.

Allen, J., Fonagy, P., & Bateman, A. (2008). *Mentalizing in clinical practice.* Washington, DC: American Psychiatric Association.

Allen, N. B., & Knight, W. E. J. (2005). Mindfulness, compassion for self and compassion for others: Implications for understanding the psychopathology and treatment of depression. In P. Gilbert (Ed.), *Compassion: Conceptualisations, research and use in psychotherapy* (pp. 239–262). London: Routledge.

Allione, T. (2008). *Feeding your demons.* New York: Little, Brown.

American Psychiatric Association. (2000). *Diagnostic and statistical manual of mental disorders* (4th ed.). Washington, DC: Author.

Amodio, D. M., Harmon-Jones, E., Devine, P. G., Curtin, J. J., Hartley, S. L., & Covert, A. E. (2004). Neural signals for the detection of unintentional race bias. *Psychological Science, 15,* 88–93.

Analayo, V. (2003). *Satipatthana: The direct path to realization.* Cambridge, UK: Windhorse.

Ano, G. A., & Vasconcelles, E. B. (2005). Religious coping and psychological adjustment to stress: A meta-analysis. *Journal of Clinical Psychology, 61,* 1–20.

Arch, J. J., & Craske, M. G. (2008). Acceptance and commitment therapy and cognitive behavioral therapy for anxiety disorders: Different treatments, similar mechanisms? *Clinical Psychology: Science and Practice, 15*, 263–279.

Ardelt, M. (2000a). Antecedents and effects of wisdom in old age. *Research on Aging, 22*(4), 360–394.

Ardelt, M. (2000b). Intellectual versus wisdom-related knowledge: The case for a different kind of learning in the later years of life. *Educational Gerontology, 26*, 771–789.

Ardelt, M. (2003). Empirical assessment of a three-dimensional wisdom scale. *Research on Aging, 25*, 275–324.

Ardelt, M. (2004). Wisdom as expert knowledge system: A critical review of a contemporary operationalization of an ancient concept. *Human Development, 47*, 257–285.

Armstrong, K. (2010). *Twelve steps to a compassionate life*. New York: Knopf.

Aron, A. R., Fletcher, P. C., Bullmore, E. T., Sahakian, B. J., & Robbins, T. W. (2003). Stop-signal inhibition disrupted by damage to right inferior frontal gyrus in humans. *Nature Neuroscience, 6*, 115–116.

Aronson, H. (1980). *Love and sympathy in Theravada Buddhism*. Delhi: Motilal Banarsidass.

Assagioli, R. (1975). *Psychosynthesis: A manual of principles and techniques*. London: Turnstone Press. (Original work published 1965)

Avants, S. K., Beitel, M., & Margolin, A. (2005). Making the shift from "addict self" to "spiritual self": Results from a stage I study of spiritual self-schema (3-S) therapy for the treatment of addiction and HIV risk behavior. *Mental Health, Religion and Culture, 8*(3), 167–177.

Baer, R. A. (2003). Mindfulness training as a clinical intervention: A conceptual and empirical review. *Clinical Psychology: Science and Practice, 10*, 125–143.

Baer, R. A. (Ed.). (2006). *Mindfulness-based treatment approaches: Clinician's guide to evidence base and applications*. Burlington, MA: Academic Press.

Baer, R. A. (Ed.). (2010a). *Assessing mindfulness and acceptance processes in clients: Illuminating the theory and practice of change*. Oakland, CA: New Harbinger Press.

Baer, R. A. (2010b). Self-compassion as a mechanism of change in mindfulness and acceptance-based treatments. In R. Baer (Ed.), *Assessing mindfulness and acceptance processes in clients: Illuminating the theory and practice of change* (pp. 135–153). Oakland, CA: Context Press/New Harbinger.

Baker, E. (2003). *Caring for ourselves: A therapist's guide to personal and professional well-being*. Washington, DC: American Psychological Association.

Bale, T. L., Baram, T. Z., Brown, A. S., Goldstein, J. M., Insel, T. R., McCarthy, M. M., et al. (2010). Early life programming and neurodevelopmental disorders. *Biological Psychiatry, 68*, 314–319.

Baltes, P. B. (2004). *Wisdom as orchestration of mind and virtue*. Berlin: Max Planck Institute for Human Development.

Baltes, P. B., Gluck, J., & Kunzmann, U. (2002). Wisdom: Its structure and function in regulating successful life span development. In C. R. Snyder & S. J. Lopez (Eds.), *Handbook of positive psychology* (pp. 327–347). Oxford, UK: Oxford University Press.

Baltes, P. B., & Smith, J. (1990). Toward a psychology of wisdom and its ontogenesis. In R. Sternberg (Ed.), *Wisdom: Its nature, origins and development* (pp. 87–120). Cambridge, UK: Cambridge University Press.

Baltes, P. B., Smith, J., & Staudinger, U. M. (1992). Wisdom and successful aging. In T. Sonderegger (Ed.), *Nebraska Symposium on Motivation* (Vol. 39, pp. 123–167). Lincoln: University of Nebraska Press.

Baltes, P. B., & Staudinger, U. M. (1993). The search for a psychology of wisdom. *Current Directions in Psychological Science, 2,* 75–80.

Baltes, P. B., & Staudinger, U. M. (2000). Wisdom: A metaheuristic (pragmatic) to orchestrate mind and virtue toward excellence. *American Psychologist, 55*(1), 122–136.

Banks, A. (2010). The neurobiology of connecting. *Work in Progress.* Wellesley, MA: Stone Center Working Paper Series.

Barasch, M. I. (2005, March). Desmond Tutu on compassion. *Psychology Today.* Available at: *www.psychologytoday.com/articles/200504/desmond-tutu-compassion.*

Barlow, D. H. (2002). *Anxiety and its disorders: The nature and treatment of anxiety and panic.* New York: Guilford Press.

Barks, C., with Moyne, J. (Trans.). (1995). *The essential Rumi.* San Francico: Harper.

Barnhofer, T., Chittka, T., Nightingale, H., Visser, C., & Crane, C. (2010). State effects of two forms of meditation in prefrontal EEG asymmetry in previously depressed individuals. *Mindfulness, 1,* 21–27.

Barret, W. (Ed.). (1996). *Zen Buddhism.* New York: Doubleday.

Bartlett, J. (2002). *Bartlett's familiar quotations: A collection of passages, phrases, and proverbs traced to their sources in ancient and modern literature* (17th ed.). New York: Little, Brown.

Bateson, M. C. (1994). *Peripheral visions: Learning along the way.* New York: HarperCollins.

Batson, C. (1991). *The altruism question: Towards a social-psychological answer.* Hillsdale, NJ: Erlbaum.

Batson, C. (2002). Addressing the altruism question experimentally. In S. G. Post, L. G. Underwood, J. P. Schloss, & W. B. Hurlbut (Eds.), *Altruism and altruistic love: Science, philosophy, and religion in dialogue* (pp. 89–105). New York: Oxford University Press.

Baumeister, R. F., Bratslavsky, E., Finkenauer, C., & Vohs, K. D. (2001). Bad is stronger than good. *Review of General Psychology, 5,* 323–370.

Baumeister, R. F., Smart, L., & Boden, J. M. (1996). Relation of threatened egotism to violence and aggression: The dark side of high self-esteem. *Psychological Review, 103,* 5–33.

Bayda, E. (with Bartok, J.). (2005). *Saying yes to life (even the hard parts).* Boston: Wisdom.

Beck, S. (2002). Dao de jing. *Wisdom Bible.* Retrieved April 20, 2010, from *www.san.beck.org/Laotzu.html#1.*

Begley, S. (2007). *Train your mind, change your brain.* New York: Ballantine Books.

Belin, D., & Everitt, B. J. (2008). Cocaine seeking habits depend upon dopamine-dependent serial connectivity linking the ventral and dorsal striatum. *Neuron, 57,* 432–441.

Bell, D. C. (2001). Evolution of care giving behavior. *Personality and Social Psychology Review, 5,* 216–229.

Ben Ze'ev, A. (2000). Why do I feel bad when you feel bad?: Pity, compassion, and mercy. In *The subtlety of emotions* (pp. 327–352.). Cambridge, MA: MIT Press.

Bennett-Goleman, T. (2001). *Emotional alchemy: How the mind can heal the heart.* New York: Three Rivers Press.

Berger, A., Kofman, O., Livneh, U., & Henik, A. (2007). Multidisciplinary perspectives on attention and the development of self-regulation. *Progress in Neurobiology, 82*(5), 256–286.

Berlin, A., Brettler, M., & Fishbane, M. (2004). *The Jewish study bible.* Oxford, UK: Oxford University Press.

Bernanos, G. (2002). *Diary of a country priest.* Cambridge, MA: Da Capo Press.

Berry, W. (2005). Poetry and marriage. In *Standing by words* (pp. 92–105). Berkeley, CA: Counterpoint.

Beyer, S. (Ed. and Trans.). (1974a). *The Buddhist experience: Sources and interpretations.* Encino, CA: Dickenson.

Beyer, S. (Trans.). (1974b). *The meditations of a bodhisattva: Kamalashila's Bhavanakrama.* Encino, CA: Dickenson.

Birnie, K., Speca, M., & Carlson, L. (2010). Exploring self-compassion and empathy in the context of mindfulness-based stress reduction (MBSR). *Stress and Health, 26,* 359–371.

Birren, J. E., & Fisher, L. M. (1990). The elements of wisdom: Overview and integration. In R. J. Sternberg (Ed.), *Wisdom: Its nature, origins, and development* (pp. 317–332). New York: Cambridge University Press.

Birren, J. E., & Svensson, C. M. (2005). Wisdom in history. In R. J. Sternberg & J. Jordan (Eds.), *A handbook of wisdom: Psychological perspectives* (pp. 3–31). New York: Cambridge University Press.

Bishop, S. R., Lau, M., Shapiro, S., Carlson, L., Anderson, N. D., Carmody, J., et al. (2004). Mindfulness: A proposed operational definition. *Clinical Psychology: Science and Practice, 11,* 191–206.

Blaine, B., & Crocker, J. (1993). Self-esteem and self-serving biases in reactions to positive and negative events: An integrative review. In R. F. Baumeister (Ed.), *Self-esteem: The puzzle of low self-regard* (pp. 55–85). Hillsdale, NJ: Erlbaum.

Blatt, S. J. (1995). Representational structures in psychopathology. In D. Cicchetti & S. Toth (Eds.), *Rochester Symposium on Developmental Psychopathology: Emotion, cognition, and representation* (Vol. 6, pp. 1–34). Rochester, NY: University of Rochester Press.

Block-Lerner, J., Adair, C., Plumb, J. C., Rhatigan, D. L., & Orsillo, S. M. (2007). The case for mindfulness-based approaches in the cultivation of empathy: Does nonjudgmental, present-moment awareness increase capacity for perspective-taking and empathic concern? *Journal of Marital and Family Therapy, 33*(4), 501–516.

Bluck, S., & Glück, J. (2005). From the inside out: People's implicit theories of wisdom. In R. J. Sternberg & J. Jordan (Eds.), *A handbook of wisdom: Psychological perspectives* (pp. 84–109). New York: Cambridge University Press.

Bluth, K., & Wahler, R. G. (2011). Does effort matter in mindful parenting? *Mindfulness, 2,* 175–178.

Bobrow, J. (2010). *Zen and psychotherapy: Partners in liberation.* New York: Norton.

Bodhi, B. (Trans.). (2000). *The connected discourses of the Buddha.* Boston: Wisdom.

Bodhi, B. (2005). *In the Buddha's words: An anthology of discourses from the Pali Canon.* Boston: Wisdom.

Bögels, S., Hoogstad, B., van Dun, L., de Schutter, S., & Restifo, K.(2008). Mindfulness training for adolescents with externalizing disorders and their parents. *Behavioural and Cognitive Psychotherapy, 36,* 193.

Bögels, S. M., Lehtonen, A., & Restifo, K. (2010). Mindful parenting in mental health care. *Mindfulness, 1,* 107–120.

Bohart, A., Elliot, R., Greenberg, L., & Watson, J. (2002). Empathy. In J. C. Norcross (Ed.), *Psychotherapy relationships that work: Therapist contributions and responsiveness to patients* (pp. 89–108). New York: Oxford University Press.

Bohart, A., & Greenberg, L. (1997). Empathy and psychotherapy: An introductory overview. In A. C. Bohart & L. S. Greenberg (Eds.), *Empathy reconsidered: New directions in psychotherapy* (pp. 3–31). Washington, DC: American Psychological Association.

Bokar Rinpoche. (1991). *Chenrezig, lord of love: Principles and methods of deity meditation.* San Francisco: ClearPoint Press.

Bolla, K., Ernst, M., Kiehl, K., Mouratidis, M., Eldreth, D., Contoreggi, C., et al. (2004). Prefrontal cortical dysfunction in abstinent cocaine abusers. *Journal of Neuropsychiatry and Clinical Neuroscience, 16,* 456–464.

Borkovec, T. D., Alcaine, O. M., & Behar, E. (2004). Avoidance theory of worry. In R. G. Heimberg, C. L. Turk, & D. S. Mennin (Eds.), *Generalized anxiety disorder: Advances in research and practice* (pp. 77–108). New York: Guilford Press.

Borkovec, T. D., & Sharpless, B. (2004). Generalized anxiety disorder: Bringing cognitive-behavioral therapy into the valued present. In S. C. Hayes, V. M. Follette, & M. M. Linehan (Eds.), *Mindfulness and acceptance: Expanding the cognitive-behavioral tradition* (pp. 209–242). New York: Guilford Press.

Borofsky, R. M. (2011). Marriage as a path of compassion. In A. Miller (Ed.), *Right here with you: Bringing mindful awareness into our relationships* (pp. 169–179). Boston: Shambhala.

Borofsky, R. M., & Borofsky, A. K. (1994). Giving and receiving. In G. Wheeler & S. Bachman (Eds.), *On intimate ground: A Gestalt approach to working with couples.* San Francisco: Jossey-Bass.

Bowen, S., Chawla, N., & Marlatt, G. A. (2011). Mindfulness-based relapse prevention for addictive behaviors. New York: Guilford Press.

Bowen, S., & Marlatt, G. A. (2009). Surfing the urge: Brief mindfulness-based intervention for college student smokers. *Psychology of Addictive Behaviors, 23,* 666–671.

Bowlby, J. (1969). *Attachment and loss: Vol. 1. Attachment.* London: Hogarth Press.

Bowlby, J. (1973). *Attachment and loss: Vol. 2. Separation.* London: Hogarth Press.

Bowlby, J. (1980). *Attachment and loss: Vol. 3. Loss, sadness, and depression.* New York: Basic Books.

Bowlby, J. (1988). *A secure base: Parent–child attachment and healthy human development.* New York: Basic Books.

Brach, T. (2003). *Radical acceptance: Embracing your life with the heart of a Buddha.* New York: Bantam Books.

Brach, T. (2012). *True refuge: Three gateways to a fearless heart.* New York: Bantam Books.

Brawer, P. A., Handal, P. J., Fabricatore, A. N., Roberts, R., & Wajda-Johnston, V. A. (2002). Training and education in religion/spirituality within APA-accredited clinical psychology programs. *Professional Psychology: Research and Practice, 33,* 203–206.

Brefczynski-Lewis, J. A., Lutz, A., Schaefer, H. S., Levinson, D. B., & Davidson, R. J. (2007). Neural correlates of attentional expertise in long-term meditation practitioners. *Proceedings of the National Academy of Sciences of the United States of America, 104,* 11483–11488.

Bretherton, I., & Beeghly, M. (1982). Talking about internal states: The acquisition of an explicit theory of mind. *Developmental Psychology, 18*(6), 906–921.

Brickman, P., & Campbell, D. T. (1971). Hedonic relativism and the good society. In M. H. Appley (Ed.), *Adaptation-level theory: A symposium.* New York: Academic Press.

Briere, J. (1992). *Child abuse trauma: Theory and treatment of the lasting effects.* Newbury Park, CA: Sage.

Briere, J. (2002). Treating adult survivors of severe childhood abuse and neglect: Further development of an integrative model. In J. E. B. Myers, L. Berliner, J. Briere, C. T. Hendrix, T. Reid, & C. Jenny (Eds.), *The APSAC handbook on child maltreatment* (2nd ed., pp. 175–202). Newbury Park, CA: Sage.

Briere, J. (2004). *Psychological assessment of adult posttraumatic states: Phenomenology, diagnosis, and measurement* (2nd ed.). Washington, DC: American Psychological Association.

Briere, J. (in press). When people do bad things: Evil, suffering, and dependent origination. In A. Bohart, E. Mendelowitz, B. Held, & K. Schneider (Eds.), *Humanity's dark side: Explorations in psychotherapy and beyond.* Washington, DC: American Psychological Association.

Briere, J., Hodges, M., & Godbout, N. (2010). Traumatic stress, affect dysregulation, and dysfunctional avoidance: A structural equation model. *Journal of Traumatic Stress, 23,* 767–774.

Briere, J., & Scott, C. (in press). *Principles of trauma therapy: A guide to symptoms, evaluation, and treatment* (2nd ed.). Thousand Oaks, CA: Sage.

Brody, A. L., Saxena, S., Mandelkern, M. A., Fairbanks, L. A., Ho, M. L., & Baxter, L. R. (2001). Brain metabolic changes associated with symptom factor improvement in major depressive disorder. *Biological Psychiatry, 50,* 171–178.

Brown, S., Nesse, R., Vinokur, A., & Smith, D. (2003). Providing social support may be more beneficial than receiving it: Results from a prospective study of mortality. *Psychological Science, 14*(4), 320–327.

Brugman, G. M. (2006). *Wisdom and aging.* Amsterdam: Elsevier.

Brunet, E., Sarfati, Y., Hardy-Bayle, M. C., & Decety, J. (2000). A PET investigation of the attribution of intentions with a nonverbal task. *NeuroImage, 11*, 157–166.

Bryan, T., & Bryan, J. (1991). Positive mood and math performance. *Journal of Learning Disabilities, 24*, 490–494.

Buddhaghosa. (1975). *The path of purification (Visuddhi Magga)* (Bhikkhu Nanamoli, Trans.). Kandy, Sri Lanka: Buddhist Publication Society.

Burns, A. B., Brown, J. S., Sachs-Ericsson, N., Plant, E. A., Curtis, J. T., Fredrickson, B. L., et al. (2008). Upward spirals of positive emotion and coping: Replication, extension, and initial exploration of neurochemical substrates. *Personality and Individuals Differences, 44*, 360–370.

Buss, D. M. (2000). The evolution of happiness. *American Psychologist, 55*, 15–23.

Cacioppo, J., & Patrick, W. (2008). *Loneliness: Human nature and the need for social connection*. New York: Norton.

Cahn, B. R., & Polich, J. (2006). Meditation states and traits: EEG, ERP, and neuroimaging studies. *Psychological Bulletin, 132*(2), 180–211.

Caplan, M. (2009). *Eyes wide open: Cultivating discernment on the spiritual path*. Louisville, CO: Sounds True.

Carlson, L. E., Speca, M., Patel, K. D., & Goodey, E. (2003). Mindfulness-based stress reduction in relation to quality of life, mood, symptoms of stress, and immune parameters in breast and prostate cancer outpatients. *Psychosomatic Medicine, 65*, 571–581.

Carlson, L. E., Speca, M., Patel, K. D., & Goodey, E. (2004). Mindfulness-based stress reduction in relation to quality of life, mood, symptoms of stress and levels of cortisol, dehydroepiandrosterone sulfate (DHEAS), and melatonin in breast and prostate cancer outpatients. *Psychoneuroendocrinology, 29*, 448–474.

Carmody, J., & Baer, R. A. (2008). Relationships between mindfulness practice and levels of mindfulness, medical and psychological symptoms and well-being in a mindfulness-based stress reduction program. *Journal of Behavioral Medicine, 31*, 23–33.

Carnelley, K., & Rowe, A. (2007). Repeated priming of attachment security influences later views of self and relationships. *Personal Relationships, 14*, 307–320.

Carnelley, K., & Rowe, A. (2010). Priming a sense of security: What goes through people's minds. *Journal of Social and Personal Relationships, 27*(2), 253–261.

Carson, J., Carson, K., Gil, K., & Baucom, D. (2004). Mindfulness-based relationship enhancement. *Behavior Therapy, 35*(3), 471–494.

Carter, C. S. (1998). Neuroendocrine perspectives on social attachment and love. *Psychoneuroendorinlogy, 23*, 779–818.

Cassell, E. J. (2005). Compassion. In C. R. Snyder & S. J. Lopez (Eds.), *Handbook of positive psychology* (pp. 434–445). Oxford, UK: Oxford University Press.

Cassidy, J., & Shaver, P. R. (Eds.). (2010). *Handbook of attachment: Theory, research, and clinical applications* (2nd ed.). New York: Guilford Press.

Cattaneo, L., & Rizzolatti, G. (2009). The mirror neuron system. *Archives of Neurology, 66*, 557–560.

Cattell, R. B. (1971). *Abilities: Their structure, growth, and action*. New York: Houghton Mifflin.

Center for Ethical Deliberation. (2011). *Ancient Greek ethics*. Greeley: University of Northern Colorado. Retrieved from *mcb.unco.edu/ced/perspectives/ancient-greek.cfm*.

Chambers, R., Gullone, E., & Allen, N. B. (2009). Mindful emotion regulation: An integrative review. *Clinical Psychology Review, 29*, 560–572.

Charney, D. S., Friedman, M. J., & Deutch, A. Y. (1995). *Neurobiological and clinical consequences of stress: From normal adaption to PTSD*. Philadelphia: Lippincott Williams & Wilkins.

Cheung, M. S. P., Gilbert, P., & Irons, C. (2004). An exploration of shame, social rank, and rumination in relation to depression. *Personality and Individual Differences, 36*, 1143–1153.

Chödrön, P. (2000). *When things fall apart: Heart advice for difficult times*. Boston: Shambhala.

Chödrön, P. (2001a). *Start where you are: A guide to compassionate living*. Boston: Shambhala.

Chödrön, P. (2001b). *Tonglen*. Halifax, NS, Canada: Vajradhatu.

Christopher, J. C., Chrisman, J. A., Trotter-Mathison, M. J., Schure, M. B., Dahlen, P., & Christopher, S. B. (2011). Perceptions of the long-term influence of mindfulness training on counselors and psychotherapists: A qualitative inquiry. *Journal of Humanistic Psychology, 51*, 318–349.

Clarkin, J. F., Levy, K. N., Lenzenweger, M. F., & Kernberg, O. F. (2007). Evaluating three treatments for borderline personality disorder: A multiwave study. *American Journal of Psychiatry, 164*, 922–928.

Clayton, V. P. (1975). Erickson's theory of human development as it applies to the aged: Wisdom as contradictory cognition. *Human Development, 18*, 119–128.

Clayton, V. P. (1982). Wisdom and intelligence: The nature and function of knowledge in the later years. *International Journal of Aging and Development, 15*, 315–321.

Clayton, V. P., & Birren, J. E. (1980). The development of wisdom across the life span: A reexamination of an ancient topic. In P. B. Baltess & O. G. Brim, Jr. (Eds.), *Life-span development and behavior* (Vol. 3, pp. 103–135). New York: Academic Press.

Cloitre, M., Stovall-McClough, K. C., Miranda, R., & Chemtob, C.M. (2004). Therapeutic alliance, negative mood regulation, and treatment outcome in child abuse-related posttraumatic stress disorder. *Journal of Consulting and Clinical Psychology, 72*, 411–416.

Cloitre, M., Stovall-McClough, K. C., Nooner, K., Zorba, P., Cherry, S., Jackson, C. L., et al. (2010). Treatment for PTSD related to childhood abuse: A randomized controlled trial. *American Journal of Psychiatry, 167*, 915–924.

Cohn, M. A., & Fredrickson, B. L. (2010). In search of durable positive psychology interventions: Predictors and consequences of long-term positive behavior change. *Journal of Positive Psychology, 5*, 355–366.

Cohn, M. A., Fredrickson, B. L., Brown, S. L., Mikels, J. A., & Conway, A. M. (2009). Happiness unpacked: Positive emotions increase life satisfaction by building resilience. *Emotion, 9*, 361–368.

Collins, N. (1996). Working models of attachment: Implications for explanation, emotion, and behavior. *Journal of Personality and Social Psychology, 71,* 810–832.

Collins, N., & Feeney, B. (2000). A safe haven: An attachment theory perspective on support seeking and caregiving in intimate relationships. *Journal of Personality and Social Psychology, 78,* 1053–1073.

Collins, P. (1990). *Black feminist thought: Knowledge, consciousness and the politics of empowerment.* Boston: Unwin Hyman.

Congdon, E., & Canli, T. (2005). The endophenotype of impulsivity: Reaching consilience through behavioral, genetic, and neuroimaging approaches. *Behavioral and Cognitive Neuroscience Reviews, 4,* 262–281.

Connors, G. J., Maisto, S. A., & Donovan, D. M. (1996). Conceptualizations of relapse: A summary of psychological and psychobiological models. *Addiction, 91,* 5–13.

Conze, E. (1958). *Buddhist wisdom: The diamond Sutra and the heart sutra.* London: Allen & Unwin.

Conze, E. (Trans.). (1973). *The perfection of wisdom in eight thought lines and its verse summary.* Bolinas, CA: Four Seasons Foundation.

Conze, E. (Trans.). (1979). *The large sutra on perfect wisdom with the divisions of the Abhisamayalankara.* Delhi: Motilal Banarsidass.

Cooney, R. E., Joormann, J., Atlas, L. Y., Eugène, F., & Gotlib, I. H. (2007). Remembering the good times: Neural correlates of affect regulation. *NeuroReport, 18,* 1771–1774.

Coopersmith, S. (1967). *The antecedents of self-esteem.* San Francisco: Freeman.

Cosley, B., McCoy, S., Saslow, L., & Epel, E. (2010). Is compassion for others stress buffering? Consequences of compassion and social support for physiological reactivity to stress. *Journal of Experimental Social Psychology, 46,* 816–823.

Courtois, C. A. (2010). *Healing the incest wound: Adult survivors in therapy* (2nd ed.). New York: Norton.

Coxhead, N. (1985). *The relevance of bliss.* London: Wildwood House.

Cozolino, L. (2008). *The healthy aging brain: Sustaining attachment, attaining wisdom.* New York: Norton.

Cozolino, L. (2010). *The neuroscience of psychotherapy: Healing the social brain.* New York: Norton.

Cree, M. (2010). Compassion-focused therapy with perinatal and mother–infant distress. *International Journal of Cognitive Therapy, 3*(2), 159–171.

Creswell, J. D., Way, B. M., Eisenberger, N. I., & Lieberman, M. D. (2007). Neural correlates of dispositional mindfulness during affect labeling. *Psychosomatic Medicine, 69,* 560–565.

Crocker, J., & Canevello, A. (2008). Creating and undermining social support in communal relationships: The role of compassionate and self-image goals. *Journal of Personality and Social Psychology, 95,* 555–575.

Crocker, J., & Park, L. E. (2004). The costly pursuit of self-esteem. *Psychological Bulletin, 130,* 392–414.

Csikszentmihalyi, M. (1990). *Flow: The psychology of optimal experience.* New York: Harper & Row.

Cunningham, W. A., Johnson, M. K., Raye, C. L., Chris, G. J., Gore, J. C., & Banaji,

M. R. (2004). Separable neural components in the processing of black and white faces. *Psychological Science, 15,* 806–813.

Dae Soen Su Nim. (1987). *The whole world is a single flower.* Lecture at the First International Conference, Sudeoksa Temple, Korea.

Dahl, J., Wilson, K. G., & Nilsson, A. (2004). Acceptance and commitment therapy and the treatment of persons at risk for long-term disability resulting from stress and pain symptoms: A preliminary randomized trial. *Behavior Therapy, 35,* 785–801.

Dahlsgaard, K., Peterson, C., & Seligman, M. (2005). Shared virtue: The convergence of valued human strengths across culture and history. *Review of General Psychology, 9*(3), 203–213.

Dalai Lama, XIV. (1995). *The power of compassion.* New York: HarperCollins.

Dalai Lama, XIV. (1999). Love, compassion, and tolerance. In R. Carlson & B. Shield (Eds.), *For the love of God.* Novato, CA: New World Library.

Dalai Lama, XIV. (2000). *Transforming the mind.* New York: Thorsons/Element. Retrieved February 19, 2011, from *www.dalailama.com/teachings/training-the-mind/verse-7.*

Dalai Lama, XIV. (2001a). *Ethics for a new millennium.* New York: Riverhead Books.

Dalai Lama, XIV. (2001b). *An open heart: Practicing compassion in everyday life.* Boston: Little, Brown.

Dalai Lama, XIV. (2003). *Lighting the path: The Dalai Lama teaches on wisdom and compassion.* South Melbourne, Australia: Thomas C. Lothian.

Dalai Lama, XIV. (2005, November). *Science at the crossroads.* Presentation at the annual meeting of the Society for Neuroscience, Washington, DC. Retrieved February 5, 2011, from *www.dalailama.com/messages/buddhism/science-at-the-crossroads.*

Dalai Lama, XIV. (2008). *Worlds in harmony: Compassionate action for a better world* (2nd ed.). Berkeley, CA: Parallax Press.

Dalai Lama, XIV. (2009a). *The art of happiness in a troubled world.* New York: Random House/Crown.

Dalai Lama, XIV. (2009b, May). *Meditation and psychotherapy: Cultivating compassion and wisdom.* Panel discussion at Harvard Medical School conference, Boston.

Dalai Lama, XIV. (2010a). *Freedom must for human creativity.* Retrieved April 10, 2011, from *www.dalailama.com/news/post/508-freedom-must-for-human-creativity.*

Dalai Lama, XIV. (2010b, May 25). Many faiths, one truth. *New York Times,* Op-Ed, p. A27. Available at: *www.nytimes.com/2010/05/25/opinion/25gyatso.html?scp=1&sq=many+faiths%2C+one+truth&st=nyt.*

Dalai Lama, XIV. (2010c). *Training the mind: Verse 1.* Retrieved December 18, 2010, from *www.dalailama.com/teachings/training-the-mind/verse-1.*

Dalai Lama, XIV. (2011). Compassion and the individual. Retrieved September 9, 2011, from *www.dalailama.com/messages/compassion.*

Dalai Lama, XIV, & Cutler, H. (2009). Preface to the 10th anniversary edition by His Holiness the Dalai Lama, *The art of happiness: A handbook for living.* New York: Riverhead Books.

Dalenberg, C. (2000). *Countertransference and the treatment of trauma*. Washington, DC: American Psychological Association.

Darwin, C. (2010). *The works of Charles Darwin: Vol. 21. The descent of man, and selection in relation to sex (part one)*. New York: NYU Press. (Original work published 1871)

Davidson, R. J. (2007, October). *Changing the brain by transforming the mind: The impact of compassion training on the neural systems of emotion*. Paper presented at the Mind and Life Institute Conference, Emory University, Atlanta, GA.

Davidson, R. J. (2009, May). *Neuroscientifc studies of meditation*. Paper presented at the Harvard Medical School conference Meditation and Psychotherapy: Cultivating Compassion and Wisdom, Boston.

Davidson, R. J., & Harrington, A. (2001). *Visions of compassion: Western scientists and Tibetan Buddhists examine human nature*. Oxford, UK: Oxford University Press.

Davidson, R. J., & Kabat-Zinn, J. (2004). Alterations in brain and immune function produced by mindfulness meditation: Three caveats. Response to letter by J. Smith. *Psychosomatic Medicine, 66*(1), 149–152.

Davidson, R. J., Kabat-Zinn, J., Schumacher, J., Rosenkranz, M., Muller, D., Santorelli, S. F., et al. (2003). Alterations in brain and immune function produced by mindfulness meditation. *Psychosomatic Medicine, 65*, 564–570.

de Carvalho, M. R., Dias, C. P., Cosci, F., de-Melo-Neto, V. L., Bevilaqua, M. C., Gardino, P. F., et al. (2010). Current findings of fMRI in panic disorder: Contributions for the fear neurocircuitry and CBT effects. *Expert Review of Neurotherapeutics, 10*, 291–303.

Decety, J., & Jackson, P. L. (2004). The functional architecture of human empathy. *Behavioral and Cognitive Neuroscience Reviews, 3*, 71–100.

Deci, E. L., & Ryan, R. M. (1995). Human autonomy: The basis for true self-esteem. In M. H. Kernis (Ed.), *Efficacy, agency, and self-esteem* (pp. 31–49). New York: Plenum Press.

Delton, A., Krasnow, M., Cosmides, L., & Tody, J. (in press). Evolution of direct reciprocity under uncertainty can explain human generosity in one-shot encounters. *Proceedings of the National Academy of Sciences*.

Depue, R. A., & Morrone-Strupinsky, J. V. (2005). A neurobehavioral model of affiliative bonding. *Behavioral and Brain Sciences, 28*, 313–395.

Descartes, R. (1988). *Descartes: Selected philosophical writings* (J. Cottingham, R. Stoothoff, & D. Murdoch, Trans.). New York: Cambridge University Press. (Original work published 1641)

de Silva, P. (2000). Buddhism and psychotherapy: The role of self-control strategies. *Journal of Humanistic Buddhism, 1*, 171.

de Vignemont, F., & Singer, T. (2006). The empathic brain: How, when and why? *Trends in Cognitive Sciences, 10*, 435–441.

Diener, E., & Biswas-Diener, R. (2002). Will money increase subjective well-being? *Social Indicators Research, 57*, 119–169.

Dilgo Khyentse Rinpoche. (1992). *The heart treasure of the enlightened ones*. Boston: Shambhala.

Dimeff, L. A., Comtois, K. A., & Linehan, M. M. (1998). Dialectical behavior therapy for substance abusers with borderline personality disorder: Applications in primary care. In B. H. Graham & T. K. Schultz (Eds.), *Principals of addiction medicine* (pp. 1063–1079). Arlington, VA: American Society of Addiction Medicine.

DiNoble, A. (2009). *Examining the relationship between adult attachment style and mindfulness traits.* Unpublished doctoral dissertation, California Graduate Institute of the Chicago School of Professional Psychology.

Dreimeyer, J., Boyke, J., Gaser, C., Büchel, C., & May, A. (2008). Changes in gray matter induced by learning–revisited. *PLoS One, 3*(7), e2669.

Dunn, E. W., Aknin, L. B., & Norton, M. L. (2008). Spending money on others promotes happiness. *Science, 319,* 1687–1688.

Dunn, J. R., & Schweitzer, M. E. (2005). Feeling and believing: The influence of emotion on trust. *Journal of Personality and Social Psychology, 88,* 736–748.

Durant, W. (1935) *Our oriental heritage.* New York: Simon & Schuster.

Dweck, C. S. (1986). Motivational processes affecting learning. *American Psychologist, 41,* 1040–1048.

Easterbrook, G. (2003). *The progress paradox: How life gets better while people feel worse.* New York: Random House.

Eisenberg, N., Fabes, R., Bustamante, D., Mathy, R., Miller, P., & Lindholm, E. (1988). Differentiation of vicariously induced emotional reactions in children. *Developmental Psychology, 24,* 237–246.

Eisenberg, N., Fabes, R., Schaller, M., Carlo, G., & Miller, P. A. (1991). The relations of parental characteristics and practices to children's vicarious emotional responding. *Child Development, 62,* 1393–1408.

Eisenberg, N., Fabes, R. A., Murphy, B., Karbon, M., Maszk, P., Smith, M., et al. (1994). The relations of emotionality and regulation to dispositional and situational empathy-related responding. *Journal of Personality and Social Psychology, 66,* 776–797.

Eisenberger, N., & Lieberman, M. (2004). Why rejection hurts: A common neural alarm system for physical and social pain. *Trends in Cognitive Sciences, 8,* 294–300.

Eisenberg, N., & Miller, P. (1987). The relation of empathy to prosocial and related behaviors. *Psychological Bulletin, 101,* 91–119.

Ekman, P. (2010). Darwin's compassionate view of human nature. *Journal of the American Medical Association, 303*(6), 557–558.

Engel, A. K., Fries, P., Konig, P., Brecht, M., & Singer, W. (1999). Temporal binding, binocular rivalry, and consciousness. *Consciousness and Cognition, 8*(2), 128–151.

Epstein, M. (1995). *Thoughts without a thinker.* New York: Basic Books.

Epstein, M. (2007). *Psychotherapy without the self: A Buddhist perspective.* New Haven, CT: Yale University Press.

Ericsson, A. (1998). The scientific study of expert levels of performance: General implications for optimal learning and creativity. *High Ability Studies, 9*(1), 75–100.

Ericsson, A., Prietula, M., & Cokely, E. (2007, July–August). The making of an expert. *Harvard Business Review,* pp. 1–7.

Erikson, E. H. (1950). *Childhood and society.* New York: Norton.

Erikson, E. H. (1959). Identity and the life cycle. *Psychological Issues, 1*, 1–173.

Erikson, E. H., & Erikson, J. M. (1998). *The life cycle completed.* New York: Norton. (Original work published 1982)

Estrada, C. A., Isen, A. M., & Young, M. J. (1997). Positive affect facilitates integration of information and decreases anchoring in reasoning among physicians. *Organizational Behavior and Human Decision Processes, 72*, 117–135.

Everitt, B. J., Belin, D., Economidou, D., Pelloux, Y., Dalley, J. W., & Robbins, T. W. (2008). Neural mechanisms underlying the vulnerability to develop compulsive drug-seeking habits and addiction. *Philosophical Transactions of the Royal Society of London: Series B, Biological Sciences, 12*(363), 3125–3135.

Fain, J. (2011). *The self-compassion diet.* Boulder, CO: Sounds True.

Farb, N. A., Anderson, A. K., Mayberg, H., Bean, J., McKeon, D., & Segal, Z. V. (2010). Minding one's emotions: Mindfulness training alters the neural expression of sadness. *Emotion, 10*(1), 25–33.

Farb, N. A., Segal, Z. V., Mayberg, H., Bean, J., McKeon, D., Fatima, Z., et al. (2007). Attending to the present: Mindfulness meditation reveals distinct neural modes of self-reference. *Social Cognitive and Affective Neuroscience, 2*(4), 313–322.

Faulkner, W. (1975). *Requiem for a nun.* New York: Vintage. (Original work published 1951)

Feeney, B. C., & Thrush, R. L. (2008). Relationship influences on exploration in adulthood: The characteristics and functions of a secure base. *Journal of Personality and Social Psychology, 98*, 57–76.

Fehr, B., Sprecher, S., & Underwood, L. (2009). *The science of compassionate love: Theory, research, and applications.* West Sussex, UK: Wiley-Blackwell.

Feshbach, N. (1997). Empathy: The formative years–implications for clinical practice. In A. C. Bohart & L. S. Greenberg (Eds.), *Empathy reconsidered: New directions in psychotherapy* (pp. 33–59). Washington, DC: American Psychological Association.

Figley, C. (2002). Compassion fatigue: Psychotherapists' chronic lack of self-care. *Journal of Clinical Psychology, 58*, 1433–1441.

Fischer, N., Drolma, L. P., & Olendzki, A. (2010, Summer). Forum: Sex, lies, and Buddhism. *Buddhadharma.* Available at: *http://bdtest1.squarespace.com/web-archive/2010/8/8/forum-sex-lies-and-buddhism.html.*

Fiske, S., Cuddy, A., Glick, P., & Xu, J. (2002). A model of (often mixed) stereotype content: Competence and warmth respectively follow from perceived status and competition. *Journal of Personality and Social Psychology, 82*, 878–902.

Fledderus, M., Bohlmeijer, E., & Pieterse, M. (2010). Does experiential avoidance mediate the effects of maladaptive coping styles on psychopathology and mental health? *Behavior Modification, 34*(6), 503–519.

Fletcher, P. C., Happe, F., Frith, U., Baker, S. C., Dolan, R. J., Frackowiak, R. S., et al. (1995). Other minds in the brain: A functional imaging study of "theory of mind" in story comprehension. *Cognition, 57*, 109–128.

Foa, E. B., Ehlers, A., Clark, D. M., Tolin, D. F., & Orsillo, S. M. (1999). The

Posttraumatic Cognitions Inventory (PTCI): Development and validation. *Psychological Assessment, 11*, 303–314.

Foa, E. B., & Rothbaum, B. O. (1998). *Treating the trauma of rape: Cognitive-behavioral therapy for PTSD*. New York: Guilford Press.

Fonagy, P., Gergely, G., Jurist, E. L., & Target, M. (2002). *Affect regulation, mentalization, and the development of the self*. New York: Other Press.

Fonagy, P., & Target, M. (1997). Attachment and reflective function: Their role in self-organization. *Development and Psychopathology, 9*, 679–700.

Fossati, P., Hevenor, S. J., Graham, S. J., Grady, C., Keightley, M. L., Craik, F., et al. (2003). In search of the emotional self: An fMRI study using positive and negative emotional words. *American Journal of Psychiatry, 160*, 1938–1945.

Franklin, B. (2005). *The autobiography of Benjamin Franklin, including Poor Richard's Almanac, and familiar letters*. New York: Cosimo Classics. (Original work published 1793)

Franklin, T. R., Acton, P. D., Maldjian, J. A., Gray, J. D., Croft, J. R., Dackis, C. A., et al. (2002). Decreased gray matter concentration in the insular, orbitofrontal, cingulated, and temporal cortices of cocaine patients. *Biological Psychiatry, 51*, 134–142.

Frederick, C., & McNeal, S. (1999). *Inner strengths: Contemporary psychotherapy and hypnosis for ego strengthening*. Mahwah, NJ: Erlbaum.

Fredrickson, B. L. (1998). What good are positive emotions? *Review of General Psychology, 2*, 300–319.

Fredrickson, B. L. (2001). The role of positive emotions in positive psychology: The broaden-and-build theory of positive emotions. *American Psychologist, 56*, 218–226.

Fredrickson, B. L. (2009). *Positivity*. New York: Three Rivers Press.

Fredrickson, B. L., & Branigan, C. (2005). Positive emotions broaden the scope of attention and thought–action repertoires. *Cognition and Emotion, 19*, 313–332.

Fredrickson, B. L., Cohn, M. A., Coffey, K. A., Pek, J., & Finkel, S. M. (2008). Open hearts build lives: Positive emotions, induced through loving-kindness meditation, build consequential personal resources. *Journal of Personality and Social Psychology, 95*, 1045–1062.

Fredrickson, B. L., & Joiner, T. (2002). Positive emotions trigger upward spirals toward emotional well-being. *Psychological Science, 13*, 172–175.

Fredrickson, B. L., Mancuso, R. A., Branigan, C., & Tugade, M. M. (2000). The undoing effect of positive emotions. *Motivation and Emotion, 24*, 237–258.

Freud, S. (1933). *New introductory lectures on psychoanalysis*. New York: Norton

Freud, S. (1957). Remembering, repeating and working-through (further recommendations on the technique of Psycho-Analysis II). In J. Strachey (Ed.), *The standard edition of the complete psychological works of Sigmund Freud: Vol. 14 (1911–1913): The case of Schreber, papers on technique and other works* (pp. 145–156). London: Hogarth Press.

Fulton, P. R. (2005). Mindfulness as clinical training. In C. K. Germer, R. D. Siegel, & P. R. Fulton (Eds.), *Mindfulness and psychotherapy* (pp. 55–72). New York: Guilford Press.

Fulton, P. R., & Siegel, R. D. (2005). Buddhist and Western psychology: Seeking common ground. In C. K. Germer, R. D. Siegel, & P. R. Fulton (Eds.), *Mindfulness and psychotherapy* (pp. 28–52). New York: Guilford Press.

Gallagher, H. L., Happé, F., Brunswick, N., Fletcher, P. C., & Frith, C. D. (2000). Reading the mind in cartoons and stories: An fMRI study of "theory of mind" in verbal and nonverbal tasks. *Neuropsychologia, 38*, 11–21.

Gallup, G., Jr., & Lindsay, D. M. (1999). *Surveying the religious landscape: Trends in U. S. beliefs*. Harrisburg, PA: Morehouse.

Gambrel, L., & Keeling, M. (2010). Relational aspects of mindfulness: Implications for the practice of marriage and family therapy. *Contemporary Family Therapy: An International Journal, 32*(4), 412–426.

Gardner, H. (1983). *Frames of mind: The theory of multiple intelligences*. New York: Basic Books.

Gardner, H. (1999). Are there additional intelligences?: The case for naturalist, spiritual, and existential intelligences. In J. Kane (Ed.), *Education, information, and transformation* (pp. 111–131). Upper Saddle River, NJ: Prentice-Hall.

Gardner, H. (2006). *Multiple intelligences: New horizons in theory and practice*. New York: Basic.

Garland, E. L., Fredrickson, B. L., Kring, A. M., Johnson, D. P., Meyer, P. S., & Penn, D. L. (2010). Upward spirals of positive emotions counter downward spirals of negativity: Insights from the broaden-and-build theory and affective neuroscience on the treatment of emotion dysfunctions and deficits in psychopathology. *Clinical Psychology Review, 30*, 849–864.

Garland, E. L., Gaylord, S., & Park, J. (2009). The role of mindfulness in positive reappraisal. *Journal of Science and Healing, 5*, 37–44.

Gehart, D., & McCollum, E. (2007). Engaging suffering: Towards a mindful revisioning of family therapy practice. *Journal of Marital and Family Therapy, 33*(2), 214–226.

Gendlin, E. (1981). *Focusing*. New York: Bantam Books.

Germer, C. K. (2005a). Anxiety disorders: Befriending fear. In C. K. Germer, R. D. Siegel, & P. R. Fulton (Eds.), *Mindfulness and psychotherapy* (pp. 152–172). New York: Guilford Press.

Germer, C. K. (2005b). Mindfulness: What is it? What does it matter? In C. K. Germer, R. D. Siegel, & P. R. Fulton (Eds.), *Mindfulness and psychotherapy* (pp. 3–27). New York: Guilford Press.

Germer, C. K. (2005c). Teaching mindfulness in therapy. In C. K. Germer, R. D. Siegel, & P. R. Fulton (Eds.), *Mindfulness and psychotherapy* (pp. 113–119). New York: Guilford Press.

Germer, C. K. (2009). *The mindful path to self-compassion: Freeing yourself from destructive thoughts and emotions*. New York: Guilford Press.

Germer, C. K., & Neff, K. (2011, July). *Mindful self-compassion training (MSC)*. Paper presented at the Max-Planck Institute for Human and Cognitive Brain Sciences conference, Berlin, Germany.

Germer, C. K., Siegel, R. D., & Fulton, P. R. (Eds.). (2005). *Mindfulness and psychotherapy*. New York: Guilford Press.

Gifford, E. V., Kohlenberg, B. S., Hayes, S. C., Antonuccio, D. O., Piasecki, M. M., Rasmussen-Hall, M. L., et al. (2004). Acceptance-based treatment for smoking cessation. *Behavior Therapy, 35*, 689–705.

Gilbert, P. (1984). *Depression: From psychology to brain state*. London: Erlbaum.

Gilbert, P. (1989). *Human nature and suffering*. Hove, UK: Erlbaum.

Gilbert, P. (1992). *Depression: The evolution of powerlessness*. Hove, UK: Erlbaum.

Gilbert, P. (1993). Defence and safety: Their function in social behaviour and psychopathology. *British Journal of Clinical Psychology, 32*, 131–153.

Gilbert, P. (2000). Social mentalities: Internal "social" conflicts and the role of inner warmth and compassion in cognitive therapy. In P. Gilbert & K. G. Bailey (Eds.), *Genes on the couch: Explorations in evolutionary psychotherapy* (pp. 118–150). Hove, UK: Brenner-Routledge.

Gilbert, P. (2005). *Compassion: Conceptualisations, research and use in psychotherapy*. London: Routledge.

Gilbert, P. (2007a). Evolved minds and compassion in the therapeutic relationship. In P. Gilbert & R. Leahy (Eds.), *The therapeutic relationship in the cognitive behavioural psychotherapies* (pp. 106–142). London: Routledge.

Gilbert, P. (2007b). *Psychotherapy and counselling for depression* (3rd ed.). London: Sage.

Gilbert, P. (2009a). *The compassionate mind: A new approach to life's challenges*. Oakland, CA: New Harbinger Press.

Gilbert, P. (2009b). Introducing compassion focused therapy. *Advances in Psychiatric Treatment, 15*, 199–208.

Gilbert, P. (2009c). *Overcoming depression* (3rd ed.). New York: Basic Books.

Gilbert, P. (2010a). Compassion focused therapy. *International Journal of Cognitive Therapy, 3*, 95–210.

Gilbert, P. (2010b). *Compassion focused therapy: The CBT distinctive features series*. London: Routledge.

Gilbert, P. (2010c). An introduction to compassion focused therapy in cognitive behavior therapy. *International Journal of Cognitive Therapy, 3*(2), 97–112.

Gilbert, P., & Bailey, K. (Eds.). (2000). *Genes on the couch: Explorations in evolutionary psychotherapy*. Hove, UK: Brunner-Routledge.

Gilbert, P., & Irons, C. (2005a). Focused therapies and compassionate mind training for shame and self-attacking. In P. Gilbert (Ed.), *Compassion: Conceptualisations, research and use in psychotherapy* (pp. 263–325). London: Routledge.

Gilbert, P., & Irons, C. (2005b). Therapies for shame and self-attacking, using cognitive, behavioural, emotional imagery and compassionate mind training. In P. Gilbert (Ed.), *Compassion: Conceptualisations, research and use in psychotherapy* (pp. 263–325). London: Routledge.

Gilbert, P., McEwan, K., Matos, M., & Rivis, A. (2011). Fears of compassion: Development of three self-report measures. *Psychology and Psychotherapy: Theory, Research and Practice, 84*, 239–255.

Gilbert, P., & Procter, S. (2006). Compassionate mind training for people with high shame and self-criticism: Overview and pilot study of a group therapy approach. *Clinical Psychology and Psychotherapy, 13*, 353–379.

Gilboa, A. (2004). Autobiographical and episodic memory—one and the same?:

Evidence from prefrontal activation in neuroimaging studies. *Neuropsychologia, 42*, 1336–1349.

Gillath, O., Shaver, P., & Mikulincer, M. (2005). An attachment-theoretical approach to compassion and altruism. In P. Gilbert (Ed.), *Compassion: Conceptualisations, research and use in psychotherapy* (pp. 121–147). London: Routledge.

Gilligan, C. (1982). *In a different voice*. Cambridge, MA: Harvard University Press.

Glaser, A. (2005). *A call to compassion: Bringing Buddhist practices of the heart into the soul of psychology*. Lake Worth, FL: Nicolas-Hays.

Glück, J. (2008). Wisdom project descriptions. In *Defining wisdom: A project of the University of Chicago*. Retrieved October 15, 2010, from *wisdomresearch.org/Arete/gluck.aspx*.

Glück, J., & Bluck, S. (2011). Laypeople's conceptions of wisdom and its development: Cognitive and integrative views. *Journal of Gerontology. Series B, Psychological Sciences and Social Sciences, 66*(3), 321–324.

Goel, V., Grafman, J., Sadato, N., & Hallett, M. (1995). Modeling other minds. *NeuroReport, 6*, 1741-1746.

Goetz, J. (2010). *Buddhist conceptions of compassion: Annotated bibliography*. Berkeley: University of California. Retrieved February 10, 2011, from *greatergood.berkeley.edu/research/research_compassion_goetz2.html*.

Goetz, J., Keltner, D., & Simon-Thomas, S. (2010). Compassion: An evolutionary analysis and empirical review. *Psychological Bulletin, 136*(3), 351–374.

Goldin, P. R., & Gross, J. J. (2010). Effects of mindfulness-based stress reduction (MBSR) on emotion regulation in social anxiety disorder. *Emotion, 10*, 83–91.

Goldin, P. R., Manber-Ball, T., Werner, K., Heimberg, R., & Gross, J. J. (2009). Neural mechanisms of cognitive reappraisal of negative self-beliefs in social anxiety disorder. *Biological Psychiatry, 66*, 1091–1099.

Goldin, P. R., McRae, K., Ramel, W., & Gross, J. J. (2008). The neural bases of emotion regulation: Reappraisal and suppression of negative emotion. *Biological Psychiatry, 63*, 577–586.

Goldstein, J. (2010, May). *The meditative journey*. Paper presented at the Harvard Medical School conference on meditation and psychotherapy, Boston.

Goldstein, J., & Kornfield, J. (1987). *Seeking the heart of wisdom: The path of insight meditation*. Boston: Shambhala.

Goleman, D. (2003). *Destructive emotions: How can we overcome them?* New York: Bantam Dell.

Goleman, D. (2006). *Social intelligence: The new science of human relationships*. New York: Bantam Books.

Gombrich, R. (1992). Dating the Buddha: A red herring revealed. In H. Betchert (Ed.), *The dating of the historical Buddha, Part 2* (pp. 237–259). Gottingen, Germany: Vandenhoeck & Ruprecht.

Goss, K., & Allen, S. (2010). Compassion focused therapy for eating disorders. *International Journal of Cognitive Therapy, 3*(2), 141–158.

Greenberg, L. S. (1983). Toward a task analysis of conflict resolution in Gestalt Therapy. *Psychotherapy: Theory, Research and Practice, 20*(2), 190–201.

Greene, J. D., Nystrom, L. E., Engell, A. D., Darley, J. M., & Cohen, J. D. (2004). The neural bases of cognitive conflict and control in moral judgment. *Neuron, 44*, 389–400.

Greene, J. D., Sommerville, R. B., Nystrom, L. E., Darley, J. M., & Cohen, J. D. (2001). An fMRI investigation of emotional engagement in moral judgment. *Science, 293*, 2105–2108.

Grepmair, L., Mitterlehner, F., Lowe, T., Bachler, E., Rother, W., & Nickel, M. (2007). Promoting mindfulness in psychotherapists in training influences the treatment results of their patients: A randomized, double blind, controlled study. *Psychotherapy Psychosomatics, 76*, 332–338.

Grienenberger, J., Slade, A., & Kelly, K. (2005). Maternal reflective functioning, mother–infant affective communication, and infant attachment: Exploring the link between mental states and observed caregiving behavior in the intergenerational transmission of attachment. *Attachment and Human Development,* 7(3), 299–311.

Grof, S. (1975). *Realms of the human unconscious*. New York: Viking.

Grof, S. (1998). *The cosmic game*. Albany: State University of New York Press.

Gumley, A., Braehler, C., Laithwaite, H., MacBeth, A., & Gilbert, P. (2010). A compassion focused model of recovery after psychosis. *International Journal of Cognitive Therapy, 3*(2), 186–201.

Gunaratana, H. (1991). *Mindfulness in plain English*. Boston: Wisdom.

Gusnard, D. A., Akbudak, E., Shulman, G. L., & Raichle, M. E. (2001). Medial prefrontal cortex and self-referential mental activity: Relation to a default mode of brain function. *Proceedings of the National Academy of Sciences of the United States of America, 98*, 4259–4264.

Gusnard, D. A., & Raichle, M. E. (2001). Searching for a baseline: Functional imaging and the resting human brain. *Nature Reviews Neuroscience, 2*, 685–694.

Halifax, J. (1993). The road is your footsteps. In T. N. Hanh, *For a future to be possible: Commentaries on the five wonderful precepts*. Berkeley, CA: Parallax Press.

Hall, S. S. (2007, May 6). The new middle ages: The older-and-wiser hypothesis. *New York Times Magazine*. Available at *www.nytimes.com/2007/05/06/magazine/06Wisdom-t.html?scp=1&sq=the%20new%20middle%20ages:%20the%20older-and-wiser%20hypothesis&st=cse*.

Hangartner, D. (2011, July). *Cultivating compassion from a Buddhist perspective*. Paper presented at the How to Train Compassion conference, Max-Planck Institute, Berlin.

Hanh, T. N. (1976). *The miracle of mindfulness: A manual on meditation*. Boston: Beacon Press.

Hanh, T. N. (1998). *The heart of the Buddha's teachings*. Berkeley, CA: Parallax Press.

Hanh, T. N. (1999). *The heart of the Buddha's teaching: Transforming suffering into peace, joy and liberation*. New York: Three Rivers Press.

Hanh, T. N. (2000). *Creating true peace: Ending violence in yourself, your family, your community and the world*. New York: Free Press.

Hanh, T. N. (2003). *Joyfully together: The art of building a harmonious community*. New York: Parallax Press.

Hanh, T. N. (2007). *For a future to be possible: Buddhist ethics for everyday life.* Berkeley, CA: Parallax Press.

Hanson, R., & Mendius, R. (2009). *Buddha's brain: The practical neuroscience of happiness, love, and wisdom.* New York: New Harbinger.

Harbaugh, W. T., Mayr, U., & Burghart, D. R. (2007). Neural responses to taxation and voluntary giving reveal motives for charitable donations. *Science, 316,* 1622–1625.

Harderwijk, R. (2011). The wisdom of emptiness. Retrieved from *viewonbuddhism.org/wisdom_emptiness.html.*

Hariri, A. B., Bookheimer, S. Y., & Mazziotta, J. C. (2000). Modulating emotional responses: Effects of a neocortical network on the limbic system. *NeuroReport, 11,* 43–48.

Harris, R. (2009). *ACT made simple: An easy-to-read primer on acceptance and commitment therapy.* Oakland, CA: New Harbinger.

Harter, S. (1999). *The construction of the self: A developmental perspective.* New York: Guilford Press.

Hartmann, H. (1958). *Ego psychology and the problem of adaptation.* New York: International Universities Press.

Harvey, P. (1990). *An introduction to Buddhism: Teachings, history and practices.* New York: Cambridge University Press.

Harvey, P. (2000). *An introduction to Buddhist ethics.* New York: Cambridge University Press.

Hayes, S. C. (2004). Acceptance and commitment therapy and the new behavior therapies: Mindfulness, acceptance, and relationship. In S. C. Hayes, V. M. Follette, & M. M. Linehan (Eds.), *Mindfulness and acceptance: Expanding the cognitive-behavioral tradition.* New York: Guilford Press.

Hayes, S. C., Follette, V. M., & Linehan, M. M. (Eds.). (2004). *Mindfulness and acceptance: Expanding the cognitive-behavioral tradition.* New York: Guilford Press.

Hayes, S. C., Strosahl, K. D., & Wilson, K. G. (1999). *Acceptance and commitment therapy: An experiential approach to behavior change.* New York: Guilford Press.

Hayes, S. C., Villatte, M., Levin, M., & Hildebrandt, M. (2011). Open, aware, and active: Contextual approaches as an emerging trend in the behavioral and cognitive therapies [Online posting]. *Reviews in Advance, 16*(51).

Hayes, S. C., Wilson, K. G., Gifford, E. V., Follette, V. M., & Strosahl, K. (1996). Experiential avoidance and behavioral disorders: A functional dimensional approach to diagnosis and treatment. *Journal of Consulting and Clinical Psychology, 64,* 1152–1168.

Heatherton, T. F., & Polivy, J. (1990). Chronic dieting and eating disorders: A spiral model. In J. H. Crowther, D. L. Tennenbaum, S. E. Hobfoll, & M. A. P. Stephens (Eds.), *The etiology of bulimia nervosa: The individual and familial context* (pp. 133–155). Washington, DC: Hemisphere.

Hein, G., & Singer, T. (2008). I feel how you feel but not always: The empathic brain and its modulation. *Current Opinion in Neurobiology, 18*(2), 153–158.

Heine, S. J., Lehman, D. R., Markus, H. R., & Kitayama, S. (1999). Is there a universal need for positive self-regard? *Psychological Review, 106,* 766–794.

Hick, S. F., & Bien, T. (Eds.). (2008). *Mindfulness and the therapeutic relationship.* New York: Guilford Press.

Hillman, J. (2003). Foreword. In Heraclitus, *Fragments* (pp. xi–xviii). New York: Penguin Classics.

Hirshfield, J. (2008). *Hiddenness, uncertainty, surprise: Three generative energies of poetry*. Northumberland, UK: Bloodaxe Books.

Hobbes, T. (1962). *Leviathan* (T. Oakeshott, Ed.). New York: Oxford University Press. (Original work published 1651)

Hoffman, M. (1981). Is altruism part of human nature? *Journal of Personality and Social Psychology, 40,* 121–137.

Hofmann, S., & Asmundson, G. (2008). Acceptance and mindfulness-based therapy: New wave or old hat? *Clinical Psychology Review, 28*(1), 1–16.

Hofmann, S., Grossman, P., & Hinton, D. (2011). Loving-kindness and compassion meditation: Potential for psychological interventions. *Clinical Psychology Review, 31,* 1126–1132.

Holliday, S. G., & Chandler, M. J. (1986). *Wisdom: Explorations in adult competence.* Basel, Switzerland: Karger.

Hollis-Walker, L., & Colosimo, K. (2011). Mindfulness, self-compassion, and happiness in non-meditators: A theoretical and empirical examination. *Personality and Individual Differences, 50*(2), 222–227.

Hölzel, B. K., Carmody, J., Vangel, M., Congleton, C., Yerramsetti, S. M., Gard, T., et al. (2011). Mindfulness practice leads to increases in regional brain gray matter density. *Psychiatry Research: Neuroimaging, 191,* 36–42.

Hölzel, B. K., Lazar, S. W., Gard, T., Schuman-Olivier, Z., Vago, D. R., & Ott, U. (2011). How does mindfulness meditation work?: Proposing mechanisms of action from a conceptual and neural perspective. *Perspectives on Psychological Science, 6,* 537–559.

Hölzel, B. K., Ott, U., Gard, T., Hempel, H., Weygandt, M., Morgen, K., et al. (2008). Investigation of mindfulness meditation practitioners with voxed-based morphometry. *SCAN, 3,* 55–61.

Hooker, T., & Hooker, L. (2004). Sumer: Origins, civilisation and myths. *Bath Royal Literary and Scientific Institution Proceedings*. Retrieved from *www.brlsi.org/proceed05/antiquity1104.html.*

Horn, N. R., Dolan, M., Elliott, R., Deakin, J. F., & Woodruff, P. W. (2003). Response inhibition and impulsivity: An fMRI study. *Neuropsychologia, 41,* 1959–1966.

Horney, K. (1950). *Neurosis and human growth: The struggle toward self-realization.* New York: Norton.

Horney, K. (1967). The flight from womanhood. In H. Kelman (Ed.), *Feminine psychology* (pp. 54–70). New York: Norton. (Original work published 1926)

Huettel, S. A., Stowe, C. J., Gordon, E. M., Warner, B. T., & Platt, M. L. (2006). Neural signatures of economic preferences for risk and ambiguity. *Neuron, 49,* 765–775.

Hui, H. C., & Yee, C. (1994). The shortened individualism and collectivism scale: Its relationship to demographic and work-related variables. *Journal of Research in Personality, 28,* 409–424.

Hume, D. (1978). *A treatise of human nature.* New York: Oxford University Press. (Original work published 1888)

Hutcherson, C. A., Seppala, E. M., & Gross, J. J. (2008). Loving-kindness meditation increases social connectedness. *Emotion, 8,* 720–724.

Hyde, K. L., Lerch, J., Norton, A., Forgeard, M., Winner, E., Evans, A. C., et al (2009). Musical training shapes structural brain development. *Journal of Neuroscience, 29*(10), 3019–3025.

Iacoboni, M. (2008). *Mirroring people.* New York: Farrar, Giroux & Strauss.

Immordino-Yang, M., McColl, A., Damasio, H., & Damasio, A. (2009). Neural correlates of admiration and compassion. *Proceedings of the National Academy of Sciences, 106*(19), 8021–8026.

Izard, C. E. (1977). *Human emotion.* New York: Plenum Press.

Jackson, S. W. (1990). *Melancholia and depression: From Hippocratic times to modern times.* New Haven, CT: Yale University Press.

Jager, W. (1994). *Contemplation: A Christian path.* Liguori, MO: Liguori.

Jager, W., & Quarch, C. (2000). *Die Welle ist das Meer: Mystische Spiritualität* [The wave is the sea: Mystical spirituality]. Freiburg, Germany: Herder.

James, W. (2007). *The principles of psychology, Vol. 1.* New York: Cosimo. (Original work published 1890)

James, W. (2010). *The varieties of religious experience.* Seattle: Pacific Publishing Studio. (Original work published 1902)

Jeste, D. V., Ardelt, M., Blazer, D., Kraemer, H. C., Vaillant, G., & Meeks, T. W. (2010). Expert consensus on the characteristics of wisdom: A Delphi method study. *Gerontologist, 50,* 668–680.

Jeste, D. V., & Harris, J. C. (2010). Commentary: Wisdom—a neuroscience perspective. *Journal of the American Medical Association, 304,* 1602–1603.

Jeste, D. V., & Vahia, I. (2008). Comparison of the conceptualization of wisdom in ancient Indian literature with modern views: Focus on the Bhagavad Gita. *Psychiatry, 71,* 197–209.

Jinpa, T., Rosenberg, E., McGonigal, K., Cullen, M., Goldin, P., & Ramel, W. (2009). *Compassion cultivation training (CCT): An eight-week course on cultivating compassionate heart and mind.* Unpublished manuscript, Center for Compassion and Altruism Research and Education, Stanford University, Stanford, CA.

Johanson, G. (2009). Nonlinear science, mindfulness, and the body in humanistic psychotherapy. *The Humanistic Psychologist, 37*(2), 159–177.

Johnson, D. P., Penn, D. L., Fredrickson, B. L., Kring, A. M., Meyer, P. S., Catalino, L. I., et al. (2011). A pilot study of loving-kindness meditation for the negative symptoms of schizophrenia. *Schizophrenia Research, 129,* 137–140.

Johnson, D. P., Penn, D. L., Fredrickson, B. L., Meyer, P., Kring, A., & Brantley, M. (2009). Loving-kindness meditation to enhance recovery from negative symptoms of schizophrenia. *Journal of Clinical Psychology, 65*(5), 1–11.

Johnson, K. J., & Fredrickson, B. L. (2005). We all look the same to me: Positive emotions eliminate the own-race bias in face recognition. *Psychological Science, 16,* 875–881.

Johnson, S. (2004). *The practice of emotionally focused couples therapy: Creating connection* (2nd ed.). New York: Brunner-Routledge.

Johnson, S. (2009). Extravagant emotion: Understanding and transforming love relationships in emotionally focused therapy. In D. Fosha, D. J. Siegel, & M. Solomon (Eds.), *The healing power of emotion: Affective neuroscience, development, and clinical practice* (pp. 257–279). New York: Norton.

Jones, E. E., & Nisbett, R. E. (1971). *The actor and the observer: Divergent perceptions of the causes of behavior.* New York: General Learning Press.

Jones, J. M. (2007). Exposure to chronic community violence: Resilience in African American children. *Journal of Black Psychology, 33*(2), 125–149.

Jordan, J. (1995). Relational awareness: Transforming disconnection. *Work in Progress, No. 76.* Wellesley, MA: Stone Center Working Paper Series.

Jordan, J. (2005). The quest for wisdom in adulthood: A psychological perspective. In R. J. Sternberg & J. Jordan (Eds.), *A handbook of wisdom: Psychological perspectives* (pp. 160–188). New York: Cambridge University Press.

Jordan, J. (2010). *Relational–cultural therapy.* Washington, DC: American Psychological Association.

Jordan, J. V. (1997). (Ed.). *Women's growth in diversity: More writings from the Stone Center.* New York: Guilford Press.

Jordan, J. V., Kaplan, A. G., Miller, J. B., Stiver, I. P., & Surrey, J. L. (Eds.). (1991). *Women's growth in connection: Writings from the Stone Center.* New York: Guilford Press.

Jordan, J. V., Walker, M., & Hartling, L. M. (Eds.). (2004). *The complexity of connection: Writings from the Stone Center's Jean Baker Miller Training Institute.* New York: Guilford Press.

Jung, C. G. (1938). *The collected works of C. G. Jung, Vol. 11: Psychology and religion: West and East* (R. F. C. Hull, Trans.). Princeton, NJ: Princeton University Press.

Jung, C. G. (1969). *The collected works of C. G. Jung, Vol. 8: The structure and dynamics of the psyche* (2nd ed.). (R. F. C. Hull, Trans.). Princeton, NJ: Princeton University Press.

Jung, C. G. (1981). *The collected works of C. G. Jung, Vol. 9: The archetypes and the collective unconscious* (R. F. C. Hull, Trans.). Princeton, NJ: Princeton University Press.

Kabat-Zinn, J. (1982). An outpatient program in behavioral medicine for chronic pain patients based on the practice of mindfulness meditation: Theoretical considerations and preliminary results. *General Hospital Psychiatry, 4,* 33–47.

Kabat-Zinn, J. (1990). *Full catastrophe living: Using the wisdom of your body and mind to face stress, pain and illness.* New York: Dell.

Kabat-Zinn, J. (1994). *Wherever you go, there you are.* New York: Hyperion.

Kabat-Zinn, J. (2003). Mindfulness-based interventions in context: Past, present, and future. *Clinical Psychology: Science and Practice, 10*(2), 144–156.

Kabat-Zinn, J., Lipworth, L., & Burney, R. (1985). The clinical use of mindfulness meditation for the self-regulation of chronic pain. *Journal of Behavioral Medicine, 8,* 163–190.

Kabat-Zinn, J., Massion, A. O., Kristeller, J., Peterson, L. G., Fletcher, K. E., Pbert, L., et al. (1992). Effectiveness of a meditation-based stress reduction program in the treatment of anxiety disorders. *American Journal of Psychiatry, 149*, 936–943.

Kabat-Zinn, M. (1998). *Mindful parenting: Interview with Jon and Myla Kabat-Zinn*. Yes! blog. Retrieved April 10, 2011, from *www.yesmagazine.org/issues/millennium-survival-guide/mindful-parenting*.

Kahill, S. (1988). Symptoms of professional burnout: A review of the empirical evidence. *Canadian Psychology/Psychologie Canadienne, 59*, 284–297.

Kaiser Greenland, S. (2010). *The mindful child*. New York: Free Press.

Kane, A. (2010). A grounded theory study of mindfulness and self-compassion as they relate to clinical efficacy and clinician self-care. *Dissertation Abstracts International, 70*(9-B), 5826.

Karcher, S. (2001). *The Kuan Yin oracle: The voice of the goddess of compassion*. London: Piatkus.

Kauer, J. A., & Malenka, R. C. (2007). Synaptic plasticity and addiction. *Nature Reviews Neuroscience, 8*, 844–858.

Keats, J. (1987). Letter to "my darling brothers." In R. Gittings (Ed.), *The letters of John Keats*. Oxford, UK: Oxford University Press. (Original letter dated 1818)

Kelly, A. C., Suroff, D., & Shapira, L. (2009). Soothing oneself and resisting self-attacks: The treatment of two intrapersonal deficits in depression vulnerability. *Cognitive Therapy and Research, 33*, 301–313.

Kelly, A. C., Zuroff, D. C., Foa, C. L., & Gilbert, P. (2009). Who benefits from training in self-compassionate self-regulation?: A study of smoking reduction. *Journal of Social and Clinical Psychology, 29*, 727–755.

Keltner, D. (2009). *Born to be good: The science of a meaningful life*. New York: Norton.

Kennedy, S. H., Konarski, J. Z., Segal, Z. V., Lau, M. A., Bieling, P. J., McIntyre, R. S., et al. (2007). Differences in brain glucose metabolism between responders to CBT and venlafaxine in a 16-week randomized controlled trial. *American Journal of Psychiatry, 164*, 778–788.

Kernis, M. H., Cornell, D. P., Sun, C. R., Berry, A., & Harlow, T. (1993). There's more to self-esteem than whether it is high or low: The importance of stability of self-esteem. *Journal of Personality and Social Psychology, 65*, 1190–1204.

Kessler, R. C., Sonnega, A., Bromet, E., Hughes, M., & Nelson, C. B. (1995). Posttraumatic stress disorder in the National Comorbidity Survey. *Archives of General Psychiatry, 52*, 1048–1060.

Khong, B., & Mruk, C. (2009). Editor's introduction to special issue on mindfulness in psychology. *The Humanistic Psychologist, 37*(2), 109–116.

Kim, J., Kim, S., Kim, J., Joeng, B., Park, C., Son, A., et al. (2011). Compassionate attitude towards others' suffering activates the mesolimbic neural system. *Neuropsychologia, 47*, 2073–2081.

Kim, S. H., & Hamann, S. (2007). Neural correlates of positive and negative emotion regulation. *Journal of Cognitive Neuroscience, 19*, 776–798.

Kingston, J., Clarke, S., & Remington, B. (2010). Experiential avoidance and problem behavior: A meditational analysis. *Behavior Modification, 34*(2), 145–163.

Kipling, R. (1999). If. In *The Collected Poems of Rudyard Kipling* (p. 605). London:Wordsworth Editions. (Original work published 1910)

Kirsch, P., Esslinger, C., Chen, Q., Mier, D., Lis, S., Siddhanti, S., et al. (2005). Oxytocin modulates neural circuitry for social cognition and fear in humans. *Journal of Neuroscience, 25,* 11489–11493.

Kitchener, K. S., & Brenner, H. G. (1990). Wisdom and reflective judgment: Knowing in the face of uncertainty. In R. J. Sternberg (Ed.), *Wisdom: Its nature, origins, and development* (pp. 212–229). New York: Cambridge University Press.

Klimecki, O., & Singer, T. (in press). Empathic distress fatigue rather than compassion fatigue?: Integrating findings from empathy research in psychology and social neuroscience. In B. Oakley, A. Knafo, G. Madhavan, & D. S. Wilson (Eds.), *Pathological altruism.* New York: Oxford University Press.

Knutson, B. (2004). Behavior: Sweet revenge? *Science, 305,* 1246–1247.

Kok, B. E., Coffey, K., Cohn, M. A., Algoe, S. B., Catalino, L. I., Vacharkulksemsuk, T., et al. (2011). *Made for loving: Vagal tone predicts responsiveness to loving-kindness meditation and loving-kindness meditation increases vagal tone.* Manuscript in preparation.

Kok, B. E., & Fredrickson, B. L. (2010). Upward spirals of the heart: Autonomic flexibility, as indexed by vagal tone, reciprocally and prospectively predicts positive emotions and social connections. *Biological Psychology, 85,* 432–436.

Koons, C. R., Robins, C. J., Tweed, J. L., Lynch, T. R., Gonzalez, A. M., Morse, J. Q., et al. (2001). Efficacy of dialectical behavior therapy in women veterans with borderline personality disorder. *Behavior Therapy, 32,* 371–390.

Kopelman, S., Rosette, A. S., & Thompson, L. (2006). The three faces of Eve: Strategic displays of negative, positive, and neutral emotions in negotiations. *Organizational Behavior and Human Decision Processes, 99,* 81–101.

Kornfield, J. (2008a, February). Lecture at Spirit Rock Meditation Center, Woodacre, CA.

Kornfield, J. (2008b). *The wise heart: A guide to the universal teachings of Buddhist psychology.* New York: Bantam.

Krain, A. L., Wilson, A. M., Arbuckle, R., Castellanos, F. X., & Milham, M. P. (2006). Distinct neural mechanisms of risk and ambiguity: A meta-analysis of decision-making. *NeuroImage, 32,* 477–484.

Kramer, D. A. (1990). Conceptualizing wisdom: The primacy of affect–cognition relations. In R. J. Sternberg (Ed.), *Wisdom: Its nature, origins, and development* (pp. 279–313). New York: Cambridge University Press.

Kramer, D. A. (2000). Wisdom as a classical source of human strength: Conceptualization and empirical inquiry. *Journal of Social and Clinical Psychology, 19,* 83–101.

Kramer, G. (2007). *Insight dialogue: The interpersonal path to freedom.* Boston: Shambhala.

Krause, N. (2006). Exploring the stress-buffering effects of church-based and secular social support on self-rated health in late life. *Journal of Gerontology: Social Sciences, 61B,* S35–S43.

Kristeller, J., & Johnson, T. (2005). Science looks at spirituality: Cultivating loving kindness–a two-stage model of the effects of meditation on empathy, compassion, and altruism. *Zygon, 4*(2), 391–407.

Krüger, E. (2010). *Effects of a meditation-based programme of stress reduction on levels of self-compassion.* Master's thesis, School of Psychology, Bangor University, Wales, UK.

Kruger, J., & Dunning, D. (1999). Unskilled and unaware of it: How difficulties in recognizing one's own incompetence lead to inflated self-assessments. *Journal of Personality and Social Psychology, 77*(6), 1121–1134.

Kunzmann, U., & Baltes, P. B. (2005). The psychology of wisdom: Theoretical and empirical challenges. In R. J. Sternberg & J. Jordan (Eds.), *A handbook of wisdom: Psychological perspectives* (pp. 110–135). New York: Cambridge University Press.

Kupperman, J. J. (1990). Morality, ethics, and wisdom. In R. J. Sternberg & J. Jordan (Eds.), *A handbook of wisdom: Psychological perspectives* (pp. 245–271). New York: Cambridge University Press.

Kuyken, W., Watkins, E., Holden, E., White, K., Taylor, R. S., Byford, S., et al. (2010). How does mindfulness-based cognitive therapy work? *Behaviour Research and Therapy, 48,* 1105–1112.

Kwok, V., Niu, Z., Kay, P., Zhou, K., Mo, L., Jin, Z., et al. (2011). Learning new color names produces rapid increase in gray matter in the intact adult human cortex. *Proceedings of the National Academy of Sciences, 108*(16), 6686–6688.

Labouvie-Vief, G. (1990). Wisdom as integrated thought: Historical and developmental perspectives. In R. J. Sternberg (Ed.), *Wisdom: Its nature, origins, and development* (pp. 52–83). New York: Cambridge University Press.

Ladner, L. (2004). *The lost art of compassion: Discovering the practice of happiness in the meeting of Buddhism and psychology*. New York: HarperCollins.

Lajoie, D. H., & Shapiro, S. Y. (1992). Definitions of transpersonal psychology: The first twenty-three years. *Journal of Transpersonal Psychology, 24*(1), 79–98.

Lambert, C. (2007). The science of happiness: Psychology explores humans at their best. *Harvard Magazine, 109*(3), 26.

Lambert, M. J., & Barley, D. E. (2001). Research summary on the therapeutic relationship and psychotherapy outcome. *Psychotherapy, 38,* 357–361.

Langemann, R., & Yamaner, S. (2011, July). *How to train compassion with the model of nonviolent communication.* Paper presented at the Max-Planck Institute for Human and Cognitive Brain Sciences conference, Berlin, Germany.

Langer, E. J. (1989). *Mindfulness.* Cambridge, MA: Merloyd Lawrence Books.

Layard, R. (2010). Measuring subjective well-being: How should human happiness and life satisfaction be assessed? *Science, 327,* 534–353.

Lazar, S. W., Kerr, C. E., Wasserman, R. H., Gray, J. R., Greve, D. N., Treadway, M. T., et al. (2005). Meditation experience is associated with increased cortical thickness. *NeuroReport, 16,* 1893–1897.

Lazarus, R. (1991). *Emotion and adaptation.* Oxford, UK: Oxford University Press.

Leary, M. R., Tate, E. B., Adams, C. E., Allen, A. B., & Hancock, J. (2007). Self-compassion and reactions to unpleasant self-relevant events: The implications of treating oneself kindly. *Journal of Personality and Social Psychology, 92,* 887–904.

Ledi, S. (1999). *The manuals of Dhamma.* Igatpuri, India: Vipassana Research Institute.

LeDoux, J. (1998). *The emotional brain.* London: Weidenfeld & Nicolson.

Lee, D. A. (2005). The perfect nurturer: A model to develop a compassionate mind within the context of cognitive therapy. In P. Gilbert (Ed.), *Compassion: Conceptualisations, research and use in psychotherapy* (pp. 326–351). Hove, UK: Routledge.

Levitt, J. T., Brown, T. A., Orsillo, S. M., & Barlow, D. H. (2004). The effects of acceptance versus suppression of emotion on subjective and psychophysiological response to carbon dioxide challenge in patients with panic disorder. *Behavior Therapy, 35,* 747–766.

Levy, B. R., Slade, M. D., Kunkel, S. R., & Kasl, S. V. (2002). Longevity increased by positive self-perceptions of aging. *Journal of Personality and Social Psychology, 83*(2), 261–270.

Lewin, R. (1996). *Compassion: The core value that animates psychotherapy.* Lanham, MD: Jason Aronson.

Leyro, T., Zvolensky, M., & Bernstein, A. (2010). Distress tolerance and psychopathological symptoms and disorders: A review of the empirical literature among adults. *Psychological Bulletin, 136*(4), 576–600.

Lieberman, M. D. (2007). Social cognitive neuroscience: A review of core processes. *Annual Review of Psychology, 58,* 259–289.

Lieberman, M. D., Eisenberger, N. I., Crockett, M. J., Tom, S. M., Pfeifer, J. H., & Way, B. M. (2007). Putting feelings into words: Affect labeling disrupts amygdala activity in response to affective stimuli. *Psychological Science, 18,* 421–428.

Linden, M. (2008). Posttraumatic embitterment disorder and wisdom therapy. *Journal of Cognitive Psychotherapy: An International Quarterly, 22*(1), 4–14.

Lindgren, K. N., & Coursey, R. D. (1995). Spirituality and serious mental illness: A two-part study. *Psychosocial Rehabilitation Journal, 18,* 93–111.

Linehan, M. M. (1993a). *Cognitive-behavioral treatment of borderline personality disorder.* New York: Guilford Press.

Linehan, M. M. (1993b). *Skills training manual for treating borderline personality disorder.* New York: Guilford Press.

Linehan, M. M. (1994). Acceptance and change: The central dialectic in psychotherapy. In S. C. Hayes, N. S. Jacobson, V. M. Follette, & M. J. Dougher (Eds.), *Acceptance and change: Content and context in psychotherapy* (pp. 73–87). Reno, NV: Context Press.

Linehan, M. M. (1997). Validation and psychotherapy. In A. C. Bohart & L. S. Greenberg (Eds.), *Empathy reconsidered: New directions in psychotherapy* (pp. 353–392). Washington, DC: American Psychological Association.

Linehan, M. M., Armstrong, H. E., Suarez, A., Allmon, D., & Heard, H. L. (1991). Cognitive-behavioral treatment of chronically parasuicidal borderline patients. *Archives of General Psychiatry, 48,* 1060–1064.

Linehan, M. M., Comtois, K. A., Murray, A. M., Brown, M. Z., Gallop, R. J., Heard,

H. L., et al. (2006). Two-year randomized controlled trial and follow-up of dialectical behavior therapy vs. therapy by experts for suicidal behaviors and borderline personality disorder. *Archives of General Psychiatry, 63*, 757–766.

Linehan, M. M., & Dimeff, L. A. (1995, November). *Dialectical behavior therapy for women with borderline personality disorder and substance abuse*. Symposium conducted at the annual convention of the Association for the Advancement of Behavior Therapy, Washington, DC.

Linehan, M. M., Dimeff, L. A., Reynolds, S. K., Comtois, K. A., Welch, S. S., Heagerty, P., et al. (2002). Dialectical behavior therapy versus comprehensive validation therapy plus 12-step for the treatment of opioid-dependent women meeting criteria for borderline personality disorder. *Drug and Alcohol Dependence, 67*, 13–26.

Linehan, M. M., McDavid, J. D., Brown, M. Z., Sayrs, J. H., & Gallop, R. J. (2008). Olanzapine plus dialectical behavior therapy for women with high irritability who meet criteria for borderline personality disorder: A double-blind, placebo-controlled study. *Journal of Clinical Psychiatry, 69*, 999–1005.

Linehan, M. M., & Schmidt, H. I., II. (1995). The dialectics of effective treatment of borderline personality disorder. In W. O. O'Donohue & L. Krasner (Eds.), *Theories in behavior therapy: Exploring behavior change* (pp. 553–584). Washington, DC: American Psychological Association.

Linehan, M. M., Schmidt, H., III, Dimeff, L. A., Craft, J. C., Kanter, J., & Comtois, K. A. (1999). Dialectical behavior therapy for patients with borderline personality disorder and drug-dependence. *American Journal on Addiction, 8*, 279–292.

Linehan, M. M., & Shaw-Welch, S. (2002, November). *Dialectical behavior therapy (DBT) for suicidal clients meeting criteria for borderline personality disorder (BPD)*. Symposium conducted at the annual convention of the Association for Advancement of Behavior Therapy, Reno, NV.

Litz, B. T., Stein, N., Delaney, E., Lebowitz, L., Nash, W. P., Silva, C., et al. (2009). Moral injury and moral repair in war veterans: A preliminary model and intervention strategy. *Clinical Psychology Review, 29*, 695–706.

Lowens, I. (2010). Compassion focused therapy for people with bipolar disorder. *International Journal of Cognitive Therapy, 3*(2), 172–185.

Lutz, A., Brefczynski-Lewis, J., Johnstone, T., & Davidson, R. J. (2008). Regulation of the neural circuitry of emotion by compassion meditation: Effects of meditative expertise. *Public Library of Science, 3*(3), 1–5.

Lutz, A., Greischar, L. L., Perlman, D. M., & Davidson, R. J. (2009). BOLD signal in insula is differentially related to cardiac function during compassion meditation in experts vs. novices. *NeuroImage, 47*, 1038–1046.

Lutz A., Greischar, L. L., Rawlings N. B., Ricard M., & Davidson R. J., (2004). Long-term meditators self-induce high-amplitude gamma synchrony during mental practice. *Proceedings of the National Academy of Sciences of the United States of America, 101*, 16369–16373.

Lykins, E. L., & Baer, R. A. (2009). Psychological functioning in a sample of long-term practitioners of mindfulness meditation. *Journal of Cognitive Psychotherapy, 23*, 226–241.

Lynch, T. R., Trost, W. T., Salsman, N., & Linehan, M. M. (2007). Dialectical behavior therapy for borderline personality disorder. *Annual Review of Clinical Psychology, 3*, 181–205.

Lysaker, P., Gumley, A., & Dimaggio, G. (2011). Metacognitive disturbances in persons with severe mental illness: Theory, correlates with psychopathology, and models of psychotherapy. *Psychology and Psychotherapy: Theory, Research and Practice, 84*, 1–8.

Lyubomirsky, S. (2008). *The how of happiness: A scientific approach to getting the life you want.* New York: Penguin Press.

Macdonald, K., & MacDonald, T. M. (2010). The peptide that binds: A systematic review of oxytocin and its prosocial effects in humans. *Harvard Review of Psychiatry, 18*, 1–21.

Magnus, C. M. R., Kowalski, K. C., & McHugh, T.-L. F. (2010). The role of self-compassion in women's self-determined motives to exercise and exercise-related outcomes. *Self and Identity, 9*, 363–382.

Makransky, J. (2007). *Awakening through love: Unveiling your deepest goodness.* Boston: Wisdom.

Marlatt, G. A. (Ed.). (2002). *Harm reduction: Pragmatic strategies for managing high-risk behaviors.* New York: Guilford Press.

Marlatt, G. A., & Gordon, J. R. (Eds.). (1985). *Relapse prevention: Maintenance strategies in the treatment of addictive behaviors.* New York: Guilford Press.

Martin, D. J., Garske, J. P., & Davis, M. K. (2000). Relation of the therapeutic alliance with outcome and other variables: A meta-analytic review. *Journal of Consulting and Clinical Psychology, 68*, 438–450.

Maslow, A. H. (1968). *Toward a psychology of being.* New York: Van Nostrand.

Maslow, A. H., & Lowry, R. (Ed.). (1973). *Dominance, self-esteem, self-actualization: Germinal papers of A. H. Maslow.* Monterey, CA: Brooks/Cole.

Mason, M. F., Norton, M. I., Van Horn, J. D., Wegner, D. M., Grafton, S. T., & Macrae, C. N. (2007). Wandering minds: The default network and stimulus-independent thought. *Science, 315*, 393–395.

Mathalon, D. H., Pfefferbaum, A., Lim, K. O., Rosenbloom, M. J., & Sullivan, E. V. (2003). Compounded brain volume deficits in schizophrenia–alcoholism comorbidity. *Archives of General Psychiatry, 60*, 254–252.

May, G. G. (1982). *Will and spirit: A contemplative psychology.* San Francisco: Harper & Row.

McCann, I. L., & Pearlman, L. A. (1990). *Psychological trauma and the adult survivor: Theory, therapy, and transformation.* New York: Brunner/Mazel.

McCarthy, M. (1995). Estrogen modulation of oxytocin and its relation to behavior. *Advances in Experimental Medicine and Biology, 395*, 235–245.

McCullough, M. E., Sandage, S. J., & Worthington, E. L., Jr. (1997). *To forgive is human: How to put your past in the past.* Downers Grove, IL: InterVarsity Press.

McKay, M., & Fanning, P. (1987). *Self-esteem.* Oakland, CA: New Harbinger.

McLellan, A. T., Lewis, D. C., O'Brien, C. P., & Kleber, H. D. (2000). Drug dependence, a chronic mental illness: Implications for treatment, insurance, and outcomes evaluation. *Journal of the American Medical Association, 284*, 1689–1695.

McMahon, D. (2007). *The pursuit of happiness: A history from the Greeks to the present.* London: Penguin.

Mcmain, S. F., Links, P. S., Gnam, W. H., Guimond, T., Cardish, R. J., Korman, L., et al. (2009). A randomized trial of dialectical behavior therapy versus general psychiatric management for borderline personality disorder. *American Journal of Psychiatry, 166,* 1365–1374.

Meeks, T. W., & Jeste, D. V. (2009). Neurobiology of wisdom: A literature overview. *Archives of General Psychiatry, 66,* 355–365.

Meins, E., Fernyhough, C., Wainwright, R., Das Gupta, M., Fradley, E., & Tuckey, M. (2002). Maternal mind-mindedness and attachment security as predictors of theory of mind understanding. *Child Development, 73*(6), 1715–1726.

Mennin, D. S., Heimberg, R. G., Turk, C. L., & Fresco, D. M. (2005). Preliminary evidence for an emotion regulation deficit model of generalized anxiety disorder. *Behavior Research and Therapy, 43,* 1281–1310.

Merriam-Webster. (2006). Merriam-Webster On-line Dictionary. Available at *www.m-w.com/dictionary/validation.*

Merriam-Webster. (2011). *Webster's Third New International Dictionary, Unabridged.* Springfield, MA: Author.

Merton, T. (2008). *Choosing to love the world: On contemplation.* Louisville, CO: Sounds True.

Mikulincer, M., & Shaver, P. R. (2007). *Attachment in adulthood: Structure, dynamics, and change.* New York: Guilford Press.

Miller, A. L., Rathus, J. H., & Linehan, M. M. (2006). *Dialectical behavior therapy with suicidal adolescents.* New York: Guilford Press.

Miller, G. (2009). Neuroscience: A quest for compassion. *Science, 324,* 458–459.

Miller, J. (1986). *Toward a new psychology of women.* Boston: Beacon Press.

Miller, J., & Stiver, I. (1997). *The healing connection: How women form relationships in therapy and in life.* Boston: Beacon Press.

Miller, W. R., & Rollnick, S. (1991). *Motivational interviewing: Preparing people to change addictive behavior.* New York: Guilford Press.

Moll, J., Krueger, F., Zahn, R., Pardini, M., Oliveira-Souza, R., & Grafman, J. (2006). Human fronto-mesolimbic networks guide decisions about charitable donation. *Proceedings of the National Academy of Sciences, 103,* 15623–15628.

Mongrain, M., Chin, J., & Shapira, L. B. (in press). Practicing compassion increases happiness and self-esteem. *Journal of Happiness Studies.*

Monroe, K. (2002). Explicating altruism. In S. G. Post, L. G. Underwood, J. P. Schloss, & W. B. Hurlbut (Eds.), *Altruism and altruistic love: Science, philosophy, and religion in dialogue* (pp. 51–64). New York: Oxford University Press.

Montague, P. R., & Berns, G. S. (2002). Neural economics and the biological substrates of valuation. *Neuron, 36,* 265–284.

Monteiro, L., Nuttall, S., & Musten, F. (2010). Five skillful habits: An ethics-based mindfulness intervention. *Counseling and Spirituality, 29*(1), 91–104.

Morgan, W. D., & Morgan, S. T. (2005). Cultivating attention and empathy. In C. K. Germer, R. D. Siegel, & P. R. Fulton (Eds.), *Mindfulness and psychotherapy* (pp. 73–90). New York: Guilford Press.

Mosewich, A. D., Kowalski, K. C., Sabiston, C. M., Sedgwick, W. A., & Tracy, J.

L. (2011). Self-compassion: A potential resource for young women athletes. *Journal of Sport and Exercise Psychology, 33*, 103–123.

Murphy, T. J., Pagano, R. R., & Marlatt, G. A. (1986). Lifestyle modification with heavy alcohol drinkers: Effects of aerobic exercise and meditation. *Addictive Behaviors, 11*, 175–186.

Myers, D. (2000). The funds, friends, and faith of happy people. *American Psychologist, 55*, 56–67.

Nairn, R. (2009, September). *Lecture as part of foundation training in compassion.* Kagyu Samye Ling Monastery, Dumfriesshire, Scotland.

Nanamoli, B., & Bodhi, B. (Trans.). (1995). *The middle length discourses of the Buddha.* Boston: Wisdom.

Naranjo, C. (1970). Present-centeredness: Technique, prescription, and ideal. In J. Fagan & I. L. Shepherd (Eds.), *Gestalt therapy now.* Palo Alto, CA: Science and Behavior Books.

Neely, M. E., Schallert, D. L., Mohammed, S. S., Roberts, R. M., & Chen, Y. (2009). Self-kindness when facing stress: The role of self-compassion, goal regulation, and support in college students' well-being. *Motivation and Emotion, 33*, 88–97.

Neff, K. (2009). Self-compassion. In M. R. Leary & R. H. Hoyle (Eds.), *Handbook of individual differences in social behavior* (pp. 561–573). New York: Guilford Press.

Neff, K. D. (2003a). Development and validation of a scale to measure self-compassion. *Self and Identity, 2*, 223–250.

Neff, K. D. (2003b). Self-compassion: An alternative conceptualization of a healthy attitude toward oneself. *Self and Identity, 2*, 85–102.

Neff, K. D. (2011a). Self-compassion, self-esteem, and well-being. *Social and Personality Compass, 5*, 1–12.

Neff, K. D. (2011b). *Self-compassion: Stop beating yourself up and leave insecurity behind.* New York: William Morrow.

Neff, K. D., & Beretvas, S. N. (in press). The role of self-compassion in romantic relationships. *Self and Identity.*

Neff, K. D., Hseih, Y., & Dejitthirat, K. (2005). Self-compassion, achievement goals, and coping with academic failure. *Self and Identity, 4*, 263–287.

Neff, K. D., Kirkpatrick, K., & Rude, S. S. (2007). Self-compassion and its link to adaptive psychological functioning. *Journal of Research in Personality, 41*, 139–154.

Neff, K. D., & McGeehee, P. (2010). Self-compassion and psychological resilience among adolescents and young adults. *Self and Identity, 9*, 225–240.

Neff, K. D., Pisitsungkagarn, K., & Hseih, Y.-P. (2008). Self-compassion and self-construal in the United States, Thailand, and Taiwan. *Journal of Cross-Cultural Psychology, 39*, 267–285.

Neff, K. D., & Pommier, E. (in press). The relationship between self-compassion and other-focused concern among college undergraduates, community adults, and practicing meditators. *Self and Identity.*

Neff, K. D., & Rude, S. S., & Kirkpatrick, K. (2007). An examination of self-compassion in relation to positive psychological functioning and personality traits. *Journal of Research in Personality, 41*, 908–916.

Neff, K. D., & Vonk, R. (2009). Self-compassion versus global self-esteem: Two different ways of relating to oneself. *Journal of Personality, 77*, 23–50.

Neff, K. D., Yarnell, L., & Pommier, E. (2011). *The relationship between self-compassion and other-focused concern.* Unpublished manuscript.

Negi, L. (2009). *Emory compassion meditation protocol.* Unpublished manuscript, Emory University, Atlanta, GA.

Nesse, R. (2000). Is depression an adaptation? *Archives of General Psychiatry, 57*, 14–20.

Nielsen, L., & Kaszniak, A. W. (2006). Awareness of subtle emotional feelings: A comparison of long-term meditators and nonmeditators. *Emotion, 6*, 392–405.

Nietzsche, F. (2010). *Beyond good and evil.* New York: Tribeca Books. (Original work published 1923)

Nisargadatta, S. (1973). *I am that.* Durham, NC: Acorn Press.

Nishijima, G., & Cross, C. (2006). *Master Dogen's Shobogenzo.* Charleston, SC: BookSurge.

Nolen-Hoeksema, S. (1991). Responses to depression and their effects on the duration of depressive episodes. *Journal of Abnormal Psychology, 100*, 569–582.

Norcross, J. (Ed.). (2002). *Psychotherapy relationships that work: Therapist contribution and responsiveness to patient.* New York: Oxford University Press.

Nussbaum, M. (1996). Compassion: The basic social emotion. *Social Philosophy and Policy, 13*, 27–58.

Nussbaum, M. (2001). *Upheavals of thought: The intelligence of emotions.* New York: Cambridge University Press.

Nyanamoli, B. (Trans.). (1964). *The path of purification (Visuddhimagga) by Buddhaghosa.* Colombo, Ceylon: A. Semage.

Nyanatiloka, B. (1972). *Buddhist dictionary: A manual of Buddhist terms and doctrines.* Colombo, Sri Lanka: Frewin & Co.

Nye, N. S. (1995). Kindness. In *Words under the words: Selected poems.* Portland, OR: Far Corner Books.

Nyklicek, I., & Kuijpers, K. F. (2008). Effects of mindfulness-based stress reduction intervention on psychological well-being and quality of life: Is increased mindfulness indeed the mechanism? *Annals of Behavioral Medicine, 35*, 331–340.

Ochsner, K. N., Bunge, S. A., Gross, J. J., & Gabrieli, J. D. (2002). Rethinking feelings: An fMRI study of the cognitive regulation of emotion. *Journal of Cognitive Neuroscience, 14*, 1215–1229.

Olendzki, A. (2005). The roots of mindfulness. In C. K. Germer, R. D. Siegel, & P. F. Fulton (Eds.), *Mindfulness and psychotherapy* (pp. 241–261). New York: Guilford Press.

Olendzki, A. (2010). *Unlimiting mind: The radically experiential psychology of Buddhism.* Boston: Wisdom.

Oliner, S. (2002). Extraordinary acts of ordinary people: Faces of heroism and altruism. In S. G. Post, L. G. Underwood, J. P. Schloss, & W. B. Hurlbut (Eds.), *Altruism and altruistic love: Science, philosophy, and religion in dialogue* (pp. 51–64). New York: Oxford University Press.

Oliver, M. (1986). *Dream work.* Boston: Atlantic Monthly Press.

Orsillo, S. M., & Roemer, L. (2011). *The mindful way through anxiety: Break free from chronic worry and reclaim your life.* New York: Guilford Press.

Orzech, K. M., Shapiro, S. L., Brown, K. W., & McKay, M. (2009). Intensive mindfulness training-related changes in cognitive and emotional experience. *Journal of Positive Psychology, 4,* 212–222.

Osbeck, L. M., & Robinson, D. N. (2005). Philosophical theories of wisdom. In R. J. Sternberg & J. Jordan (Eds.), *A handbook of wisdom: Psychological perspectives* (pp. 61–83). New York: Cambridge University Press.

Oveis, C., Horberg, E., & Keltner, D. (2009). *Somatic markers in compassion.* Unpublished manuscript.

Oxford English Dictionary: 11th Edition. (2008). New York: Oxford University Press.

Oxford English Dictionary. (2010). New York: Oxford University Press. Retrieved February 26, 2011, from *www.oed.com.ezp-prod1.hul.harvard.edu/viewdictionaryentry/Entry/229491.*

Pagnoni, G., Cekic, M., & Guo, Y. (2008). Thinking about not-thinking: Neural correlates of conceptual processing during Zen meditation. *PLoS ONE, 3*(9), e3083.

Pani, L. (2000). Is there an evolutionary mismatch between the normal physiology of the human dopaminergic system and current environmental conditions in industrialized countries? *Molecular Psychiatry, 5,* 467–475.

Panksepp, J. (1998). *Affective neuroscience.* New York: Oxford University Press.

Panksepp, J. (2011). The neurobiology of social loss in animals: Some keys to the puzzle of psychic pain in humans. In G. MacDonald & L. Jensen-Campbell (Ed.), *Social pain: Neuropsychological and health implications of loss and exclusion* (pp. 11–51). Washington DC: American Psychological Association.

Pargament, K. I. (1997). *The psychology of religion and coping: Theory, research, practice.* New York: Guilford Press.

Pargament, K. I. (2007). *Spiritually integrated psychotherapy: Understanding and addressing the sacred.* New York: Guilford Press.

Pargament, K. I., & Sweeney, P. J. (2011). Building spiritual fitness in the military: An innovative approach to a vital aspect of human development. *American Psychologist, 66,* 58–64.

Patsiopoulos, A., & Buchanan, M. (2011). The practice of self-compassion in counseling: A narrative inquiry. *Professional Psychology: Research and Practice, 42*(4), 301–307.

Pauley, G., & McPherson, S. (2010). The experience and meaning of compassion and self-compassion for individuals with depression or anxiety. *Psychology and Psychotherapy: Theory, Research, and Practice, 83,* 129–143.

Pearlman, L. A., & Courtois, C. A. (2005). Clinical applications of the attachment framework: Relational treatment of complex trauma. *Journal of Traumatic Stress, 18,* 449–459.

Pennington, B. (1980). *Centering prayer.* Garden City, NY: Doubleday.

Perner, J., & Lang, B. (1999). Development of theory of mind and executive control. *Trends in Cognitive Sciences, 3,* 337–344.

Peterson, C., & Seligman, M. (2004). *Character strengths and virtues: A handbook and classification.* Washington, DC: American Psychological Association.

Phan, K. L., Fitzgerald, D. A., Nathan, P. J., Moore, G. J., Uhde, T. W., & Tancer, M. E. (2005). Neural substrates for voluntary suppression of negative affect: A functional magnetic resonance imaging study. *Biological Psychiatry, 57*, 210–219.

Phillips, A. (1989). *Winnicott*. Cambridge, MA: Harvard University Press.

Phillips, J. B. (1997). *Your God is too small*. New York: Touchstone Books.

Piaget, J. (1972). *The psychology of intelligence*. Totowa, NJ: Littlefield-Adams.

Pinker, S. (2008, January 13). The moral instinct. *New York Times Magazine*, pp. 32–58.

Pizer, S. (2006). Repetition, negotiation, relationship: An introduction to the work of Paul L. Russel, MD. *Contemporary Psychoanalysis, 42*, 579–587.

Poldrack, R. A. (2002). Neural systems for perceptual skill learning. *Behavioral and Cognitive Neuroscience Reviews, 1*(1), 76–83.

Pommier, E. (2010). The compassion scale. *Dissertation Abstracts International, 72*(04), UMI 3445994.

Porges, S. W. (1995). Orienting in a defensive world: Mammalian modifications of our evolutionary heritage—a polyvagal theory. *Psychophysiology, 32*, 301–318.

Porges, S. W. (2001). The polyvagal theory: Phylogenetic substrates of a social nervous system. *International Journal of Psychophysiology, 42*, 123–146.

Porges, S. W. (2007). The polyvagal perspective. *Biological Psychology, 74*, 116–143.

Post, S. (2002). The tradition of agape. In S. G. Post, L. G. Underwood, J. P. Schloss, & W. B. Hurlbut (Eds.), *Altruism and altruistic love: Science, philosophy, and religion in dialogue* (pp. 51–64). New York: Oxford University Press.

Power, M. (2004). *Mood disorders: A handbook of science and practice*. Chichester, UK: Wiley.

Powers, J. (2007). *Introduction to Tibetan Buddhism*. Ithaca, NY: Snow Lion.

Powers, T. A., Koestner, R., & Zuroff, D. C. (2007). Self-criticism, goal motivation, and goal progress. *Journal of Social and Clinical Psychology, 26*, 826–840.

Putnam, R. (2000). *Bowling alone: The collapse and revival of American community*. New York: Simon & Schuster.

Rad, G. (1972). *Wisdom in Israel*. New York: Abington Press.

Raes, F. (2010). Rumination and worry as mediators of the relationship between self-compassion and depression and anxiety. *Journal of Personality and Individual Differences, 48*, 757–761.

Raes, F. (2011). The effect of self-compassion on the development of depression symptoms in a nonclinical sample. *Mindfulness, 2*(1), 33–36.

Rahula, W. (1974). *What the Buddha taught*. New York: Grove Weidenfeld.

Raichle, M. E., MacLeod, A. M., Snyder, A. Z., Powers, W. J., Gusnard, D. A., & Shulman, G. L. (2001). A default mode of brain function. *Proceedings of the National Academy of Sciences of the United States of America, 98*, 676–682.

Raque-Bogdan, R., Ericson, S., Jackson, J., Martin, H., & Bryan, N. (2011). Attachment and mental and physical health: Self-compassion and mattering as mediators. *Journal of Consulting Psychology, 58*(2), 272–278.

Ray, R. (2001). *Secret of the vajra world: The tantric Buddhism of Tibet*. Boston: Shambhala.

Readers Digest Association. (1973). *The last two million years*. New York: Author.

Resick, P. A., & Schnicke, M. K. (1993). *Cognitive processing therapy for rape victims: A treatment manual.* Newbury Park, CA: Sage.

Ricard, M. (2010). The difference between empathy and compassion. *HuffPost Living.* Retrieved October 15, 2010, from *www.huffingtonpost.com/matthieu-ricard/could-compassion-meditati_b_751566.html.*

Rich, S. (2010, November). fMRI predicts outcome to talk therapy in children with an anxiety disorder. Paper presented at the annual meeting of the Society for Neuroscience, San Diego, CA. Available at *explore.georgetown.edu/news/?ID=54076&PageTemplateID=295.*

Rilke, R. M. (1954). *Letters to a young poet* (M. D. H. Norton, Trans.). New York: Norton.

Rilke, R. M. (1984). *Letters to a young poet* (S. Mitchell, Trans.). New York: Vintage Books.

Rilling, J., Gutman, D., Zeh, T., Pagnoni, G., Berns, G., & Kilts, C. (2002). A neural basis for social cooperation. *Neuron, 35,* 395–405.

Ringenbach, R. (2009). A comparison between counselors who practice meditation and those who do not on compassion fatigue, compassion satisfaction, burnout and self-compassion. *Dissertation Abstracts International: Section B: The Sciences and Engineering, 70*(6-B), 3820.

Rizzolatti, G., & Craighero, L. (2004). The mirror-neuron system. *Annual Review of Neuroscience, 27,* 169–192.

Rizzolatti, G., Fadiga, L., Gallese, V., & Fogassi, L. (1996). Premotor cortex and the recognition of motor actions. *Cognitive Brain Research, 3,* 131–141.

Rizzolatti, G., & Sinigaglia, C. (2010). The functional role of the parieto-frontal mirror circuit: Interpretations and misinterpretations. *Nature Reviews Neuroscience, 11*(6), 264–274.

Robb, C. (2006). *This changes everything: The relational revolution I psychology.* New York: Farrar Strauss.

Robinson, D. N. (1990). Wisdom through the ages. In R.J. Sternberg (Ed.), *Wisdom: Its nature, origins, and development.* New York: Cambridge University Press.

Robinson, D. N. (1995). *An intellectual history of psychology.* Madison, WI: University of Wisconsin Press.

Roemer, L., & Orsillo, S. M. (2009). *Mindfulness- and acceptance-based behavioral therapies in practice.* New York: Guilford Press.

Roemer, L., Orsillo, S. M., & Salters-Pedneault, K. (2008). Efficacy of an acceptance-based behavior therapy for generalized anxiety disorder: Evaluation in a randomized controlled trial. *Journal of Consulting and Clinical Psychology, 76,* 1083–1089.

Rogers, C. (1951). A research program in client-centered therapy. *Research Publications of the Association for Research in Nervous and Mental Disease, 31,* 106–113.

Rogers, C. (1957). The necessary and sufficient conditions of therapeutic personality change. *Journal of Consulting Psychology, 21,* 95–103.

Rogers, C. (1959). A theory of therapy, personality and interpersonal relationships as developed in the client-centered framework. In S. Koch (Ed.), *Psychology: A study of a science.* New York: McGraw-Hill.

Rogers, C. (1961). *On becoming a person: A therapist's view of psychotherapy*. Boston: Houghton Mifflin.

Rose, E. M., Westefeld, J. S., & Ansley, T. N. (2001). Spiritual issues in counseling: Clients' beliefs and preferences. *Journal of Counseling Psychology, 48*, 61–71.

Rothschild, B. (2000). *The body remembers: The psychophysiology of trauma and trauma treatment*. New York: Norton.

Rowe, G., Hirsh, J. B., & Anderson, A. K. (2007). Positive affect increases the breadth of attentional selection. *Proceedings of the National Academy of Sciences USA, 104*, 383–388.

Rubia, K. (2009). The neurobiology of meditation and its clinical effectiveness in psychiatric disorders. *Biological Psychology, 82*, 1–11.

Rudd, M. D., Joiner, T. E., & Rajab, M. H. (2001). *Treating suicidal behavior: An effective time-limited approach*. New York: Guilford Press.

Rumi, J. (1996). *The essential Rumi* (C. Barks, Trans.). New York: HarperCollins.

Rumi, J., Green, M., & Barks, C. (1997). *The illuminated Rumi*. New York: Broadway Books.

Rumi, J., & Helminski, K. (Trans.). (2000). *Love is a stranger: Selected lyric poetry of Jelaluddin Rumi*. Boston: Shambhala Press.

Russell, P. (1996). Process with involvement: The interpretation of affect. In L. E. Lifson (Ed.), *Understanding therapeutic action: Psychodynamic concepts of cure*. Hillsdale, NJ: Analytic Press.

Safer, D. L., Telch, C. F., & Chen, E. Y. (2009). *Dialectical behavior therapy for binge eating and bulimia*. New York: Guilford Press.

Safran, J. D. (Ed.). (2003). *Psychoanalysis and Buddhism: An unfolding dialogue*. Boston: Wisdom.

Safran, J. D. (1998). *Widening the scope of cognitive therapy: The therapeutic relationship, emotion, and the process of change*. Northvale, NJ: Jason Aronson.

Salmivalli, C., Kaukiainen, A., Kaistaniemi, L., & Lagerspetz, K. M. J. (1999). Self-evaluated self-esteem, peer-evaluated self-esteem, and defensive egotism as predictors of adolescents' participation in bullying situations. *Personality and Social Psychology Bulletin, 25*, 1268–1278.

Salzberg, S. (1997). *Lovingkindness: The revolutionary art of happiness*. Boston: Shambhala.

Salzberg, S. (2011). *Real happiness: The power of meditation*. New York: Workman.

Samson, D., Apperly, I. A., & Humphreys, G. W. (2007). Error analyses reveal contrasting deficits in "theory of mind": Neuropsychological evidence from a 3-option false belief task. *Neuropsychologia, 45*, 2561–2569.

Samson, D., Apperly, I. A., Kathirgamanathan, U., & Humphreys, G. W. (2005). Seeing it my way: A case of a selective deficit in inhibiting self-perspective. *Brain, 128*, 1102–1111.

Sanderson, C., & Linehan, M. M. (1999). Acceptance and forgiveness. In W. R. Miller (Ed.), *Integrating spirituality into treatment: Resources for practitioners* (pp. 199–216). Washington, DC: American Psychological Association.

Sanford, K. (2010, May). Lecture at the Hammer Museum, University of California, Los Angeles.

Schanche, E., Stiles, T., McCollough, L., Swartberg, M., & Nielsen, G. (in press). The relationship between activating affects, inhibitory affects, and self-compassion in patients with cluster C personality disorders. *Psychotherapy: Theory, Research, Practice, Training.*

Schaef, A. W. (2000). *Meditations for living in balance: Daily solutions for people who do too much.* New York: HarperCollins.

Schmitz, T. W., De Rosa, E., & Anderson, A. K. (2009). Opposing influences of affective state valence on visual cortical encoding. *Journal of Neuroscience, 29,* 7199–7207.

Schopenhauer, A. (1966). *The world as will and representation.* New York: Dover. (Original work published 1844)

Schore, A. N. (1994). *Affect regulation and the origin of the self: The neurobiology of emotional development.* Mahwah, NJ: Erlbaum.

Schroevers, M. J., & Brandsma, R. (2010). Is learning mindfulness associated with improved affect after mindfulness-based cognitive therapy? *British Journal of Psychology, 101,* 95–107.

Schwartz, R. C. (2001). *Introduction to the internal family systems model.* Oak Park, IL: Trailheads Publications, The Center for Self-Leadership.

Schwartz, R. C. (1995). *Internal family systems therapy.* New York: Guilford Press.

Sedikides, C. (1993). Assessment, enhancement, and verification determinants of the self-evaluation process. *Journal of Personality and Social Psychology, 65,* 317–338.

Segal, Z. V., Williams, J. M. G., & Teasdale, J. D. (2002). *Mindfulness-based cognitive therapy for depression: A new approach to preventing relapse.* New York: Guilford Press.

Seitz, R. J., Nickel, J., & Azari, N. P. (2006). Functional modularity of the medial prefrontal cortex: Involvement in human empathy. *Neuropsychology, 20,* 743–751.

Seitz, R. J., Schäfer, R., Scherfeld, D., Friederichs, S., Popp, K., Wittsack, H. J., et al. (2008). Valuating other people's emotional face expression: A combined functional magnetic resonance imaging and electroencephalography study. *Neuroscience, 152,* 713–722.

Sephton, S. E., Sapolsky, R. M., Kraemer, H. C., & Spiegel, D. (2000). Diurnal cortisol rhythm as a predictor of breast cancer survival. *Journal of the National Cancer Institute, 92,* 994–1000.

Shafranske, E. P. (2001). Religious beliefs, attitudes, and personal and professional practices of physicians and psychologists specializing in rehabilitation medicine. In T. G. Plante & A. C. Sherman (Eds.), *Faith and health: Psychological perspectives* (pp. 311–338). New York: Guilford Press.

Shankaracharya. (2004). *The Bhagavad Gita with the commentaries of Adi Sri Shankaracharya.* Chennai, India: Samata Books.

Shapira, L., & Mongrain, L. (2010). The benefits of self-compassion and optimism exercises for individuals vulnerable to depression. *Journal of Positive Psychology, 5*(5), 377–389.

Shapiro, S. L., Astin, J. A., Bishop, S. R., & Cordova, M. (2005). Mindfulness-based stress reduction for health care professionals: Results from a randomized trial. *International Journal of Stress Management, 12,* 164–176.

Shapiro, S. L., Brown, K. W., & Biegel, G. M (2007). Teaching self-care to caregivers: Effects of mindfulness-based stress reduction on the mental health of therapists in training. *Training and Education in Professional Psychology, 1,* 105–115.

Shapiro, S. L., & Carlson, L. E. (2009). *The art and science of mindfulness: Integrating mindfulness into psychology and the helping professions.* Washington, DC: American Psychological Association.

Shapiro, S. L., Carlson, L. E., Astin, J. A., & Freedman, B. (2006). Mechanisms of mindfulness. *Journal of Clinical Psychology, 62,* 373–386.

Shapiro, S. L., & Izett, C. D. (2008). Meditation: A universal tool for cultivating empathy. In S. F. Hick & T. Bien (Eds.), *Mindfulness and the therapeutic relationship* (pp. 161–175). New York: Guilford Press.

Sharpe, E. J. (1986). *Comparative religion: A history.* London: Duckworth.

Shaver, P., Schwartz, J., Kirson, D., & O'Connor, C. (1987). Emotion knowledge: Further exploration of a prototype approach. *Journal of Personality and Social Psychology, 52,* 1061–1086.

Shem, S., & Surrey, J. (1998). *We have to talk: Healing dialogues between women and men.* New York: Basic Books.

Siegel, D. J. (1999). *The developing mind: How relationships and the brain interact to shape who we are.* New York: Guilford Press.

Siegel, D. J. (2001). Toward an interpersonal neurobiology of the developing mind: Attachment relationships, "mindsight," and neural integration: *Infant Mental Health Journal, 22,* 67–94.

Siegel, D. J. (2007). *The mindful brain: Reflection and attunement in the cultivation of well-being.* New York: Norton.

Siegel, D. J. (2010a). *The mindful therapist: A clinician's guide to mindsight and neural integration.* New York: Norton.

Siegel, D. J. (2010b). *Mindsight: The new science of personal transformation.* New York: Bantam.

Siegel, D. J., & Hartzell, M. (2003). *Parenting from the inside out: How a deeper self-understanding can help you raise children who thrive.* New York: Tarcher/Penguin.

Siegel, R. D. (2005). Psychophysiological disorders: Embracing pain. In C. K. Germer, R. D. Siegel, & P. R. Fulton (Eds.), *Mindfulness and psychotherapy* (pp. 173–196). New York: Guilford Press.

Siegel, R. D. (2009). *Positive psychology: Harnessing the power of happiness, personal power and mindfulness.* Boston: Harvard Medical School.

Siegel, R. D. (2010). *The mindfulness solution: Everyday practices for everyday problems.* New York: Guilford Press.

Siegel, R. D., Allison, K. C., & Allison, S. M. (Eds.). (2009). *Positive psychology: Harnessing the power of happiness, personal strength, and mindfulness.* Boston: Harvard Health.

Siff, J. (2010). *Unlearning meditation: What to do when the instructions get in the way.* Boston: Shambhala.

Singer, T., Kiebel, S. J., Winston, J. S., Dolan, R. J., & Frith, C. D. (2004). Brain responses to the acquired moral status of faces. *Neuron, 41,* 653–662.

Singer, W. (2005, November). Paper presented at the Mind and Life Institute conference, Washington, DC.

Singer, T., & Decety, J. (2011). Social neuroscience of empathy. In J. Decety & J. T.

Cacioppo (Eds.), *The Oxford handbook of social neuroscience*. New York: Oxford University Press.

Sinha, R., Lacadie, C., Skudlarski, P., Fulbright, R. K., Rounsaville, B. J., Kosten, T. R., et al. (2005). Neural activity associated with stress-induced cocaine craving: A functional magnetic resonance imaging study. *Psychopharmacology, 183*, 171–180.

Smith, J., & Baltes, P. B. (1990). Wisdom-related knowledge: Age/cohort differences in response to life-planning problems. *Developmental Psychology, 26*, 494–505.

Smith, J., Staudinger, U. M., & Baltes, P. B. (1994). Occupational settings facilitative of wisdom-related knowledge: The sample case of clinical psychologists. *Journal of Consulting and Clinical Psychology, 64*, 989–1000.

Smith, T. B., Bartz, J., & Richards, P. S. (2007). Outcomes of religious and spiritual adaptations to psychotherapy: A meta-analytic review. *Psychotherapy Research, 17*(6), 643–655.

Soeng, M. (2007, Fall). How deep (and sad) is your love? *Buddhadharma*, p. 65.

Soeng, M. (2010). *The heart of the universe*. Somerville, MA: Wisdom.

Sogyal Rinpoche. (2002). *The Tibetan book of living and dying*. New York: HarperCollins.

Soler, J., Pascual, J. C., Campins, J., Barrachina, J., Puigdemont, D., Alvarez, E., et al. (2005). Double-blind, placebo-controlled study of dialectical behavior therapy plus olanzapine for borderline personality disorder. *American Journal of Psychiatry, 162*, 1221–1224.

Solomon, J. L., Marshall, P., & Gardner, H. (2005). Crossing boundaries to generative wisdom. In R. J. Sternberg & J. Jordan (Eds.), *A handbook of wisdom: Psychological perspectives* (pp. 272–296). New York: Cambridge University Press.

Sommerville, J. A., & Decety, J. (2006). Weaving the fabric of social interaction: Articulating developmental psychology and cognitive neuroscience in the domain of motor cognition. *Psychonomic Bulletin and Review, 13*, 179–200.

Soto, D., Funes, M. J., Guzman-Garcia, A., Warbrick, T., Rotshtein, P., & Humphreys, G. W. (2009). Pleasant music overcomes the loss of awareness in patients with visual neglect. *Proceedings of the National Academy Science USA, 106*, 6011–6016.

Stahl, B., & Goldstein, E. (2010). *A mindfulness-based stress reduction workbook*. Oakland, CA: New Harbinger Press.

Staudinger, U. M. (1999). Older and wiser?: Integrating results on the relationship between age and wisdom-related performance. *International Journal of Behavioral Development, 23*(3), 641–664.

Staudinger, U. M., & Baltes, P. B. (1996). Interactive minds: A facilitative setting for wisdom-related performance. *Journal of Personality and Social Psychology, 71*, 746–762.

Staudinger, U. M., & Glück, J. (2011). Psychological wisdom research: Commonalities and differences in a growing field. *Annual Review of Psychology, 62*, 215–241.

Staudinger, U. M., Smith, J., & Baltes, P. B. (1992). Wisdom-related knowledge in a life review task: Age differences and the role of professional specialization. *Psychology and Aging, 7*(2), 271–281.

Staw, B. M., & Barsade, S. G. (1993). Affect and managerial performance: A test of the sadder-but-wiser vs. happier-and-smarter hypothesis. *Administrative Science Quarterly, 38*, 304–331.

Steptoe, A., Wardle, J., & Marmot, M. (2005). Positive affect and health-related neuroendocrine, cardiovascular, and inflammatory processes. *Proceedings of the National Academy of Sciences of the United States of America, 102*(18), 6508–6512. Retrieved May 21, 2010, from *www. pnas.org*.

Sternberg, E. (2011). *Approaches to defining mechanisms by which altruistic love affects health*. Stony Brook, NY: The Institute for Research on Unlimited Love. Retrieved April 15, 2011, from *www.unlimitedloveinstitute.org/publications/pdf/whitepapers/Mechanisms_Altruistic.pdf*.

Sternberg, R. J. (1990a). Understanding wisdom. In R. J. Sternberg (Ed.), *Wisdom: Its nature, origins, and development*. New York: Cambridge University Press.

Sternberg, R. J. (Ed.). (1990b). *Wisdom: Its nature, origins, and development*. New York: Cambridge University Press.

Sternberg, R. J. (1998). A balance theory of wisdom. *Review of General Psychology, 2*(4), 347–365.

Sternberg, R. J. (2001). Why schools should teach for wisdom: The balance theory of wisdom in educational settings. *Educational Psychologist, 36*, 227–245.

Sternberg, R. J. (2002). Smart people are not stupid, but they sure can be foolish: The imbalance theory of foolishness. In R. J. Sternberg (Ed.), *Why smart people can be so stupid* (pp. 232–242). New Haven, CT: Yale University Press.

Sternberg, R. J. (2003). *Wisdom, intelligence, and creativity, synthesized*. New York: Cambridge University Press.

Sternberg, R. J. (2005a). Foolishness. In R. J. Sternberg & J. Jordan (Eds.), *A handbook of wisdom: Psychological perspectives* (pp. 331–352). New York: Cambridge University Press.

Sternberg, R. J. (2005b). Older but not wiser?: The relationship between age and wisdom. *Ageing International, 30*(1), 5–26.

Sternberg, R. J. (2005c). What is wisdom and how can we develop it? In D. L. Evans, E. Foa, R. Gur, H. Hendin, C. O'Brien, M. E. P. Seligman, et al. (Eds.), *Treatments that work for adolescents* (pp. 664–674). New York: Oxford University Press.

Sternberg, R. J. (in press). Personal wisdom in the balance. In M. Ferrari & N. Weststrate (Eds.), *Personal wisdom*. Amsterdam: Springer.

Sternberg, R. J., & Jordan, J. (Eds.). (2005). *A handbook of wisdom: Psychological perspectives*. New York: Cambridge University Press.

Sternberg, R. J., & Lubart, T. (2001). Wisdom and creativity. In J. E. Birren & K. W. Schaie (Eds.), *Handbook of the psychology of aging* (pp. 500–522). New York: Academic Press

Stewart, P. (1964). *Jacobellis v. Ohio*, 378 U.S. 184.

Stopa, L. (2009). *Imagery and the threatened self: Perspective on mental imagery and the self in cognitive therapy*. London: Routledge.

Stosny, S. (1995). *Treating attachment abuse: A compassionate approach*. New York: Springer.

Stott, R. (2007). When the head and heart do not agree: A theoretical and clinical analysis of rational–emotional dissociation (RED) in cognitive therapy. *Journal of Cognitive Psychotherapy, 21*, 37–50.

Sullivan, W. (1972, March 29). The Einstein papers: A man of many parts. *New York Times*, p. 1.

Surrey, J. L. (2005). Relational psychotherapy, relational mindfulness. In C. K. Germer, R. D. Siegel, & P. R. Fulton (Eds.), *Mindfulness and psychotherapy* (pp. 91–110). New York: Guilford Press.

Surya Das, L. (2011). Wisdom in Buddhism. In *New dharma talks of Lama Surya Das*. Unpublished manuscript.

Sussman, R., & Cloninger, C. (Eds.). (2011). *Origins of altruism and cooperation*. New York: Springer.

Suzuki, D. T. (1998). *The Buddha of infinite light*. Boston: Shambhala.

Suzuki, S. (1973). *Zen mind, beginner's mind*. New York: John Weatherhill.

Suzuki, S. (2007). *Zen is right here: Teaching stories and anecdotes of Shunryu Suzuki*. Boston: Shambhala.

Sy, T., Cote, S., & Saavedra, R. (2005). The contagious leader: Impact of the leader's mood on the mood of group members, group affective tone, and group process. *Journal of Applied Psychology, 90*, 295–305.

Takahashi, M., & Overton, W. F (2005). Cultural foundations of wisdom: An integrated developmental approach. In R. J. Sternberg & J. Jordan (Eds.), *A handbook of wisdom: Psychological perspectives* (pp. 32–60). New York: Cambridge University Press.

Talarico, J. M., Berntsen, D., & Rubin, D. C. (2009). Positive emotions enhance recall of peripheral details. *Cognition and Emotion, 23*, 380–398.

Tang, W., Geng, X., Stein, E., Yang, Y., & Posner, M. (2010). Short-term meditation induces white matter changes in the anterior cingulate. *Proceedings of the National Academy of Sciences, 107*(35), 15649–15652.

Tarchin, S. (1999). *Achieving bodhichitta: Instructions of two great lineages combined into a unique system of eleven categories* (pp. 63–98). Howell, NJ: Mahhayana Sutra and Tantra Press.

Taris, T. W. (2000). Dispositional need for cognitive closure and self-enhancing beliefs. *Journal of Social Psychology, 140*, 35–50.

Tarrier, N. (2010). Broad minded affective coping (BMAC): A "positive" CBT approach to facilitating positive emotions. *International Journal of Cognitive Therapy, 3*, 64–76.

Taylor, S. E., Klein, L. C., Lewis, B. P., Gruenewald, T. L., Gurung, R. A., & Updegraff, J. A. (2000). Biobehavioral responses to stress in females: Tend-and-befriend, not fight-or-flight. *Psychological Review, 107*, 411–429.

Taymiyyah, I., Al-Ani, S., & Tel, A. (1999). *Kitab al-Iman: Book of faith*. Bloomington, IN: Iman.

Teasdale, J. D., Segal, Z. V., Williams, J. M., Ridgeway, V. A., Soulsby, J. M., & Lau, M. A. (2000). Prevention of relapse/recurrence in major depression by mindfulness-based cognitive therapy. *Journal of Consulting and Clinical Psychology, 68*, 615–623.

Teasdale, J. D., Segal, Z. V., & Williams, M. G. (1995). How does cognitive therapy prevent depressive relapse and why should attentional control (mindfulness training) help? *Behaviour Research and Therapy, 33*, 25–39.

Terence. (2001). *The woman of Andros, the self-tormentor, the eunuch* (Vol. I). Cambridge, MA: Harvard University Press.

Tesser, A. (1999). Toward a self-evaluation maintenance model of social behavior. In R. F. Baumeister (Ed.), *The self in social psychology* (pp. 446–460). New York: Psychology Press.

Thakar, V. (2003). *Blossoms of friendship*. Berleley, CA: Rodmell Press.

Thanissaro Bhikku. (Trans.). (2011). *Ogha-tarana Sutta: Crossing over the flood*. Retrieved April 10, 2011, from *www.accesstoinsight.org/tipitaka/sn/sn01/sn01.001.than.html*.

Thayer, J. F., & Sternberg, E. (2006). Beyond heart rate variability: Vagal regulation of allostatic systems. *Annals of New York Academy of Sciences, 1088*, 361–372.

Thompson, B. L., & Waltz, J. (2008). Self-compassion and PTSD symptom severity. *Journal of Traumatic Stress, 21*, 556–558.

Thondup, T. (1995). *Enlightened journey: Buddhist practice as daily life*. Boston: Shambhala.

Tiberius, V. (2010). The Rosewood report: Questions about wisdom, part 1. *Defining wisdom: A project of the University of Chicago*. Retrieved from *wisdomresearch.org/forums/t/846.aspx*.

Tick, E. (2005). *War and the soul: Healing our nation's veterans from post-traumatic stress disorder*. Wheaton, IL: Quest Books.

Tirch, D. (2011). *The compassionate mind guide to overcoming anxiety*. London: Constable.

Tononi, G., & Edelman, G. M. (1998). Consciousness and complexity. *Science, 282*, 1846–1851.

Trilling, D. (1982). *Mrs. Harris: Death of the Scarsdale diet doctor*. New York: Penguin.

Trivers, R. (1971). The evolution of reciprocal altruism. *Quarterly Review of Biology, 46*, 35–57.

Tsoknyi Rinpoche. (2004). *Carefree dignity: Discourses on training the mind*. Berkeley, CA: North Atlantic Books.

Tugade, M. M., & Fredrickson, B. L. (2004). Resilient individuals use positive emotions to bounce back from negative emotional experiences. *Journal of Personality and Social Psychology, 86*, 320–333.

Turner, R. M. (2000). Naturalistic evaluation of dialectical behavioral therapy-oriented treatment for borderline personality disorder. *Cognitive and Behavioral Practice, 7*, 413–419.

Twenge, J. M., & Campbell, W. K. (2009). *The narcissism epidemic: Living in the age of entitlement*. New York: Free Press.

Twenge, J. M., Gentile, B., DeWall, C. N., Ma, D., Lacefield, K., & Schurtz, D. R. (2010). Birth cohort increases in psychopathology among young Americans, 1938–2007: A cross-temporal meta-analysis of the MMPI. *Clinical Psychology Review, 30*, 145–154.

Uddin, L. Q., Iacoboni, M., Lange, C., & Keenan, J. P. (2007). The self and social cognition: The role of cortical midline structures and mirror neurons. *Trends in Cognitive Sciences, 11*, 153–157.

Underwood, L. (2009). Compassionate love: A framework for research. In B.

Fehr, S. Sprecher, & L.G. Underwood (Eds.), *The science of compassionate love* (pp. 3–26). West Sussex, UK: Wiley-Blackwell.

Urry, H. L., van Reekum, C. M., Johnstone, T., Kalin, N. H., Thurow, M. E., Schaefer, H. S., et al. (2006). Amygdala and ventromedial prefrontal cortex are inversely coupled during regulation of negative affect and predict the diurnal pattern of cortisol secretion among older adults. *Journal of Neuroscience, 26*, 4415–4425.

Vaillant, G. (2003). *Aging well: Surprising guideposts to a happier life from the landmark Harvard study of adult development*. New York: Little, Brown.

Van Dam, T., Sheppard, S., Forsyth, J., & Earleywine, M. (2011). Self-compassion is a better predictor than mindfulness of symptom severity and quality of life in mixed anxiety and depression. *Journal of Anxiety Disorders, 25*, 123–130.

van den Heuvel, O. A., Veltman, D. J., Groenewegen, H. J., Cath, D. C., van Balkom, A. J., van Hartskamp, J., et al. (2005). Frontal–striatal dysfunction during planning in obsessive–compulsive disorder. *Archives of General Psychiatry, 62*, 301–309.

van der Oord, S., Bögels, S., & Peijnenburg, D. (2011). The effectiveness of mindfulness training for children with ADHD and mindful parenting for their parents. *Behavioural and Cognitive Psychotherapy, 39*, 193.

Veenhoven, R. (2008). Healthy happiness: Effects of happiness on physical health and the consequences for preventive health care. *Journal of Happiness Studies, 9*, 449–464.

Verheul, R., van den Bosch, L. M. C., Koeter, M. W. J., de Ridder, M. A. J., Stijnen, T., & van den, B. W. (2003). Dialectical behaviour therapy for women with borderline personality disorder: 12-month, randomised clinical trial in The Netherlands. *British Journal of Psychiatry, 182*, 135–140.

Vessantara. (1993). *Meeting the Buddhas: A guide to Buddhas, bodhisattvas and tantric deities*. New York: Windhorse.

Viorst, J. (1986). *Necessary losses*. New York: Simon & Schuster.

Vivino, B., Thompson, B., Hill, C., & Ladany, N. (2010). Compassion in psychotherapy: The perspective of therapists nominated as compassionate. *Psychotherapy Research, 19*(2), 157–171.

Wachholz, A., & Pearce, M. (2007). Compassion and health. In T. G. Plante & C. E. Thoresen (Eds.), *Spirit, science, and health* (pp. 115–128). Westport, CT: Praeger.

Wadlinger, H. A., & Isaacowitz, D. M. (2006). Positive mood broadens visual attention to positive stimuli. *Motivation and Emotion, 30*, 87–99.

Wallace, A., & Wallace, V. (Trans.). (1997). *A guide to the bodhisattva way of life by Santideva*. Ithaca, NY: Snow Lion.

Wallace, D. F. (2008, September 19). David Foster Wallace on life and work. *Wall Street Journal*.

Wallin, D. J. (2007). *Attachment in psychotherapy*. New York: Guilford Press.

Wang, S. (2005). A conceptual framework for integrating research related to the physiology of compassion and the wisdom of Buddhist teachings. In P. Gilbert (Ed.), *Compassion: Conceptualisations, research and use in psychotherapy* (pp. 75–120). London: Brunner-Routledge.

Warkentin, J. (1972). The paradox of being alive and intimate. In A. Burton (Ed.), *Twelve therapists*. San Francisco: Jossey-Bass.

Watkins, E. (2008). Constructive and unconstructive repetitive thought. *Psychological Bulletin, 134*, 163–206.

Watson, B. (1993). *The lotus sutra*. New York: Columbia University Press.

Waugh, C. E., & Fredrickson, B. L. (2006). Nice to know you: Positive emotions, self–other overlap, and complex understanding in the formation of a new relationship. *Journal of Positive Psychology, 1*, 93–106.

Wei, M., Liao, K., Ku, T., & Shaffer, P. (in press). Attachment, self-compassion, empathy, and subjective well-being among college students and community adults. *Journal of Personality*.

Weibel, D. T. (2007). *A loving-kindness intervention: Boosting compassion for self and others*. Doctoral dissertation, Ohio University.

Welford, M. (2010). A compassion focused approach to anxiety disorders. *International Journal of Cognitive Therapy, 3*(2), 124–140.

Wells, A. (1999). A metacognitive model and therapy for generalized anxiety disorder. *Clinical Psychology and Psychotherapy, 6*, 86–95.

Wells, H. K. (1972). Alienation and dialectical logic. *Kansas Journal of Sociology, 3*, 7–32.

West, M. L. (1963). *Shoes of the fisherman*. New York: Morrow.

Williams, D. C., & Levitt, H. M. (2007). A qualitative investigation of eminent therapists' values within psychotherapy: Developing integrative principles for moment-to-moment psychotherapy practice. *Journal of Psychotherapy Integration, 17*, 159–184.

Williams, J., & Lynn, S. (2010). Acceptance: An historical and conceptual review. *Imagination, Cognition, and Personality, 30*(1), 5–56.

Williams, J. G., Stark, S. K., & Foster, E. E. (2008). Start today or the very last day?: The relationships among self-compassion, motivation, and procrastination. *American Journal of Psychological Research, 4*, 37–44.

Williams, J. M. (2010). Mindfulness and psychological process. *Emotion, 10*, 1–7.

Williams, J. M. G., Teasdale, J. D., Segal, Z. V., & Kabat-Zinn, J. (2007). *The mindful way through depression: Freeing yourself from chronic unhappiness*. New York: Guilford Press.

Wilson, K. G., & Murrell, A. R. (2004). Values work in acceptance and commitment therapy. In S. C. Hayes, V. M. Follette, & M. M. Linehan (Eds.), *Mindfulness and acceptance: Expanding the cognitive-behavioral tradition* (pp. 120–151). New York: Guilford Press.

Winnicott, D. (1960). The theory of the parent–child relationship. *International Journal of Psychoanalysis, 41*, 585–595.

Witkiewitz, K., & Bowen, S. (2010). Depression, craving and substance use following a randomized trial of mindfulness-based relapse prevention. *Journal of Consulting and Clinical Psychology, 78*, 362–374.

Wolman, B. B. (1973). *Handbook of general psychology*. New York: Prentice Hall.

Woodward, F. L. (1979). *The book of the gradual sayings*. London: Pali Text Society.

World Health Organization. (2011). Depression. Geneva: Author. Available at *www.who.int/mental_health/management/depression/definition/en/*.

Yarnell, L. M., & Neff, K. D. (in press). Self-compassion, interpersonal conflict resolutions, and well-being. *Self and Identity.*

Yeats, W. B. (2004). *The Celtic twilight.* Mineola, NY: Dover. (Original work published 1902)

Ying, Y. (2009). Contribution of self-compassion to competence and mental health in social work students. *Journal of Social Work Education, 45*, 309–323.

Young, J. E., Klosko, J. S., & Weishaar, M. E. (2003). *Schema therapy: A practitioner's guide.* New York: Guilford Press.

Zayas, V., Mischel, W., Shoda, Y., & Aber, J. L. (2011). Roots of adult attachment: Maternal caregiving at 18 months predicts adult peer and partner attachment. *Social Psychological and Personality Science, 2*, 289–297.

Author Index

Subject Index

Page numbers followed by *f* indicate figure